FRITZ SPIEGL'S
SICK NOTES

FRITZ SPIEGL'S
SICK NOTES

*An Alphabetical Browsing-Book of Medical
Derivations, Abbreviations, Mnemonics and Slang
for the Amusement and Edification of
Medics, Nurses, Patients and Hypochondriacs*

With a Foreword by Lord Smith of Marlow

President, Royal College of Surgeons, 1973–1977

and an

Introduction by
Stephen Lock

Editor, British Medical Journal, 1975–1991

The Parthenon Publishing Group

International Publishers in Medicine, Science & Technology

NEW YORK   LONDON

Published in Europe by:
The Parthenon Publishing Group Ltd.
Casterton Hall, Carnforth, Lancs. LA6 2LA, UK

Published in the USA and Canada by:
The Parthenon Publishing Group Inc.
One Blue Hill Plaza, PO Box 1564, Pearl River, New York 10965, USA

British Library Cataloguing in Publication Data
Spiegl, Fritz
    Fritz Spiegl's Sicknotes: Alphabetical
    Browsing-book of Medical Derivations,
    Abbreviations, Mnemonics and Slang for
    the Amusement and Edification of Medics,
    Nurses, Patients and Hypochondriacs
    I. Title II. Tidy, Bill
    610.014

ISBN 1-85070-627-1

Library of Congress Cataloging-in-Publication Data
Spiegl, Fritz.
    Fritz Spiegl's sick notes: an alphabetical browsing book of medical derivations,
abbreviations, mnemonics, and slang for the amusement and edification of
medics, nurses, patients, and hypochondriacs/with a foreword by
Lord Smith of Marlow: an introduction by Stephen Lock.
      p. cm.
    Includes bibliographical references.
    ISBN 1-85070-627-1
    1. Medicine--Terminology   2. Medicine--Humor.
I. Title
    [DNLM: 1. Medicine--terminology. 2. Medicine--humor. W 15 S755f 1995]
R123.S645   1995
610'.14--dc20
DNLM/DLC
for Library of Congress   95-41861
                                             CIP

Typeset by H&H Graphics, Blackburn
Printed and bound by Bookcraft (Bath) Ltd., Midsomer Norton

FOREWORD

by Lord Smith of Marlow

President of the Royal College of Surgeons
1973–1977

In common with others, I admit to being flattered by a request to write a foreword to a book. I qualified in medicine in the distant past, in 1937, and have been engaged in surgical practice since 1939. It is inevitable that almost all the books, where my help was asked, were textbooks upon surgical subjects. I always regarded the invitation with mixed feelings: one cannot write a foreword without reading the book. If the subject was dull or if the author was illiterate, boring or incompetent, it might be a chore, and to write a foreword might be without profit and dull in the extreme. On the other hand, if the author was a master of the English language, with a subject of abiding interest, one might, in reading the book, experience instruction, delight and fascination beyond one's wildest dreams.

I have written forewords for many surgical textbooks but now I break new ground, having read this book with growing appreciation and with profitable instruction and delight. The subject is not one which you would automatically grab from the bookshelf and say 'I must read this' – unless you had perhaps listened to the discourses by Fritz Spiegl on the BBC. This would have alerted you to the situation. Fritz is a master of the English language, and always the subject is described with a style of simplicity and instruction.

Many of the older doctors were brought up with a groundwork of classical tuition at school, and many of them will know most of the classical derivations of abbreviations with which the medical literature is dotted. Nowadays, in younger doctors, the reverse is the case, and many are woefully unaware of the debt we owe to the classical languages for medical words.

This book fills a gap in the knowledge of every doctor, but it is more than a dictionary. Each derivation and origin is described in a way that combines superb English with a style and attraction that enthrals the reader. Fritz says that the book is written 'for medical students, nurses, patients and hypochondriacs' but I am none of these. In reading the work, I started at the beginning and thought that I should skip one or two entries. Not a bit of it. I read every word, and I think it ought to be compulsory reading for every medical student. This is not a chore, because when you read the first few entries you will clamour for more and will persist in your thirst for knowledge – and enjoy yourself immensely, as I did.

INTRODUCTION

by Dr Stephen Lock

Editor of *The British Medical Journal*
1975–1991

'Take a subject of the utmost seriousness and treat it with the utmost triviality'. A glance at this dictionary might suggest that Fritz Spiegl had followed Bernard Shaw's advice. Moreover, few devotees of the arcane could fail to be fascinated, for instance by the suggestion that the composer Luigi Albinoni was 'probably' descended from an albino (I like the scholarship of that 'probably'), or by the exegesis on the four major types of fart. But, like all major humorists, Spiegl is at heart a moralist and, I suspect, a disillusioned idealist. His message is much more profound than might appear at first: to paraphrase Lord Acton, it is that all language can corrupt, but that, correctly tailored, language can be used to corrupt absolutely.

Part of Spiegl's intention, then, is to dispel the clouds of medical obfuscation (obfuscate, darken, obscure. XVI. f. pp. stem of late L. obfuscare, f. OB + fuscare, darken. *Oxford Dictionary of English Etymology*). To be sure, 'all professions are conspiracies against the laity', to quote Shaw again, but is that any reason why the doctor should hide his ignorance behind 'chlorosis' when the parent has already said that she's worried that her daughter has an unhealthy green look? And doctors themselves need reminding of the necessity of using language as scrupulously as they would a cardiac catheter or an autoanalyser: the dangers of confusing 'hypo' with 'hyper' are self-evident, those of doing the same with 'alternate' and 'alternative' less so. All too often as Editor of *The British Medical Journal* I found that many articles submitted for publication were atrociously written. Even tabloid journalists are taught not only to find out what's new, true and important about a story but also to leave their readers with a message.

Alas, articles for medical journals often do little to inform the readers at all; as a result, conscientious editors and their referees spend time trying to find out whether the research project was worthwhile, and if so, preparing an intelligible version for publication. Those with a more relaxed temperament, or less time, go ahead and publish the text unchanged. Few people read this, surveys show, and even fewer cite the paper as a reference. To an author all this doesn't matter too much. Read or not, the paper can now swell his curriculum vitae, as part of the current 'arms race' for publication – which has led to some doctors publishing articles carrying their names every few weeks of their lives (how they get time to write them, read them, and help their co-workers do the research, let alone live any outside life, nobody has ever been able to explain). Never mind, in the world after Thatcher, funding-councils for research and teaching give grants for quantity rather than quality, so that they can now weigh them rather than read them for content. To the reader, also, this doesn't matter too much: he (and I was delighted to see Spiegl adopting the Scots saying 'here man embraceth woman') has one less paper to read. But to the community at large a poorly written paper is a disaster. It has failed to do what has been expected of it for almost 350 years: communicate new facts to fellow-scientists, who can then weigh them in the balance. Articles may be bad because they report bad science, or they may be bad because they are so poorly written that nobody reads them. In either case they represent a waste of resources – laboratories, animals, people. Bad articles, then, are one form of unethical scientific behaviour.

Nevertheless, the use of distorted language by Government departments can have even worse results, and where more so than in the National Health Service? The fourth reorganization since it began was prompted by public concern about long hospital waiting lists and delays in operating-theatres. The new Men in Grey Suits (as Spiegl terms them in chronicling their activities) have not only raised administrative costs – once the leanest in the developed world – with no perceptible 'health gain' (their jargon): they have also introduced the flabby vocabulary of business management and economics, as if caring for patients was the same as brewing lager. (That said, though, some authorities have shortened waiting-lists, by removing the names of all those waiting for over two years). And presiding over all this, in a country that prides itself on its democratic institutions, including the 'mother of Parliaments', is a system of health authorities working in secret. Its decisions are taken by paid, politically-appointed members who discuss in secret a secret agenda devoted to spending money provided by our taxes.

As Orwell reminded us in his essay 'Politics and the English Language', there are only two defences against all this: vigilance and humour. The rapier wit of a Jonathan Swift or of a Fritz Spiegl may be effective where the bludgeon of righteous indignation achieves nothing. English is a particularly rich language – a civilised speaker has perhaps two-and-a-half times the vocabulary of his Latin counterpart – and we should suspect any new term that is vague or unnecessary. Fritz Spiegl's new book will help enormously; I hope that he will now do the same for the other professions.

AUTHOR'S NOTE

Doctors are obliged to learn a huge vocabulary. They need to have more words at their command than any philosopher, mathematician, engineer or astronomer. It is a daunting prospect for the medical student that apart from the manual and observational skills he must learn he is also required to be a polyglot linguist – for most of the essential words of his trade are foreign. While the chef in his kitchen can get by on a handful of French terms, the musician with a smattering of Italian, German and French (everyday words, mostly, such as they might encounter on holiday), the doctor's professional vocabulary is constructed chiefly from Latin and Greek (or a mixture of the two) – languages which only a couple of generations ago were pronounced dead by misguided 'educationists' (fortunately there have been no 'medicalists') who removed them from the required British curriculum. Yet until only comparatively recently it would have been unthinkable for anyone to embark on a medical career without Latin and perhaps a little Greek. Instead of making things easier for students (not only of medicine) the abolition of the classics actually created obstacles to understanding and comprehension. The 'tone' of this book, not to mention the numerous asides and digressions, disqualify it from any pretension to the status of a scientific treatise, let alone a medical textbook (which it would hardly be appropriate for a non-medical person to write).

I have concentrated, first, on the classical 'building-blocks', like essential pre- and suffixes and other word-elements which reveal the meaning of numerous medical terms constructed from them. To take an extreme example, cited in Robertson's *Words for a Modern Age*, pneumonoultramicroscopisilicovolcanoconiosis, which should by rights mean a tapeworm but which, says Robertson, when divided into its component parts, pneu/mono/ultra/micro/scopi/silico/volcano/coni/osis, turns out to be the unabbreviated name for the miners' and stone-workers' lung

disease more sensibly shortened to silicosis (though Robert-son was doubtless teasing).

I have tried to gather together the 'real' meanings behind many medical and anatomical terms, some harking back to Greek and Roman architecture and other aspects of the ancients' everyday life, their gods and superstitions. Many words which may startle the reader as sexually suggestive were in fact the everyday words of the ancients. I also list abbreviations in common use, a few mnemonics that help the learning of lists, and numerous trade nicknames kindly divulged by friends in the medical profession. Also those mysterious abbreviations – if you can decipher them from the traditionally-illegible handwriting – with which doctors tell chemists what to prescribe: strange that chemists are still expected to know their everyday Latin.

A little space is devoted to the British National Health Service and its wider manifestation, the Welfare State, a remarkable humanitarian innovation in its time which, during the half-century of its existence, has developed its own language – that of bureaucracy as well as the slang of the fraudsters and false claimants who try to exploit 'the system'. American and other non-British English-speakers may find some of the Welfare State traditions and practices quaint but, I hope, interesting, and shedding some light on what remains of the British national character. All opinions are my own, and – unusual for a reference work, I have not hesitated to express them – even at the risk of contravening what is now called 'political correctness'. When I write 'he', 'him' or 'man' I mean not a male but a person, a member of mankind or humankind – *Homo sapiens*, a description from which surely no woman would wish to be excluded (though of course I have written 'she' or 'her' when these words are anatomically and exclusively correct). When, under 'almoner', I state that this usually voluntary hospital post was often occupied by 'a friendly lady of mature years' that is precisely what I mean: a *lady* as opposed to a woman (akin to the gentleman/man difference), which is neither patronising nor discriminatory. Indeed the name of the post was formerly 'Lady Almoner'. Nor have I been nervous about using 'English' where English rather than British is meant; 'England', 'Britain' and 'UK' are not always necessarily synonymous. Classical prefixes and suffixes oc-cassionally pose an Anglo-American problem, making it sometimes necessary to wave a danger-flag at certain spelling-simplifications that have taken root on both sides of the Atlantic. For example, when *paed-* is simplified to *ped-* it acquires a different meaning: strictly, a paediatrician deals with children, a pediatrician with feet. Worse, in Latin a *paedicator* is 'one given to unnatural practices' (as the dictionaries delicately put it) and a pedicator is presumably therefore a foot-fetishist – and what is more, I see that the dictionary-adjacent *pediculosus* is the word for 'one who is infested with lice'. So it can be dangerous to meddle with classical spellings. Drastic confusions may arise if the *-rexi* suffix is confused with *-rhexi*; and the *haema-* 'blood' prefix when simplified to *hema-* turns into a 'day' prefix – so that 'hematology' should really mean 'the study of the day', not of the blood (Greek *haima*). Such differences could be as important as the failure to distinguish between *ante* and *anti*, and *hyper* and *hypo*. The accidental omission of the letter r from 'parthenogenesis' would produce 'pathenogenesis', a different thing altogether; and anyone who spells synovitis (an inflammation of a synovial membrane) 'sinovitis' would be referring to an as yet undescribed condition called 'inflam-mation of the Chinese'. It is perhaps significant that the word 'dissect', from the Latin *dissecare*, to cut apart, is now often pronounced 'die-sect', which suggests a different word with different spelling and meaning.

I have concentrated chiefly on the linguistic and historical aspects of medical terms, not their clinical explanations, which are more reliably learned from specialised medical treatises. When I feel obliged to offer them they are presented with the learning of a parrot or magpie, and I rely on my sources for their accuracy. I have omitted most syndromes, and diseases that have their discoverers' names attached. Medical eponyms may be found in several excellent books from Parthenon Publishing. In spite of the seriousness of my original intentions, cheerfulness kept breaking in, because many slang and jargon expressions clamoured to be included, especially those normally kept from us patients. A book like this can never be complete, and every reader will look for things in vain. If there are errors, medical or semantic, I would like to be put right. I am deeply grateful to the friends listed below for suggestions and amendments, for rescuing me from my ignorance and, on some pages, for keeping me in order. Some of these friends examined the typescript with such close and constructively critical attention that Sick Notes has become their book as much as mine. In transcribing Greek terms I have omitted diaereses over letters which classicists would probably expect them to carry. My cross-referencing (indicated in small bold capitals) is not always consistent: sometimes I point to a related formation, e.g. 'agoraphobic', when the actual entry may be 'agoraphobia'; or, in some cases, I omit cross-references as altogether too obvious. As this is an alphabetical browsing-book and not a real dictionary for serious reference, many obvious entries may have been omitted; and I have also necessarily been inconsistent by sometimes giving the Greek, Latin, etc., words as main entries, followed by the English derivatives, while sometimes the English word is given first, followed by its classical or foreign origins. Suggestions and corrections for future editions will be gratefully received and, of course, acknowledged.

Fritz Spiegl

Special gratitude is due to the following, who (some after painstakingly going through the manuscript) made numerous valuable suggestions:

Dr Eleanor Ashton (General Practitioner)
Miss Delia Bethell (Student)
Dr Alison Callister (General Practitioner)
Dr George Cook (General Practitioner)
Mr Robert Connolly (Anatomist)
Mr Reg Cox (Designer)
Dr Peter Dangerfield (Medical Educationalist)
Dr Scott Frazer (Consultant Anaesthetist)
Dr Erich Geiringer (General Practitioner)
Dr Sian Gilchrist (General Practitioner)
Dr Liz Hare (Anatomist)
Mr Graham Hayes (Consultant Orthopaedic Surgeon)
Dr David Heaf (Consultant Paediatrician)
Dr Douglas D.C. Howat (Consultant Anaesthetist)
Professor Arthur Jacobs (Musicologist and Lexicomaniac)
Miss Lisa Knight (Medical Representative)
Dr Simon La Frenaix (General Practitioner)
Dr Stephen Lock (Editor, *British Medical Journal*, 1975–1991)
Dr Stuart Marshall-Clarke (Immunologist)
Mr John McFarland (Consultant Surgeon)
Dr Penelope Murray (Classicist)
Dr Dermot O'Hara (General Practitioner)
Mr Michael Reilly (Consultant Surgeon and Classicist)
Dr Janet Robertson (Bacteriologist)
Dr Ian Rodgers (General Practitioner)
Mr Robert Sells (Consultant Surgeon)
Lord Smith of Marlow (Past President, Royal College of Surgeons of England)
Mrs Ingrid Spiegl (Housewife, Picture Researcher and Stern Critic)
Dr Cyril Taylor (General Practitioner)
Miss Lucy Wood (Art Historian)

Lern Yerself Scouse (Scouse Press) 4 vols.
(How to talk Proper in Liverpool) ed.

Scally Scouse
The Language of Law and Disorder on Merseyside (Scouse Press)

A Small Book of Grave Humour (Pan Books)

Dead Funny (Pan Books)

Lives, Wives, and Loves of the Composers (Marion Boyars)
(1995)

Choked, Chuffed or Over the Moon?
The Jargon of Football, A Word-by-Word Commentary
(in preparation)

The Guinness Book of Musical Blunders
(1996)

The Joy of Words (Elm Tree – Hamish Hamilton)
(A Bedside Book for English Lovers)

Keep taking the Tabloids (Pan Books)
(What the Papers say and how they say it)

Music through the Looking Glass (RKP)
(Musicians' Shoptalk and Jargon)

InWords and OutWords (Elm Tree Books)

MediaWrite / MediaSpeak (Elm Tree Books) *(The Jargon of the Media)*

The Medical Muse (Sick Notes)
A Collection of Songs and Verse for Doctors and Patients,
about Lotions, Potions, Motions, Urges and Purges
(unpublished medical concert material 17th – 20th centuries), etc.

A*a*

A & E Accident and Emergency (Department, Ward, etc.)

A(N)- The Greek prefix element, originally a negative, now variously denoting off, from, away from, not, lacking, absent, missing, without – one of the most useful in medical terminology, e.g. aphasia, absence of speech; acephalic, lacking a head; acholia, absence of bile, or too little; an(a)emia, lack of blood; analgesic, painless or a painkiller (see **ALGIA**, below), asphyxia, etc. See also **ANA-** and **IM-/IN-**.

AA Latin for ana, pharmacists' abbreviation for 'of each', i.e. of each prescribed drug. See also **ANA-**.

Ab Abbreviation standing for abortion.

AB- The Latin 'from, away from' prefix. In Latin it is a separate preposition, with its other form a-, and should not be confused with the Greek a-, above, under **A(N)**.

ABDOMEN That part of the belly that lies below the **DIAPHRAGM**. Latin, but of uncertain origin: dictionaries suggest either *adeps*, fat (see ADIPOSE, below), or *abdo*, I hide away, *abdere* to hide away (see under **GILLES DE LA TOURETTE SYNDROME** for a hidden-away, imaginary place called *Abdera*): the 'hiding-away' may refer to the concealed vital organs contained in the belly. The classical Romans called a hiding-place an *abditorium* – and 17th-century English doctors described pot-bellied persons as abdominous – a description that might be revived to describe men with a **BEER-BELLY** or general **OBESITY**. There is occasional conflict between those who say 'AB-domen' and those who prefer to stress the middle syllable, 'ab-DO-men'.

ABDOMIN(O)- The 'belly' prefix: see above.

ABDUCERE Latin, to lead away, hence to abduct, whereas *adducere* means to lead towards – one of many medical words illustrating the need for clear speech and good handwriting. The difference could be vital.

ABLEIST, ABLEISM Recently coined words belonging to the growing vocabulary of **PC**, or 'Political Correctness'. This unlovely coinage is meant to convey the idea of discrimination against the disabled, and by implication *for* the 'abled' (another deplorable new word). See also under **CRIPPLE**.

ABLEPSY Old-fashioned word for blindness, from the Greek *ablepsia*, itself created from *blepein*, to see, preceded by the **A-** negating letter.

ABORT(I)- The abortion prefix, from the negating prefix *ab* + *ortus*, a birth, an arising. This also means the rising of the sun, and thus *abortus* is its setting.

AB(O)ULIA In Greek, the word for thoughtlessness, but in psychiatric medicine specifically the absence or impairment of will-power, a common symptom of disorders like **SCHIZOPHRENIA**.

ABRADE/ABRASION From Latin *abradere*, to tear or scrape off.

ABSCESS From Latin *abscessus*, *abscedere*, 'a going-away' – from the **PUS** that has formed on part of the body and separates from the flesh. Not to be confused with:–

ABSCISSION Latin *abscissum*, 'a cutting-away'. A further source for confusion might be *abscido*, *abscisum*, a cutting away with a sharp instrument – perhaps scissors? Note the **-CID(E)** element denoting cutting (*cf* incision) and killing (suicide, matricide, regicide, etc.), as the most common way of being murdered or put to death was with a knife.

(THE) ABSENT FRIEND General practitioners' code for a **FAF**, or **PHANTOM PATIENT**. See also under **(IT'S) FOR A FRIEND**.

ABUSE 'Most parents abuse their children at some time or another'. Up to the mid-1980s this statement would have been accepted as an almost universal truth; for what parent has not spoken sharply to, smacked, or even shouted abuse at, an errant offspring, to bring it to its senses? Even as recently as 1982, in the *Oxford English Dictionary*, the only kind of abuse that could possibly be interpreted as a socio-sexual assault is defined as 'violation, defilement, now only in *self-abuse*' (for which see **MASTURBATION**); and

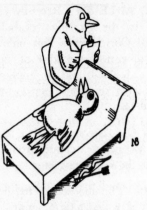

"Yes, I killed Cock Robin – he
abused me when I was an egg"

The Times Saturday Magazine, January 18, 1994
(with permission)

that definition appears next to one defining abuse as 'injurious speech, reviling, execration' (for which see under **CATACHRESIS**). By the end of that decade, however, 'abuse' had become one of the most widely and inaccurately applied catch-all terms, usually with sensationalised connotations of shameful sex and sadism. Members of the **CARING** professions (and therefore also journalists) now cry 'abuse' at the slightest opportunity – sexual abuse, drug abuse, alcohol abuse, solvent abuse, child abuse, geriatric abuse – the list seems almost endless (and what is often meant is, of course, misuse, e.g. of solvents or drugs). Furthermore, this polarisation of 'abuse' has rendered all but useless the verb 'to disabuse'. American laws and court proceedings are bristling with instances of alleged abuse cases, trailing in numbers only to claims for 'harassment'. In court cases concerning offences from serial killing to embezzlement, from personal violence, cruelty or sexual assault, to indecent exposure, the standard legal defence put forward is now almost always the unprovable 'My client was himself abused as a child'.

AC Pharmacists' abbreviation: *ante cibum*, Latin for 'before meals'.

ACCOUCHEMENT Euphemism for the birth-delivery of a child, from the French *accoucher*, to put to bed; an alternative for (and equivalent of) the English term, 'lying-in', or 'being brought to bed'. It was long current in popular English, especially among people who spoke, or newspapers which wrote, of the con-

finement of royal or grand ladies, but has been kept in circulation by the office of the Resident Accoucheur at St. Thomas' Hospital in London.

ACETABULUM Originally a cup-shaped vessel for holding vinegar, from Latin *acetum*, sour wine, vinegar; in anatomy, the hip socket. Many parts of the body were named in allusion to everyday objects or the structures of dwellings – see **ARCHITECTURAL TERMS**.

ACHILLES' TENDON See **TENDO ACHILLIS**.

ACHROMATOPSIA Colour-blindness. Taking the word apart backwards, one finds the elements ops-, sight, *chrom*-, colour + *a*- the 'absence' prefix (see above).

ACOUSMA An imagined, hallucinatory impression of speech, music, etc. Joan of Arc presented a clear case of it, and some murderers claim it as a defence or justification for their crime. The Greek word *akousma*, means something heard.

ACROMION The point of the shoulder. Greek *acros*, point, summit + *omos*, shoulder.

ACROPHOBIA A fear of heights such as mountain-tops, tall buildings, etc., from Greek *akros*, the topmost, the highest, the outermost – which has also given us acronyms – the craze for making new words from initials or syllables of older ones. Acrophobia is not to be confused with **AGORAPHOBIA**. See also **VERTIGO** and **CLAUSTROPHOBIA**.

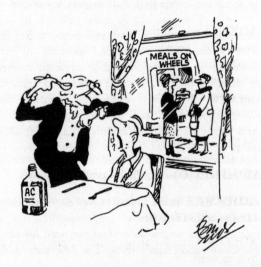

AC – Latin for before meals

ACTH Adrenocorticotrophic hormone, discovered in 1927 by Evans and Long in the United States of America.

ACU- The prefix of sharpness, from Latin *acer, acr-* sharp or bitter, *acerbus*, bitter and sour (which some remarks may be) and *acus*, a needle: hence a great number of pointed words, like acid; exacerbate, to make worse; and acupuncture, the old Chinese art of treating illness by puncturing the body with needles. Also **ACROPHOBIA**, above. In addition, there is both acme, as in the peak of perfection, as well as acne (those troublesome **MACULA** or **ZIT**, with little points or centres). See also **AGUE** – and:–

ACUTUS Latin for sharp, acute, as in pain, perhaps of short duration, as opposed to **CHRONIC** pain. The Greek is *oxys*, as in paroxysm.

ADD Attention Deficit Disorder. The afflicted are usually children with learning difficulties and a low attention span who display a variety of other signs and symptoms long familiar to parents but only recently named as a **SYNDROME** – for details of which see a specialist publication. With the customary eye for a memorable acronym the ADD 'support group' has named itself 'LADDER', which somehow manages to stand for the National Learning and Attention Deficit Disorders Association. No doubt **COUNSELLING** is available for sufferers and their parents – and, I hope, for compulsive acronymists.

ADEN Greek for a gland. Thus adenoid (with the addition of **-OID**, the 'in the shape of' suffix) means gland-shaped. The Latin equivalent is **GLANS**.

ADEPS Latin for the soft fat, grease or lard in animals and humans, hence the now modish euphemism 'adipose tissue' when unwanted body-fat is meant (usually so called by the fashion and slimming industries to make women feel better). Some authorities say this word also provided the origin of the word **ABDOMEN**, see above, though the 'hiding away' theory seems more convincing, since not all abdomens are adipose. The Latin word for the harder and more tallow-like fat is **SEBUM**.

ADIP(O)- The fat, grease or lard prefix. See also **LIP(O)-** and **STEAT(O)-**.

ADITUS Latin for an approach or entry, from *ad*, to + *ire*, to go.

ADJUVANT A substance used to enhance the activity of another. From Latin *adjuvo, -jutum*, to give help, to aid – think of an army adjutant, or aide.

ADRENAL Pertaining to or near the kidney, or referring to the adrenal glands: from Latin *ad*, towards, of, near or belonging to + *renes*, the kidneys.

ADRENALIN(E) A **HORMONE** secreted by the adrenal glands (though it can also be produced synthetically). It prepares the body for 'fright, flight or fight'; but when sportsmen say 'I was pumping adrenalin like mad' they are talking nonsense. The adrenalin causes the *heart* to pump harder and faster but is itself incapable of 'pumping'. See also **EPINEPHRINE**.

ADVENTITIOUS Description of a disease or condition found, or occurring, in a place other than the usual one, e.g. **MALARIA** in Edinburgh or heatstroke in Alaska. From the Latin *adventicius*, 'coming to us from abroad' (*advenire*, 'to come to'). It is sometimes incorrectly written *'adventicius'* but even *'adventitious'* is an erroneous form: the *Oxford English Dictionary* says that *adventicious* is etymologically the better English spelling.

(A)EGOPHONY One of the sounds of **VOCAL RESONANCE** which, like **WHISPERING PECTRILOQUY**, the doctor hears through his stethoscope to enable him to make his diagnosis. Aegophony means a bleating sound which occurs in cases of pneumonia with pleurisy, from Greek *aigis*, goat + *phonos*, sound. Incidentally, to be 'under the aegis' of something or someone means to be under the (goatskin-covered?) shield of Zeus/Jupiter or Minerva – or simply covered by a goatskin.

-(A)EMIA A variant of the 'blood' words, **HAIMA**, **HAEMA**, used both as prefix and suffix elements. Americans prefer the simplified **-EMIA**.

AEROBIC Derived from the Greek *aer*, air (later also meaning oxygen, whose concept was not understood in ancient times). An anaerobic environment is one without oxygen – so 'aerobics', and 'aerobic exercises', are nonsense terms, intended to convey the idea that the exerciser is obliged to gasp for more air containing oxygen. All that aerobics usually means is strenuous exercise to loud pop music – a noisier form of **CALLISTHENICS**.

AEROPHAGY/AEROPHAGIA Swallowing air, usually resulting in **FLATULENCE**. From the Greek word for air + *phagein*, eating. It is done voluntarily to permit (o)esophageal speech after the removal of the larynx. This might therefore be descibed as 'ventiloquism', or 'wind-speaking', as opposed to ventriloquism, which literally means 'belly-speaking' – see under **VENTR-**.

AESCULAPIUS The Latin spelling of **ASKLEPIOS**, the Greek God of Medicine.

(A)ESTH- The feelings-related prefix, derived from the Greek word *aisthanesthai*, to feel, hence (a)esthetics and **AN**(a)esthesia, absence of feeling.

(A)ETIOLOGY The Greek word *aitia* means the cause or reason, so aetiology is simply a fancy way of speaking of the cause of a disease, though literally it means 'the knowledge of the cause'. Americans use the simplified spelling **ETIOLOGY**, risking confusion with things dried up, pale, sickly or colourless, i.e. **ETIOLATED**.

AGAR Really *agar-agar*, the Malayan word for several kinds of East-Indian seaweeds, especially the Sinhalese moss *Gracilaria lichenoides*, which the Chinese use in making soup, silk and paper, and bacteriologists find useful as a solidifying agent in culture media such as **SOUPS**. See also under **IMMUNISATION**.

AGITO Latin for 'I excite': the connection with agitation is obvious.

AGONY Sustained and powerful pain, often described by the patient as 'indescribable'. It originally meant a contest (*agon*, a meeting), the Greeks' *agonia* being usually associated with a painful struggle, for that was the nature of their games. But when used figuratively, agony was not always necessarily painful: Alexander Pope (1725) had '...cries and agonies of wild delight'. See also **-ALGIA** and **EXQUISITE**. See also under **ACUTUS**.

AGORAPHOBIA A fear of open spaces, suffered by people who are afraid of leaving the apparent security of their home (unlike those with **CLAUSTROPHOBIA**, who are frightened of being locked in and *prefer* open spaces – *claustrum*, Latin for an enclosed space, an inner room). The Greek *agora* means a marketplace, to which is added *phobos*, fear. (But see also

ACROPHOBIA, above; and **-PHOBIA**, below). According to the *Oxford English Dictionary* the earliest agoraphobic attacks to be described (in *The Lancet*) occurred in 1884. Previously, people were presumably just regarded as excessively shy, or nervous about meeting strangers. Now that the word has become part of everyday speech, sufferers from the condition have multiplied. The press occasionally prints some interesting accidental variations, like 'aggrophobia', presumably a fear of aggression; and 'agrophobia', which is almost a fear of things agricultural, except that this would be agriphobia. Yet the *Concise Oxford Medical Dictionary* includes the word *agromania*, defined as 'a pathologically strong impulse to live alone in open countryside': it is not in the big Oxford so frequently quoted here, and probably an erroneous formation for 'agrimania' (which isn't there either). Newspapers occasionally fall for the misprint 'angoraphobia', which would mean either a fear of a certain species of goat, or an aversion to hairy knitwear. A recently described condition whose sufferers have a compulsion to go shopping, and who are described as 'shopaholics', might be said to have 'agrophilia'.

AGRA Greek for a seizure or attack, e.g. *podagra*. See also **PELLAGRA**.

AGROM From Gujarati *agrun*, a rough and cracked condition of the tongue, often chronic, and accompanied by ulceration. One of the 'regional' (perhaps almost 'racist') diseases – see under **THALASS-(ANA)EMIA** and cross-references.

AGUE A sharp, acute or violent fever; later specifically malarial, with its characteristic, intermittent, cold-hot-and-sweating stages. The name comes via French from the Latin *acutus*, sharp.

AHA The American Hospital Association.

'AHA' REACTION Nothing to do with the above, at least nominally, but (says *Mosby's Pocket Dictionary of Medicine*) 'in psychology, a sudden realisation or inspiration experienced, especially during creative thinking'.

AID Artificial Insemination by Donor. See also **ONAN**.

AIDS Perhaps the most ill-chosen acronym of the 20th century (at any rate after that of the Vintners' and United Licensed Victuallers' Association). It is usually explained as the 'Acquired Immune

Deficiency Syndrome', which makes it even more inapt: first, because as an acronymic coinage it compromises an existing word (as in hearing-aids, sex aids, aid is at hand, etc.), and second, because the two middle words suggest a quite different meaning: the 'correct' term is Acquired *Immunodeficiency* Syndrome (see also under **SYN-**), but this form is used by only a few speakers and writers; among printed publications *The Lancet* was notable in always insisting on it. It is, after all, not the *deficiency* that is immune, just as the infants in **SIDS** (Sudden Infant Death Syndrome) are not 'sudden infants'. And to speak of 'the AIDS syndrome' is as tautologous as 'the HIV virus', for the last initial of each stands for 'syndrome' and 'virus', respectively, making a nonsensical 'syndrome syndrome' and 'virus virus'. At first, when it was noticed that AIDS affected mainly male homosexuals, American doctors baldly called it the Gay Compromise Syndrome – and the sensational tabloid press jumped at the chance of calling it the Gay Plague; another early name was GRID, for Gay Related Immune Deficiency, but both are offensive to homosexuals and have rightly been declared politically incorrect (see **PC**). Another early acronym was AID, the syndrome being added only later. During the late 1980s and early 1990s the United Kingdom spent millions of pounds on advertising campaigns to persuade heterosexuals that all humankind was equally at risk: even the nuns of a convent near to where I write these words received leaflets from the British government warning them to refrain from anal sexual intercourse. Nevertheless AIDS has remained a threat mainly to homosexuals and drug injecters, and apocalyptic forecasts were proved wrong. The UK at present (late 1994) has about ten 'AIDS Workers' (including **COUNSELLORS**) to every AIDS sufferer (for whose condition the word 'full-blown AIDS' appears to be obligatory). Even in Africa, where the syndrome was at first believed to have reached calamitous **EPIDEMIC** proportions (and where for insufficiently explained reasons it equally affects heterosexuals and women – possibly because **BUGGERY** is used as a form of birth-control) the projected spread, with predictions of entire nations being wiped out, has been greatly overestimated: the majority of deaths on that troubled continent are, as before, caused by tribal wars, starvation and **MALARIA**. Just as Ehrlich's **SALVARSAN** was condemned as an encouragement of sin, so has AIDS been looked upon by moralisers and religious fundamentalists as a visitation on homosexuals to punish them for their promiscuous ways. But as **HIPPOCRATES** pointed out 2500 years ago, long before Christianity began to preach eternal damnation and hellfire, disease is not sent as a miraculous punishment by the gods. In French, which uses a different word order, the AIDS acronym is turned inside-out, to become SIDA, explained by some as 'Syndrome Introduit Dans l'Anus'.

AKOUEIN Greek, to hear, *akousma* something that is heard. In Latin, to hear or listen is *auscultare*. And see **AUSCULTATION**.

ALBINO A person lacking part of or all the colouring pigment in the skin, hair and eyes, so that the first two are abnormally light, almost white, while the last named are pink and ultra-sensitive to light, and prone to errors of refraction. Albinism is also known as hypopigmentation. The word albino was coined by the Portuguese, who in the 18th century thus described white negroes they encountered in Africa, for albinism affects several races (I have seen a white 'black' man, the captain of a Trinidadian steel band, and a most impressive sight he was). Albinism is a recessive inherited condition, and the name of the Italian composer Tommaso Albinoni (1671–1751) suggests that he was probably descended from an albino. It has been said that it may be one of the causes for the unintentional **SPOONERISM**. See also **VITILIGO**.

ALBUS The Latin word for white, hence albumen, egg-white; albumin, a type of protein in the bloodstream; albino, a person of pale appearance due to a lack of pigmentation in the skin; etc. See above and also under **CANDIDA**.

ALCOHOL From Arabic, *al-kohl*, a powder with which women used to stain their eyelids (see also under **CASCARA** for a cross-reference to mascara). The transformation from a cosmetic to a distilled substance used for drinking or surgical skin cleansing is too complicated to be included in this book, and the effect of alcohol on humans too obvious. As **HIPPOCRATES** said: 'Who could have foretold, from the structure of the brain, that wine could derange its functions?'

ALCOHOLISM See **TMA**.

ALE GUT The popular name for a big belly on a man. Women tend to have **CELLULITE** instead.

ALEXIA From the **A-** prefix followed by the word-related element, from Greek *lexis*, word. An acquired inability to read, owing to disease; unlike **DYSLEXIA**, which is a developmental disorder – when it *is* a disorder and not merely the result of watching too much television and not reading enough printed matter to make words and letters familiar. Not to be confused with **ALEXO-**, the fighting, warding-off prefix, as in alexocyte (not to mention Alexander the Great). But *alecto-* produces something of a red herring: it comes from Greek *alektryon*, Latin *alectorius*, cock.

ALEXIN A class of substances found in blood serum, having the capacity of destroying bacteria, etc. From Greek *alexein*, to ward off.

ALEXIPHARMAC An antidote, from the above, and *pharmakon*, a poison. See **PHARMACY**.

-ALGIA From Greek *algos*, pain, hence the suffix indicating pain, as in cephalgia, headache, etc. Yes, and even an ache for our old never-to-be-the-same-again friend of long ago, **NOSTALGIA**. See also **AGONY** and **ANGINA**.

AL(IM)- From Latin *alere*, to feed, nourish, hence the alimentary canal.

ALKA-SELTZER A large, analgesic, alkaline, antacid pill soluble in water, long established as a remedy for indigestion. See also other **PATENT** medicines, like **ANDREWS** and **ENO'S**.

ALLANTOIS Vascular fetal membrane, from Greek *allas*, a sausage. Equally unappetising is 'mother's cake', or **PLACENTA**.

ALLERGY Invented in 1909 as a German word *Allergie* for which it was adapted from Greek *allos*, other + *ergon*, work (a like formation being 'energy'). It entered English medical language two years later, when C. E. von Pirquet's German paper was translated ('We might rightly use the word *allergy* as a clinical conception') and the word was then popularised by the English bacteriologist Sir Almroth Wright (1861–1947), who had been a pupil of the German physician and scientist Paul Ehrlich (see under **SALVARSAN**). More about Wright will be found under **IMMUNISATION**. See also (**THE DREADED**) **LURGY**.

ALLO- The 'difference' prefix, from Greek *allos* meaning 'other'. It occurs in various formations like allopathy, which is what practitioners in **HOMEOPATHY** call ordinary or traditional medical practice; and allograft, an Anglo-Greek word mixture meaning an organ transplant between non-identical members of the same species (formerly called homograft). See also under **ISO-** and **XENO-**.

ALMONER From Chaucer's time this was 'an official distributor of alms'; and, in British hospitals until the introduction of the **NHS**, the person responsible for seeing that poorer patients suffered no financial distress. The Almoner was nearly always a friendly lady of mature years who (often under the official title of 'Lady Almoner') worked voluntarily and without remuneration. At the same time she perhaps also gently persuaded those able to pay to contribute a little towards their treatment; and sometimes she inspired the really rich (or their relatives) to make a donation by way of thanksgiving: many a named ward endowed under such circumstances attests to the almoner's diplomacy and tact. The **WELFARE STATE** changed all that and the post was boringly renamed Medical Social Worker. Under **CHIEF/PRINCIPAL NURSING OFFICER** you will find a plethora of other new and grand job titles.

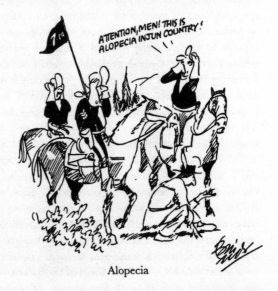

Alopecia

ALOPECIA/ALOPEX Baldness, or a dramatic and/or uneven hair-loss leading to it. From the Latin *alopex*, meaning 'a (mangy) fox' – which shows how insensitive the ancients could be about the **PHYSICALLY CHALLENGED**. See also **TERATO-**, the 'monster' prefix.

ALVEUS Latin for a cavity, a channel or hollow, e.g. in a tooth, *alveolus* a diminutive of it, a little hole. Latin *alvearium*, a beehive, hence medical words like alveated and alveolariform, honeycombed.

ALZHEIMER'S DISEASE This disorder of the brain was clinically described by a German neurologist, Dr Alois Alzheimer (1864–1916) – not 'Altzheimer' as often written. But informal descriptions abound in literature from classical times onwards. In 1726 Jonathan Swift (1667–1745) in his *Gulliver's Travels*, gave an early account of the symptoms of sufferers who '...have no remembrance of anything but what they learned in their youth and middle age, and even that is imperfect... In talking they forget the common appellation of things, and the names of persons, even those who are their nearest friends and relations. Neither are they able to hold any conversation (farther than a few general words) with their neighbours. They were the most mortifying sight I ever beheld'. Swift himself spent his last years in distress as an Alzheimer sufferer. With longer life-expectancy the condition has become more common and the word has entered every newspaper reader's vocabulary.

AMANITA Greek *amanitai*, fungus. The deceptively pretty name (see under **AMELIA**, below) for a species of mushroom of which *Amanita phalloides* is the deadliest, causing gastrointestinal upset, and possibly damage to the liver, kidney and central nervous system.

AMBROSIA The food eaten by Greek gods, and in late Latin the word for 'immortality' – the ultimate aim of **GERIATRIC** medicine. It is also the name of a patent brand of canned rice-pudding – delicious, sweetened pap food considered good for invalids and children. This was developed by an Englishman, Alfred Morris, and his American colleague (name unknown), who in 1917 discovered a way of drying milk and canning it with pudding-rice. A milk-drying process led to the formation of the pharmaceuticals company now trading as **GLAXO**. See also **PABULUM**.

AMBUL- The Latin word *ambulare*, to walk, or walk about, has acquired some confusing applications. For example, a patient who can walk is correctly described as an ambulant one; but one who cannot, is carried – in an ambulance. Babies are 'walked', i.e. pushed along, in a perambulator (Latin *perambulare*,

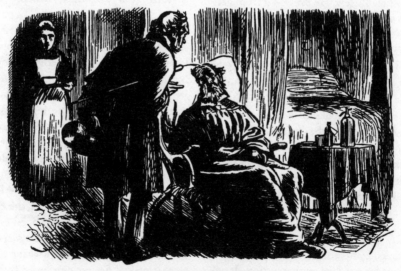

THE RULING PASSION.

Doctor. "NO, MY DEAR SIR, WE MUST KEEP OURSELVES QUIET FOR THE PRESENT. NO STIMULANTS - NOTHING MORE EXCITING THAN GRUEL. GRUEL FOR BREAKFAST, GRUEL FOR LUNCHEON, GRUEL FOR DINNER, GRUEL FOR-"
Peter Pundoleful (a noted Burlesque Writer - though you wouldn't have thought it to look at him - rousing himself suddenly). "AH! MY DEAR DOCTOR, WHY IS THERE NOT A SOCIETY FOR THE PREVENTION OF GRUELTY TO ANIMALS?"

Punch, April 12, 1884

'to amble or ramble about', which is nearly always abbreviated to 'pram' in the UK and called a baby carriage in North America. A sleep-walker is called a **NOCTAMBULIST**, which strictly means a *night-walker* (the true word for a sleepwalker being somnambulist – remember Bellini's opera *La Sonnambula*, which includes a character who claimed that she walked in her sleep and conveniently finished up in the wrong bedroom). See also **CLINIC** and **ZIMMER**.

AMBULANCE Originally a French word, which in early usage was often printed in italics to indicate its foreignness. Indeed it was a French idea to carry wounded soldiers in specialised horse-drawn vehicles rather than on shutters or stretchers: '*Ambulance*, a French word applied to moving hospitals which are attached to every French army' (*Penny Magazine*, 1833). Its inventor is said to have been Napoleon's surgeon, Baron Dominique Jean Larrey (who performed 200 operations in 24 hours after the Battle of Borodino in 1812), though the first recorded appearance of the word in print is dated 1809. But the German side was not to be outdone: Johann Gottlieb Benjamin Siegert, who served as a surgeon under von Blücher at the Battle of Waterloo, invented Angostura Bitters. He brewed it from gentian roots, rum and other ingredients, and it has ever since served to 'settle the stomachs' of British officers and colonials, especially when it was – and still is – heavily out-proportioned by gin, producing the famous Pink Gin (see also under **TONIC**). During the 1994 World Cup, which was held in the United States, a new kind of ambulance was seen on the world's television screens, the sporting Medical Cart, a kind of golf-cart adapted to hold a stretcher and one or more **PARAMEDICS**. It was used to remove the non-ambulant wounded from the soccer field and will doubtless soon come into use elsewhere.

AMBULANCE CHASER Lawyer who, sometimes accompanied by doctors, makes a business out of raising actions for medical compensation. It will surprise no-one that the term is an imaginative American coinage, as the medico-legal compensation industry was born in the USA; but the date of its probable first use may astonish even some Americans: 'In New York City there is a style of lawyers known to the profession as 'ambulance chasers', because they are on hand whenever there is a railway wreck, or a street-car collision ... with their offers of professional services' – *Congressional Records*, 24 July 1897.

AMELIA A pretty name for a girl – and the medical term for a calamitous total absence of arms or legs due to a congenital defect, from the Greek 'absence' prefix A- and *melos*, limb – and see also **PHOCOMELIA**. Other pretty female names might be **ALEXIA, AMANITA, BELLADONNA, CANDIDA, PLACENTA, PRUNELLA, QUINSY** and **SALMONELLA**. I once read somewhere of an American couple living in some isolated region who possessed only two books: one was the family Bible, the other the family's Home Doctor. Having given their first few children Biblical names, they turned to the other book and named some of those who followed after words they found in the index, including Hernia-Sue and Scarlatina (and if these why not also the ravishing young **ANGINA**, a girl who fair takes one's breath away?) Other reports speak of twins named Ireen and Urine (presumably because they were as alike as two peas); and that indefatigable researcher into language H.L. Mencken (1880–1956) knew of children christened '... Delirious, Anonymous, Neuralgia, Sterilize, Sal Hepatica, Morphine, Castor Oil, Ether, Constipation, Castile, Jingo, Vaseline and La-Urine. The name Positive Wasserman Johnson, sometime of Evanston, Ill., probably represents the indelicate humour of a medical student. The young brethren who deliver coloured mothers in the vicinity of the Johns Hopkins Hospital in Baltimore sometimes indulge the mothers to give their babies grandiose physiological and pathological names, but these are commonly expunged later on by watchful social workers and coloured pastors. Placenta, Granuloma and Gonadia, however, seem to have survived in a few cases. Medical humour probably explains the name of the coloured female twins, Roseola and Variola, born on James Island, S.C., in 1936.' (*The American Language*, Knopf, 1979). Modern composers have greater choice than the stock classical figures employed by, say, Handel or Ravel. For in addition to *Acis and Galatea* and *Daphnis and Chloe* they could write works about the marriage between *Annulus and Hymen*, about the word-blind twins, *Alexis and Alexia*, the neo-Wagnerian giants, *Myositis and Megalomania*, those perpetually frustrated lovers, *Dyspareunia and Phimosis*, and a radio/television drama about the battle between *Dysarthria and Eulalia*, which the former always wins.

AMNESIA Forgetfulness, from the Greek negating prefix *A-* + *mnemonic*, memory. See also **ANAMNESIS**.

AMNION The innermost membrane enveloping an embryo. From the Greek *amnos*, a lamb. *Amnion* means a caul – hence amniotic fluid and other derivatives; also amniocentesis, constructed with the addition of the Greek word for pricking, *kentein*: literally 'pricking a little lamb'. This is one of many instances (some of which will be found below) of Greek or Latin words for everyday objects being used as medical terms. Just as the word for an afterbirth, placenta, is the ordinary word for a cake (and many animal mothers dispose of the afterbirth by eating it as if it were one) so the cauls most often seen would have been those of new-born lambs.

AMPH(I)- Greek prefix meaning 'both' – both kinds, both sides, etc. But the drug amphetamine is based on an acronym arrived at when the persons naming it left out (or picked out) letters from its chemical components, *alpha*methyl*phe*ne*t*hyl*amine*. The naming of drugs (usually proprietary ones) is a subject beyond the scope of this book.

AMPUTARE Latin for cutting away, lopping off, pruning – in botany as well as the amputation of limbs from humans or animals. One who has suffered a loss by amputation is an *amputee*, the -ee suffix being legal in origin, from the Old French -é, as in 'lessee', 'legatee', 'garnishee', etc. and was later applied humorously to what the *Oxford English Dictionary* calls nonce-words, e.g. 'sendee', 'educatee' and 'devotee' (the last-named now respectably nonjocular) denoting that something has been done to, or suffered by, persons with an *-ee* suffix (in the Second World War people got used to 'evacuees' – and 'escapees' from places like Colditz, where presumably they were 'prisonees' of war). 'Escapee' is no improvement on 'escaper'. Some lawyers and coroners presiding over cases involving a donor refer to the recipient as a 'donee'; and employees of the British National Health Service also love -ee words. The *Oxford English Dictionary* gives a 1910 reference in verse from the *St. Bartholomew's Hospital Journal*:

> *Please put the patient both to bed*
> *And then perhaps we'll see*
> *Which is the amputated part*
> *And which the amputee.*

The most extreme form of amputation, decapitation, was invented by the French physician Joseph Ignace Guillotin (1738–1814), whose name the instrument carries. The guillotine, the most notable symbol of the excesses of the French Revolution, was in fact devised by him as a *humanitarian* innovation, to replace the messier hanging (used for commoners) or killing with the sword (reserved for the nobility). He argued that beheading by machine was quicker and less painful than the work of the rope and the sword. In 1791 the Assembly adopted beheading by machine as the state's preferred manner of execution, which continued to be the official French method of judicial murder well into the 20th century. Another beheading device was designed by Dr Antoine Louis, secretary of the French College of Surgeons, and first used on April 25, 1792, to execute a highwayman. The device was called a *louisette* or *louison* after its inventor, but Guillotin's name irrevocably stuck to the machine, whatever modifications it underwent. After Guillotin's death his children tried unsuccessfully to get the device's name changed. When their efforts failed, they changed their name instead. See also **BASKET CASE**.

AMUSIA The inability to comprehend (and therefore to reproduce or imitate by singing) musical sounds – see the long and amusing article on the subject by Natasha Spender in *Grove's Dictionary of Music*, sixth edition, commonly known as *The New Grove*.

AN Code abbreviation of **ANOREXIA**.

ANA- The Greek word for reduplication, over again, up, on, etc. Hence anabolic (e.g. as in the steroids illicitly taken by athletes), which combines *ana* with *bol*, the Greek word for a ball, literally 'a throwing up'. Such substances seem to be able to turn women athletes into near-males, with great, ball-like **BICEPS** and huge shoulder muscles. See also **EMBOLISM**; and **ANALYSIS**, definable as 'going over something again and again'; anatomy is cutting something up (see **-TOM-**). Also **-BOL**.

AN(A)EMIA A lack of blood, or blood containing less than the normal concentration of red cells.

AN(A)ESTHESIA Produced from two much-used Greek elements (see **AESTH-**) meaning, literally, 'no feeling'. The earliest known anaesthetic substance was **ALCOHOL**, and **HOUSE OFFICERS** in hospital casualty units testify to its effectiveness on **SATURDAY NIGHTS**. The first recorded anaesthetic was administered in AD 1236 by the Dominican friar Theodoric of Lucca, who taught medicine at Lucca, Italy and was the son of a surgeon to the Crusaders. Theodoric advocated the use of sponges soaked in a narcotic and applied to the nose in order to put patients to sleep before surgery, for which he favoured opiates like mandragora and opium. He also recommended mercurial ointments for skin diseases. In 1884 the New York surgeon William Stewart Halsted injected a patient with cocaine, thus pioneering the practice of local anaesthesia. He is probably the first anaesthetist reported to have succumbed to the narcotics used in his work, for during the course of his experiments he became addicted to cocaine; and although he recovered, he required morphine for the rest of his life in order to function.

ANALGESIC Tending to remove pain, or a medicine or other agent that does so. The *Oxford English Dictionary* says 'A better formation would be analgetic' – on the analogy of 'dyslectic' and 'anorectic', for which I have long fought a hopeless battle.

ANAMNESIS Greek *anamimneskein*, remembrance of the past (see also **NOSTALGIA**); also a psychiatric term for the accumulation of data; and an immunological one about the immune system's ability to remember previous infections.

ANAPHYLAXIS From the **ANA-** prefix + *phylaxis*, protection. An extreme hypersensitive reaction to a drug, food, etc. which can lead to anaphylactic shock and possibly death. Cases have been reported of such allergy to everyday foodstuffs, e.g. peanuts, in which the patients died within minutes. The most common cause of anaphylactic shock is an **ALLERGY** to **PENICILLIN**.

ANASARCA A form of dropsy, from **ANA-**, above + **SARC-**, the flesh prefix.

ANATOMIST Literally a 'cutter-up', from two Greek word-elements which are much in evidence in this book.

ANCILLARY Aiding, subservient, auxiliary: from Latin *ancilla*, a serving-maid.

ANDREWS LIVER SALTS 'Liver salts' usually denote laxatives (hence the description of anything

fast-moving as 'Like a dose of salts'). Andrews, on sale in Britain as 'health salts' (another euphemism) since 1893 is an effervescent powder to be dissolved in water. See also its sister-salts, **ENO'S** and **KRUSCHEN SALTS**.

ANDR(O)- The 'male' prefix. The female equivalent is **GYN(O)-**, (**GUNE-**). See also **-OID**.

ANDROGYNOUS From Greek *aner*, *andro-*, man (see above) and **-GYNE**, woman: having both male and female sexual characteristics. See also **HERMAPHRODITE**.

ANEURYSM A balloon-like swelling in a weakened place in the wall of an artery, from the Greek *aneurysma* for a 'widening out'. See also **HERNIA** and **DIVERTICULUM**. Most modern *-neur(o)-* words have to do with nerves, as does the neurologist – but for the sinew connection see under **NEURON**.

ANGELS A nickname for British nurses, first popularised by the title of a television 'soap'. But it goes back to William Cowper's 'ministering angels' and ultimately the Old Testament: 'Angels came and ministerd unto him' (St Matthew, iii, 11). They also minister in Shakespeare's *Hamlet*. Like all book, film and TV titles 'angels' soon entered **TABLOID** press shorthand ('Angel Strangled Baby') and was finally taken up by patients, especially when they wanted to convey their gratitude after a stay in hospital.

ANG(IO)- One of the prefixes denoting vessels, blood (or lymph – see **LYMPHA**), from Greek *aggeion*, vessel. The prefix has produced numerous formations.

ANGINA From Latin *angere*, to strangle, *angustia*, tightness or narrowness, which already in ancient French (*angoisse*, *anguisse*) and Italian (*angoscia*) took on the meaning of choking. Hence not only angina pectoris, a tightness of the chest, but also words like *anger* and *anguish* – which indeed may help to bring on an attack of angina. And, of course, the German *ANGST*, immediately below. The Greek word for strangling, or binding tight, *sphingein*, gave us the **SPHINCTER**, with its undertones of that remorseless quiz-mistress, the Sphinx.

ANGST This is the ordinary, normal, everyday German word meaning fear, anguish or anxiety and in the third sense often occurs in the writings of

Freud. For some reason, however, the German word *Angst* was never translated into English by Freud's translators, so that it has become a fully anglicised one that is pronounced in the English manner and written angst, with a small *a*. In its clinical sense it denotes the deeper states of clinical anxiety, remorse, guilt or irrational fear; but journalists have long used it indiscriminately, thus devaluing it to a cliché.

ANHEDONIA From Greek *hedon*, pleasure, preceded by the **AN-** prefix of negation: literally, 'no pleasure'. It is applied to sexual intercourse: *Merck* says that in this condition 'a patient experiences erection and ejaculation with no pleasure during orgasm', and adds that 'the cause is psychogenic penile anaesthesia'. This should please the Irish Catholic priest who told a couple that having sex on Sundays or holy days was 'all right so long as you don't enjoy it'. Female anhedonia must be much more common but appears not to figure much in the textbooks.

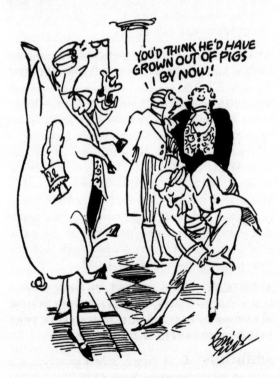

Animal baths

ANIMAL BATHS From the German *Tierbäder*. This 'cure' (described here for historical and culinary rather than practical reasons) is an ancient method of promoting healing by inserting an affected part into the carcass of a freshly-slaughtered animal. A journalist dining with Ludwig van Beethoven in 1820 wrote down for him: 'The Emperor Leopold I [1640–1705] was a 7-month baby. To make him put on weight they constantly kept him inside the carcass of a freshly-slaughtered pig. Afterwards the meat was given to the poor. That's why it's called *Kaiser Fleisch*'. (It is still a favourite Austrian delicacy: lightly-smoked lean pork, originally from a sucking-pig, which would have been about the right size for a prematurely-born baby emperor). Schumann, too, had animal baths prescribed for him, at first to speed the healing of his fingers (after having his tendons cut in hopes of achieving a bigger stretch at the piano) and again, in a different topical application, when he caught **GONORRH(O)EA** – after which, one hopes, the pork was *not* distributed to the poor.

ANKYLO- The stiffness prefix, from Greek *angkulos*, crooked; hence *ankylosis*, stiffness in the joints, from various causes. But see also **CLAUDICATION**.

ANODYNE From Greek *an* + *odune*, pain: relief from pain, or a substance or measure designed to relieve it. The **ANALGESIC** Anadin is a cleverly punning trade-name.

ANOPHELES The Greek word meaning useless, and very aptly applied to the mosquito, whose sole use seems to be to spread **MALARIA**. See also **PARASITE**.

ANOREXIA Also Anorexia nervosa. Lack of appetite, from *AN-*, the 'absence' prefix + *orexis*, which is Greek and Latin for appetite, hunger, desire or a longing (in this case for food). The 'correct' adjective is anorectic; and sufferers are anorectics, but the unpleasantly sibilant and erroneous formation 'anorexics' has taken root, and been accepted by all but a handful of medical people (who never said 'prophylaxics' or 'dyspepsics'). The same process gave us 'dyslexics' instead of dyslectics (read more about it under **DYSLEXIA**). But when the word **DYSPEPSIA** went into common usage Latin and Greek were still on the school curriculum, so that even the advertising industry got it right. See also **DYS-** and the various other food- and eating-related cross-references, from **BANTING** onwards.

ANOSMIA From Greek **AN-** + *osme*, smell, an inability to smell things, especially food (*anosmia-*

gustatoria). Loss of smell also impairs taste: see **GEUSIS** for ageusia, lack of taste sensation. Also **GUSTUS**.

ANOXIA A 'made-up' word meaning lack of oxygen, or a condition caused by such a lack.

ANTE-, ANTERO- The 'frontal' or 'before' prefixes, from the Latin *anterus*, front. Not to be confused with **ANTI-**, against. The Romans must have been good spellers and meticulous pronouncers: nowadays many people consider the difference trivial (like that between the Greek **HYPER-** and **HYPO-**). A large English hospital displayed a painted signpost reading TO THE GYNAECOLOGICAL AND ANTI-NATAL CLINICS: the latter presumably a birth-control clinic.

ANTHRAX Latin for a carbuncle, from the Greek word meaning coal (*cf* anthracite). See also **ECZEMA**.

ANTHROP(O)- Prefix denoting man – in its pre-feminist-challenged meaning, from the Greek *anthropos*, man – in the sense of mankind, humankind. Hence anthropology, the study of man; and numerous other formations.

ANTHROPOMETRY Literally, measurement of man.

ANT(I) Can mean both 'against' and 'opposite'. Both senses are much used in Latin. An antidote is a medicine given to counteract a poison – see below. See also **ANTE-**, above, and several other formations, below.

ANTIBIOTICS Latin *anti*, against + *bios*, Greek for life: a seemingly contradictory name for a group of life-*saving* drugs (beginning with **PENICILLIN**). The explanation is that the *life* which these fungus-based drugs attack is that of harmful micro-organisms. If antibiotics had been discovered earlier they would have changed the course of history, social, military and artistic – and also ruined the plots of many operas, e.g. Verdi's *La Traviata*: one shot from Dr Grenvil into Violetta's backside could have brought down the curtain on a happy ending before the close of the first act. See also **MYC-** and **PHTHISIS**. An equally oxymoronic name was given to the **ANTIBODY** – below.

ANTIBODY A translation from the German *Antikörper* (first noted in 1901) and, I suggest, not a very happy one: antibacterial, antidepressant, anti-vaccination, anti-this and anti-that – and then we are supposed to learn to love the antibody, which sounds as though it should work *against* our body. It is in fact a defensive plasma protein, either naturally present in the body or produced in response to the introduction of an antigen (below), and is a wholly Good Thing.

ANTIDOTE From Greek/Latin *anti*, against, + *dotos*, that which is given, e.g. a dose, which is derived from the latter word. A drug or other substance that opposes the action of another drug or a poison. See also **TOXI-**.

ANTIGEN From the German *Antigen*, itself taken from the French *antigène* (1899, associated with the work of Louis Pasteur). A foreign substance which, when introduced into the body, stimulates the production of an **ANTIBODY**, above.

ANTISEPTIC See **SEPSIS**.

ANTR(O)- The prefix indicating a hollow place or cavity in the body. From Latin *antrum*, a cave, itself from the Greek *antron* – perhaps a prehistoric kind of **ARCHITECTURAL** naming.

ANUS Latin for a ring; hence, in both classical and medical Latin, the lower, open end of the **RECTUM**. *An(n)ulus* is a little ring (the extra *n* was erroneously added in medieval Latin), *annular*, little-ring-shaped – one of many words now used scientifically but originally, in everyday Roman use, facetious or obscene. Like many Latin words, *anus* is inflected according to case: *ani*, of the anus, *per anum*, by the anus, etc. Not to be confused with *per annum*, once a year, though I regret to report that *The Merck Manual of Diagnosis and Therapy* (1977 edition, p. 761) asserts that wind may be passed 'per anus': an error that would have horrified every medical student of previous generations. See also **PROCTOS**.

APERIENT A laxative, from Latin *aperire*, to open, in this case the bowels. For other **GENTLE PERAMBULATORS** see **CASCARA**, **KRUSCHEN SALTS**, **PERISTALTIC PERSUADERS** and cross-references.

APHRODISIAC A drug or substance which, it is claimed, stimulates sexual desire, **CUPIDITY**, **LAGNIA** or **LIBIDO**. It is named after Aphrodite, Goddess of Love. *Institutiones Chirurgicae*, published in London in 1655, recommends the following: 'To make a man have lust to a Woman – Take Fennell-seeds and steirwith, of each 2 ounces, grind it & mingle it with new Cows Milk, and make Pellets thereof as big as beans, and take it at night and three in the morninge; (but) first of all anoint the Member with Oyle and the Juice of Morrell and Vinegar...' (though the process of anointing the member with oil, if continued long enough, would probably have been the most effective part of the treatment). One of the most powerful aphrodisiacs known to man is revealed under **GERON-TOPHILIA**. See also **CANTHARIDES** or 'Spanish Fly'.

APHRODITE The Greek Goddess of Love, mother of **EROS** and daughter of Zeus (though some said she emerged ready-made and perfectly-formed, from sea foam). The Romans identified her with **VENUS**; and both her and her family's Greek and Latin names have provided words on subjects touched on in this book.

APN(O)EA Greek *A-* + *pnein*, breath: an absence of spontaneous respiration. There are several kinds, but the one the layman is most aware of is sleep apn(o)ea.

APO- One of those multi-purpose Greek prefixes that can have various shades of meaning, such as 'off', 'from' or 'away from'. Hence apoclasm, the fracture of an extremity.

APOGLUTIC Small-buttocked: usually said of a woman. See also **GLUT(A)EUS**, **NATES** and **CALLI-**.

APONEUROSIS A fibrous membrane, sometimes serving as the sheath of a muscle, sometimes connecting a muscle and a tendon. There is nothing 'neurotic' about it in the popular sense, although most modern **NEUR(O)-** words have to do with nerves, not fibrous tissue. The confusion is explained under **NEURON**.

APOSIOPESIS In classical rhetoric this is 'an artifice in which the speaker comes to a sudden halt, as if unable or unwilling to proceed' (Greek *aposiopan*, to be quite silent, from *siope*, silence); but in a more prosaic application it is the Greek equivalent of the Latin **COITUS INTERRUPTUS** – usually not so much an inability or unwillingness to proceed but the inability to stop.

APOTHECARY A store-keeper, one who shuts away drugs for safe-keeping, from Greek *apotheke*, a storehouse – of any kind, not only for **PHARMACEU-TICALS**. In German-speaking countries you will find

APOTHEKE written above pharmacies, usually illustrated for the benefit of foreigners with a blue cross and/or a symbolic pestle-and-mortar, which is the traditional, ancient shop-sign for the trade, originally affixed for the benefit of the illiterate.

APPENDECTOMY/APPENDICECTOMY
The first is the American form, which is gaining ground in Britain, while purists maintain that the name for the operation should be appendicectomy. See **CAECUM**, **-ECTOMY**, **-TOM-** and the appendix entry below. The first recorded successful removal of a patient's appendix is said to have been performed in 1736 by the English surgeon Claudius Aymand. In recent decades the incidence of the operation has sharply declined, thus depriving trainee surgeons of one of the 'nursery' operations traditionally entrusted to them. As a newspaper implausibly put it, 'the appendix used to be what young surgeons cut their teeth on'. Another suspect formation will be found under **NOCTURIA**.

APRICOT SICKNESS Literally translated from the Afrikaans *Appelkoossiekte*, a form of **DYSENTERY** found in South Africa which often appears at the beginning of summer, when apricots are ripening. For the origin of the name of the fruit see under **PRAECOX**.

ARACHN(O)- The 'spider' prefix, hence arachnoidism, poisoning from the bite of a spider, arachnophobia, a fear of spiders, arachno-**DACTYL**y, abnormally long fingers (in the pathological, not the thieving, sense); but 'arachnoid' is also applied to various parts of the body, e.g. sections of the brain and spinal cord, which are thought to be web-like.

ARCHITECTURAL TERMS The Greeks and Romans set standards of beauty and design in architecture which have remained valid ever since, so it is not surprising that they named many parts of the human body after architectural features they thought resembled them. See individual headings, e.g. **ATRIUM**, **CLAUS-TRUM**, **CLIMA(CTERIC)**, **CUPOLA**, **FASTIGIUM**, **FAUCES**, **FOCUS**, **FORNIX**, **PALATUM**, **PHRAGMA**, **PORTA**, **TECTUM**, **TENTORIUM**, **THALAMOS**, **TRA-BECULUM**, **VESTIBULUM**, etc. Even **FORENSIC** medicine owes something to classical buildings.

AREOLA Latin for a very small space, or 'little area' (the Latin diminutive of *area*, which was originally a vacant piece of level ground in a town). It became a euphemism used by the early doctors for the circle around the human nipple (ranging in colour from the palest pale pink to almost black) but may also describe any round coloured spot.

ARISTO- Greek prefix, from *aristos*, the best, hence aristocracy, literal meaning 'rule by the best people'. This may displease **PROLES** – but do we not *want* to be ruled by the *best* people? For a sidelight on the British aristocracy see under **DOWAGER'S HUMP** – though not **LORDOSIS**.

AROMATHERAPY The first part of the word means a smell, the second, healing, so it should be self-explanatory; but this kind of alleged healing borders on the outermost fringes of fringe medicine, possibly even **CHARLATANISM**. (And yet, the Greek *therapeuein*, which gave us **THERAPY**, means not only to heal but also to cherish or cosset – so why not with pleasant odours?). 'Aromaprophylaxis', if there were such a word, might find a place here, for until the nature of antisepsis was understood the inhaling of perfumes was thought to help ward off infection, or would at any rate mask bad smells. During the 17th and 18th centuries English caricaturists and painters often depicted doctors in consultation (or concentration) holding the top of a cane or walking-stick against their (the doctors') chin or side of the face. These ornamental knobs, usually of gold or silver, were hollow, perforated pomanders which contained sweet-smelling herbs. Even today doctors report that they encounter many a **REEKER**.

ARSD Alcohol-Related Sudden Death Syndrome. See **ALCOHOL** and **HOLIDAY HEART SYNDROME**.

ARS LONGA, VITA BREVIS The First Aphorism of the Greek physician **HIPPOCRATES** (c.460–c.370 BC). Although much quoted in its four-word, abbreviated Latin form, and usually used as though it applied to the arts in general, Hippocrates meant the Art of Healing: 'Life is short, the art long, opportunity fleeting, experiment treacherous, judgment difficult'. As W.H. Auden (1907–73) wrote (in *A Certain World*, 'Medicine', 1970): A doctor, like anyone else who has to deal with human beings, each of them unique, cannot be a scientist; he is either, like the surgeon, a craftsman, or, like the physician and the psychologist, an artist. . . . This means that in order to be a good doctor a man must also have a good character, that is to say, whatever weaknesses

and foibles he may have, he must love his fellow human beings in the concrete and desire their good before his own'.

ARTERIO- Latin and Greek *arteria* mean both artery and vein (the word *aorta* is related) but other prefixes include *angio-*, *phlebo-* and *veno-*.

ARTHR- The joints prefix – from:–

ARTHRON Greek for a joint. The prefix, above, is often combined with suffixes, e.g. **-ALGIA**, **-ITIS**; and see also **GROWING-PAINS**.

ARTICULATIO The Latin equivalent of **ARTHRON**, above. It has given us words denoting articulation, i.e. moveability, of jointed limbs.

ARTIFICIAL PACEMAKER The man-in-the-waiting-room will know that a pacemaker is an electrical device used for maintaining the heart's rhythm (the idea was first postulated in about 1950) but will assume that this apparatus was named after the sports pacemaker, a rider or rower who sets the pace for another in training. But according to the textbooks the heart has its natural pacemaker, which determines the rate at which the heart contracts: 'the sinoatrial node of specialised nervous tissue located at the junction of the superior vena cava and the right atrium...'

ASH CASH Fee paid to a doctor for signing a cremation form.

ASKLEPIOS The Greek God of Medicine, *AESCULAPIUS* in Latin. Although the precepts attributed to him are doubtless rooted in primitive folk remedies they profoundly influenced later practitioners. If the classical gods 'assumed human form' it is not too fanciful to suppose that Asklepios really existed and that his transformation was in the opposite direction – that is, he may have been an intuitively clever man endowed with an uncommon degree of common-sense, who was raised to godhead for his powers as a healer: after all, the intuitive system of medicine still remains among practitioners (and so does the eventual elevation of some of the British ones). Asklepios was the son of Coronis, a mortal woman who when pregnant was killed by Apollo's sister Artemis, but he was saved by post-mortem **CAESAREAN** section. Subsequently he was struck dead by Zeus – only to be resurrected as a god himself – rehabilitation with a vengeance. Asklepios (Aesculapius, Esclapius or Asclepius, etc., – spellings vary) over-reached himself when he claimed he was so good a healer that he could restore the dead to life. It was for this that he was killed with a thunderbolt by Zeus, who resented the fact ('fact'?) that he (Asklepios) was depriving the underworld of interesting recruits. He was symbolised by the device of a snake winding round a staff, which is now the international emblem of medicine. His daughter was the Goddess **HYGIEIA**. Mr Michael Reilly writes, 'His influence is still strong in the medical world, and survives in Epidaurus. When I visited his grove there I felt a frisson: I could imagine the therapeutic effects of drama, in the magnificent theatre (where one hears a whisper on the stage in the back row of the auditorium) of music and "aromatherapy". No wonder that his symbol is a serpent – a sibilant intruder, with phallic implications, into secret places'. Grateful patients made offerings to Asklepios, often in the form of terracotta models of those parts of their body which he had healed – limbs, breasts, ears, genitals, etc. Many of these survive in museums, and in Greece and other countries touched by the Graeco-Roman civilisation these small effigies are still displayed in Christian churches by former sufferers (though not intimate body parts, which are presumably forbidden by the incumbent priests). See also **HERMES**, **GALEN** and **HIP-POCRATES** – and those altruistic doctor-twins, Saints **COSMAS AND DAMIAN**.

ASPHYXIA Greek combination-word meaning, literally, 'no breath/pulse', from Latin *spirare*, to breathe. See **A-**.

ASPIRIN A word contructed in 1899 by Dr C. Wittauer from the German words *Acetilirte Spirsäure*, acetylated spireic acid, and manufactured by the German chemicals firm Bayer. This retained the patent for many years (except in Australia: see below) but it is now a **GENERIC** preparation – and fast becoming the century's wonder-drug. Salicylates are related to the willow tree, Latin *salix*, parts of which were used by the ancients for their **ANALGESIC** properties.

ASPRO Bayer, the makers of **ASPIRIN**, above, forgot to apply for a patent for it in Australia, which from 1914 onwards made its own version and called it Aspro. The name is a combination of the surname of its Australian producer, the chemist George Nicholas, and the first syllable of the word *Pro*duct. Australia also gave **BILE BEANS** to the world. But Dispirin, i.e. *dis*solvable as*pirin*, was registered in 1944 by Roy Vickers of Liverpool.

ASR Acute Stress Reaction, which sounds more impressive to lawyers than severe shock, which is what it is – an earlier stage of **PTS**, perhaps.

ASTHENIA The Greek word for weakness, debility: strictly 'lacking in strength': *sthenos*, with the A-prefix denoting a lack of it. Hence *myasthenia*, muscle weakness (see **MYS/MUS**, the 'muscle' element); and **NEURASTHENIA**, an imprecise name for what was thought to have been a 'general weakness of the nerves'.

ASTHMA From the Greek *asthmatikos*, panting, short of breath. The standard pronunciation 'ast-ma' appears to have been joined by a new one, now increasingly used in some circles: 'azz-ma'. There is no law against new foibles, but this one is capricious and lacks any etymological basis.

ASTIGMATISM Greek *stigma*, a mark or point which, preceded by the A- prefix, creates the word for a defect of vision when the sight of the two eyes does not converge on the same point.

ASYLUM Latin for a sanctuary or place of refuge for criminals and debtors, from which they could not be removed without the commission of sacrilege by the remover. The usage gradually changed, and later it came to describe a benevolent but secure place where the afflicted, especially **LUNATICS**, were confined, so that the word 'asylum' on its own eventually took on the meaning of an institution for persons suffering from mental illness; also for the education of children of the poor: 'The Royal Military Asylum – to give the institution its official title – or the Duke of York's School, as it is both locally and generally known', as *The Graphic* of May 26, 1888 put it. Former lunatic asylums were eventually euphemised as Mental Homes, Psychiatric **CLINICS**, etc., for which see also **HOSPITAL NAMES**.

ATAXIA Unsteady, shaky or awkward movement, usually in walking; from **TAX-** the prefix for order, with the A- prefix. Hence the archaic English word ataxy, general disorder, e.g. as found in my own study.

ATHERE Greek for porridge or gruel. Used at first to describe the contents of a sebaceous cyst, then transferred, usually as the prefix *ather-*, to descriptions of vascular disease, e.g. atheroma. *See* **-OMA**.

ATHLETE'S FOOT The popular name for tinea pedis. See **TINEA**.

ATRIUM The central chamber or court of a Roman house – a feature now back in vogue, thanks to fashion-conscious modern architects, though Romans could afford to leave theirs open to the skies. It was also the place where the hearth, or focus, would be situated, so that the walls soon became blackened: and the Latin word for black is *ater*. The heart has two atria (or atriums, either is accepted) and the appropriate prefix for the resulting adjectives is *atrio-*. Meanwhile, over in Greece, the focus was on the bedroom, the inner chamber, or **THALAMOS**, which please see. For other architectural-anatomical features see **CLAUSTRUM, FAUCES, FORNIX, PHRAGMA, PORTA, TRABECULUM, VESTIBULUM,** etc.

ATROPHY Literally 'no growth' – see **TROPHE**. Also **VESTIGIUM**.

ATROPINE From Greek **A-** + *tropos*, 'no turning', that is, inflexible, which is what the **PUPIL** becomes when dilated with the alkaloid substance found in deadly nightshade (see **BELLADONNA**) or the seeds of the thorn-apple for which the botanic name is *Atropa*. Atropos was one of the Three Cruel Fates, who paid no regard to the wishes of anyone. One of the others was **LACHESIS**.

AUDIRE Latin to hear. The Greek is *akouein* or *akousma*, something that is heard.

AUR- Related to the above, the Latin *auris*, ear, has given us the 'hearing' prefix too common to need examples. Also auricle, a small ear-shaped appendage of the **ATRIUM**.

AUSCULTATION From Latin *auscultare*, to listen, especially to listen attentively: to diagnose illness by

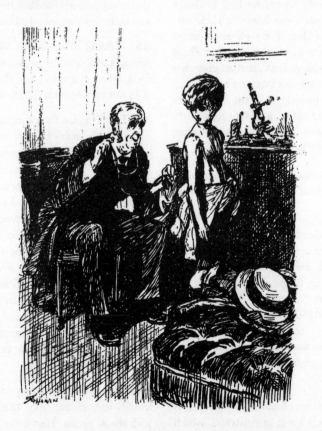

Gentle Voice from Boy. "DOCTOR, IF YOU'RE LOOKING FOR MY CHEST, I *THINK* YOU'LL FIND IT IN FRONT."

Punch, 2 August, 1909

listening, e.g. to the heart. Like palpate, from *palpare*, to feel, the word is often unnecessarily used in place of the simpler English equivalent. For more about palpation and the finger recommended for its use see under **DIGITUS**.

AUT(O)- The prefix of soleness, sameness, aloneness or even loneliness, from the Greek *autos*, self. *Autistic* people are thought to be introspective or inward-looking. There is a range of other *auto*-constructions, most of them self-explanatory, like autograft, skin taken from (and grafted to) the same body, autoeroticism, etc. But:–

AUTOPSY The viewing, examination and probably dissection of a dead body literally means 'seeing for oneself' – or else 'looking for oneself', which lends a philosophical dimension to this often unpleasant task. Purists say **NECROPSY** would be better.

AUXOLOGY The study of growth. Greek *auxesis*, growth, *auxein*, to increase – hence also the auctioneer.

A&W Alive and well.

B*b*

BABINSKI REFLEX A test relating to a response of the sole of the foot, or **PLANTAR** response.

BABY CATCHER Nickname for an obstetrician.

BACILLUS See **BACTERIUM**, below.

BACITRACIN An antibiotic named after the first syllable of **BACILLUS** + an American woman called Tracy, from whose organisms it was first obtained, by Johnson and others, in the United States in 1945.

BACTERIUM From the Greek *bakterion*, a little rod or staff, for which the Latin word is *bacillus*, a variant of *baculum*, a rod or little stick. Bacteria and bacilli come in great numbers, so it is wrong to speak of 'a bacteria' or 'a bacillus', as many journalists – and even some doctors – now do. A patient hearing this solecism from his doctor should hurry for a second opinion. See also **VIRUS**.

BALANOS The Greek word for an acorn – see under **GLANS**.

BALNEOTHERAPY The medicinal (and allegedly beneficial) use of baths for **THERAPY**. Baths used frequently to be prescribed by doctors – especially when they ran out of other ideas – and they would carefully distinguish between different kinds, e.g. in sea-water, or **THALASSOTHERAPY**; baths with or without additives in the water; hot baths, cold baths, or **PSYCHROLUSIA**, or both in alternation; or either, combined with physical exercise (which requires less effort when part of the body is submerged and therefore approaching weightlessness). Today no-one questions the beneficial effects of relaxation in warm water, but up to late Victorian times this, too, was considered dangerous unless done under strict supervision. Such thinking conveniently led men to bagnios or bath-houses – which offered 'therapy' that is beyond the scope of this book.

BANTING To most people today the word suggests – quite rightly – Sir Frederick Grant Banting (1891–1941) who with C.H. Best first used the hormone insulin in the treatment of diabetes (which he at first called 'isletin', after the islets of Langerhans). But the same name was already on most English-speaking lips from the middle of the 19th century until well into the 20th, and had connotations of food, dieting and obesity. 'Banting' and 'to bant' meant the same as 'to slim', after a weight-reduction regime devised by William Banting (1797–1878).

As a fashionable London cabinet-maker and undertaker he empirically observed the relationship between obesity and ill-health, having noticed that many of his prematurely deceased clients were much overweight. **CORPULENCE** was then considered synonymous with good health, and even regarded as an insurance against disease and guard against infection, especially **PHTHISIS**. The relationship he discovered between obesity and early death alarmed him greatly, as he himself was so stout that, he complained, his ankles were unable to support his weight, and even his personal hygiene had suffered (he was, as he delicately put it, 'unable to attend to the *little offices* which humanity requires' – in other words, he simply could not reach). Banting's regimen of physical exercise, combined with a fat-, starch- and sugar-free diet, including a little white wine, achieved national and international fame. In Britain he became a celebrity, his name was a household word and was even, as is mentioned above, turned into a verb: 'Do you bant?', people would ask each other. Several songs were inspired by his diets and the English satirical magazine *Punch* used him as a butt for its amiable jokes, thereby further helping his cause. In his dual role of undertaker and slimming-adviser he numbered among his clients members of the – then usually overweight – Royal family as well as the 15-stone (210 lb) novelist Anthony Trollope.

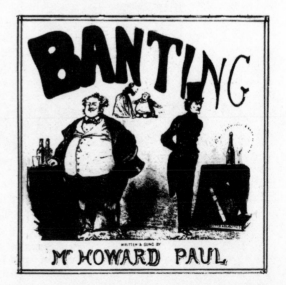

Before and after. Part of the title-page of one of numerous slimming songs composed in honour of William Banting.

BARBITURATE From the Greek *barbitos*, a many-stringed lyre, which presumably had a soothing effect on the hearers and possibly even sent them to sleep. That is one explanation. The other is given in the *Oxford English Dictionary*, which says that barbituric acid (in German *Barbitursäure*), was so named by a German chemist called Bayer who derived it 'from Barbara, a woman's name'. The substance has also been linked with St. Barbara, which is unlikely as she was the patron saint of gunners and miners, who tend to keep people awake with loud, explosive noises. For undisputed female connections see, however, **BACITRACIN** and **BELLADONNA**.

BAREFOOT DOCTOR See **FELDSHER**.

BARK A type of flatulence authoritatively defined in the *Merck Manual of Diagnosis and Therapy* (16th edition). You will find it under the heading of **FLATULENCE**.

BARTHOLIN'S GLANDS Situated on the posterior and lateral aspect of the vestibule of the vagina, they secrete mucus during sexual arousal. They were discovered – or at any rate described, as their owners doubtless knew of them first – by the Dutch anatomist Caspar T. Bartholin, born in 1655.

BART'S/BARTS The almost universal nickname-abbreviation of St. Bartholomew's Hospital, London, founded in 1123 by one Rahere. He was born in the reign of William the Conqueror and was buried in St. Bartholomew the Great in 1144. In about 1120 he went on a pilgrimage to Rome, where he contracted **MALARIA**, and on his convalescence vowed that he would make a hospital 'yn recreacioun of poure men'. In a subsequent vision or dream the apostle Bartholomew appeared to him, indicating Smithfield as the site he desired. Other ancient London hospitals include St. Thomas's and Guy's, though their future is at present (1994) uncertain. According to an old saying, young women 'Go to Thomas's to be a Lady, to Bart's to get Married and to Guy's to learn Nursing'.

BASIN GPs' diagnostic mnemonic when testing for multiple sclerosis: B for the **BABINSKI REFLEX**; A for abdominal Reflexes; S for Speech Impairment; I for **INTENTION TREMOR**; and N for **NYSTAGMUS**.

BASKET CASE American forces' name for an unfortunate patient, especially a soldier, who has lost all four limbs and whose trunk is therefore supported in a basket-like device. The expression is also (says

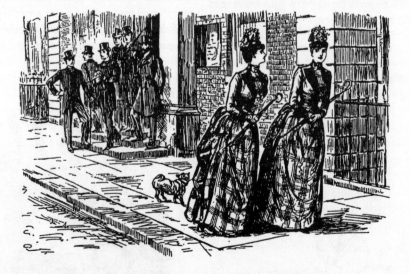

HAPPY THOUGHT - A VOCATION!

Eva. "I suppose those extremely nice-looking Young Men are the Students, or House-Surgeons, or something!"
Maud. "No doubt. Do you know, Eva, I feel I should very much like to be a Hospital-Nurse!"
Eva. "How strange! Why the very same Idea has just occurred to Me!"

Punch, May 21, 1887

the *Oxford English Dictionary*) used of someone emotionally or mentally unstable and unable to cope; or something that is no longer functional, even a country unable to pay its debts or feed its people. 'Basket' is also an informal nickname for the **SCROTUM**. And see **HEMICORPORECTOMY**.

BBA In obstetrics, abbreviation for '(Baby) Born before Arrival'; also sometimes, inevitably, Baby Born in Ambulance'. See also **DOA**.

BD Pharmacists' abbreviation of *bis die,* Latin for twice daily.

BDELLATOMY The practice of cutting leeches to empty them of blood while they continue to suck. From Greek *bdella,* a leech, for which the Latin is **HIRUDO**.

BED BLOCKERS Those who cannot be discharged from hospital, having been cured of everything except old age.

BED HOPPERS Nothing to do with sexual promiscuity among medics and nurses but a term for patients who feign illness to gain admission to hospital, where they enjoy being pampered and made the centre of attention: in other words, unfortunate people, usually, who were deprived of such treatment in their childhood. See also **MÜNCHHAUSEN SYNDROME**.

BEDLAM Now the word for any place of noise, uproar and confusion, like a casualty department on a Saturday night, but originally the contracted popular name of the Hospital of St. Mary of Bethlehem, founded as a priory in Bishopsgate, London, in 1247. Quite early in its existence it received, and attempted to cure (mostly by preaching religion), mentally deranged persons. It was in 1676 rebuilt near London Wall; and again transferred, in 1815, to St George's Fields, Lambeth, which was turned (after the last occupants were moved out in 1931) into what is now the Imperial War Museum. Early Bedlam inmates not considered dangerous were accommodated in the Abraham Ward and occasionally allowed out onto the streets (or **RELEASED INTO THE COMMUNITY**, as the British **NHS** would now describe it) to beg, provided they wore distinctive dress. They were known as Abra(ha)m-men, hence 'to sham Abram' meant to feign illness or madness while playing on the generosity of passers-by. One was described in 1561 (by Awdelay) as 'bare-armed and bare-legged, and fayneth hymselfe mad'; and an author called Head wrote in 1674, 'for all their seeming madness, they had wit enough to steal as they went along'. They are also portrayed in Shakespeare's *King Lear* and Beaumont and Fletcher's *Beggar's Bush*. In this instance no-one laments the passing of the old English **HOSPITAL NAMES**.

BEDSIDE MANNER The behaviour of a doctor (or nurse) as perceived by the patient. It is a subject to which insufficient attention is sometimes paid, especially when the patient is elderly or old. Some doctors or nurses forget that a patient may be hard-of-hearing; others automatically assume that all old people are either deaf, or stupid, or both and shouts at them. Hospital patients who in the outside world follow (or if retired have behind them) a distinguished career and are used to being treated with respect, suddenly find themselves addressed by their first name (or a diminutive of it) by nurses in their late teens who would not dream of addressing thus their

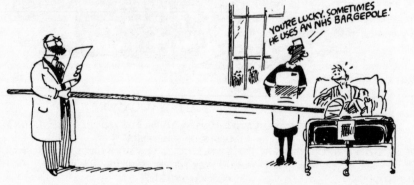

Bedside Manner

own grandparents. Conversely, an elderly spinster who never married and had no children, let alone grandchildren, may be awarded the title 'granny': a dignified old lady so addressed was once heard to say, 'The name is '*Miss* Greville-Wilkinson. I am nobody's *granny*'. Even the grandest hospital consultant who when doing his rounds had everyone jumping to attention may find himself at the receiving-end of such over-familiarity (mistaken for 'friendliness') from unknowing staff as soon as doctor turns patient. I have long treasured a set of instructions, copied by hand, and described as 'taken from a mediaeval manuscript', on how a visiting physician should conduct himself:

1. Dress soberly, like a Clerke, not like a Minstrell.
2. When called to a patient, find out from the messenger all you can about him before you arrive. Then you can impress the pacient with your knowledge of his condicioun, even if his puls and uryne tell you nothing.
3. Ensure that the pacient has confess'd *before* you examine him. If you wait until after your examinatioun, and then advise him to confess, he will suspect the worst.
4. When feeling the pacient's pulse, allow for the fact that he may be disturb'd by your presence, or the thought of the fee you will charge him.
5. Tell the patient that with God's help you hope to cure him. But to relatives say that the Case is grave. If he dies, this will save your reputatioun, if he recovers, enhaunce it.
6. Stay sober, modest and grave at all times.
7. Do not look lecherously at the pacient's wife, daughtres or servants, nor fondle theyr brestes, nor whisper to them in corners.
8. Do not dysparage your fellow-physiciouns.

BEECHAM'S PILLS Formerly Britain's most famous 19th/20th-century proprietary medicine, invented and patented in 1847 by Thomas Beecham (1820–1907). He was a successful vendor of **PATENT MEDICINES** and built factories in St. Helens, Lancashire and (in 1885) in New York, as well as on the continent of Europe, to manufacture the product. Beecham made a fortune with his pills but, as many pharmaceutical companies do to this day, became a tireless benefactor, especially in South Lancashire, where he used much of his wealth for the benefit and education of the people. He published cheap popular editions of books (by Charles Dickens, among others) and collections of music, the so-called Beecham's

Portfolios, which were interspersed with 'commercial' jingles extolling his Pills in song and verse. His good fortune enabled his grandson, Sir Thomas Beecham (1879–1961), to enter the musical profession as conductor–impresario without having to endure preliminary apprenticeships or assistantships, and to establish opera companies and orchestras (including the Royal Philharmonic Orchestra of London, in which the present writer for a time played Principal Flute). Beecham's Pills were sold under an advertising slogan which entered the quotations dictionaries: 'Worth A Guinea a Box', a claim which the British Medical Association questioned as early as 1909, in its investigative book, *Secret Remedies – What they Cost and what they Contain,* concluding that 'the prime cost of the ingredients of the 56 pills ... is about half a farthing' – a quarter of an old, pre-decimal penny. Beecham's Pills were eventually superseded by Beecham's Powders, which are aspirin-based and sold without prescription for the relief of common-cold symptoms.

BEER BELLY Also called **ALE GUT**, a form of **OBESITY** in men popularly attributed to an excessive consumption of beer but usually caused by a combination of several avoidable factors, e.g. too much of the wrong food and too little exercise. It is sometimes accompanied by **GYN(A)ECOMASTIA**. See also **ABDOMEN**.

BEHAVIO(U)RISM A school of psychology that seeks to explain behaviour in terms of observable responses to outside or environmental stimuli. The idea was suggested by **PAVLOV** and his dogs, but developed by others.

BELLADONNA The poisonous Deadly Nightshade plant (dwale to English countryfolk and *Atropa belladonna* to botanists) whose juice, distilled from the leaves and root, produces the alkali atropine. One of the properties of this substance is to dilate the pupils of the eye, and from the 16th century onwards this seems to have been employed as a rather dubious method of making women more appealing, in a wide-eyed sort of way. *Bella donna* means 'beautiful woman' in Italian, and the following explanation comes from the *Philosophical Transactions of the Royal Society* of 1757 'Bella Donna is the name which the Italians, and particularly the Venetians, apply to this plant; and Mr Ray observes, that it is so called, because the Italian ladies make a cosmetic from the juice'. A more fanciful definition is given in *The Devil's Dictionary* by Ambrose Bierce (1842–?1914), in the new, enlarged

Penguin edition: 'Belladonna: In Italian a beautiful lady; in English a deadly poison. A striking example of the essential identity of the two tongues'. As any man knows who has had atropine drops put into his eyes (or been in love with a beautiful lady) the consequent, wide-eyed dilation of the pupils does indeed make the sky look bluer and the grass greener: but the factual, unromantic reason is that the eye admits more light.

BESTIALITY See **BUGGERY**.

BEZOAR From the Arabic word *bazahr*, formerly used to denote a poisonous substance employed as a counter-poison but now means any calculus or concretion in the stomach or intestines, such as a hairball or **TRICHOBEZOAR**. Cats grooming themselves can also get them. See also **MERDA** and **PICA**. Arabs produced some of the leading physicians during what were the Dark Ages in Europe. In 986 *al-Tasrif* was compiled at Cordova and served for centuries as a manual of surgery. The surgeon Albucasis (Abul Kasim), who served as court physician to Caliph Hakam II, illustrated the résumé of Arabian medical knowledge in which he describes the position for lithotomy (the cutting of a stone out of the urinary bladder), differentiated between goitre and cancer of the thyroid gland, and instructed surgeons in the delivery of infants in abnormal positions; described the use of iron cautery, amputation of limbs, transverse tracheotomies, the removal of goitres, the tying of arteries, the repair of fistulas, the healing of aneurysms and arrow wounds, and other matters.

BID Brought In Dead: ambulancemen's and doctors' abbreviation, pronounced as separate letters, not acronymically like 'bid'. See also **DOA**. Also pharmacists' abbreviation for *bis in diem* – twice a day.

BIDET A modern **SITZBATH**. The word was originally French for a pony or small horse, i.e. something that one sat upon in an astride posture. Its use for (surely not exclusively feminine) 'personal' hygiene (i.e. washing the perineum) was first noted by the Scottish ex-doctor novelist Tobias George Smollett (1721–1771) in his *Travels in France and Italy* (1766): 'Will custom exempt from the imputation of gross indecency a French lady, who shifts her frowsy smock in presence of a male visitant, and talks to him of her *lavement*, her *medecine*, her *bidet!*' Strange how the English preferred to use foreign words for the washing of their private parts. See also **SITZBATH**.

BIFIDUS Latin for cleft in two, split (feminine *bifida*). From *bis* + *findere*. See **FINDO**.

(THE) BIG C This started as a euphemistic cipher for cancer used by doctors but was soon taken over by patients who hesitate to pronounce the dreaded word.

BILE From Latin *bilis*, the fluid (see also **CHOLE-**) secreted by the liver and poured into the duodenum as an aid to the digestive process. Its properties are encapsulated in the mnemonic

> *Bile from the liver emulsifies greases,*
> *Tinges the urine and colours the faeces,*
> *Aids peristalsis, prevents putrefaction,*
> *If you remember all this you will give satisfaction.*

BILE BEANS A laxative pill and general **TONIC**, developed by an Australian chemist, Charles Fulton, in 1898. Adrian Room says they 'claimed to stimulate the flow of **BILE** and the pill was originally oval, or bean-shaped. Bile Beans were still being produced in the 1980s'. See also other patent laxatives and salts, above and below.

BIO-/(BIOT-) The 'life' prefix, from Greek *bios*, life, which gave us hundreds of familiar English words: biology, biography ('writing about life'), biorhythm (the alleged rhythm of life), symbiosis (living together), biochemistry (the chemistry of living things), macrobiotics (long life) and microbes (i.e. very small, microbiotic things). Biopsy (see also **OP-**), the removal of a small piece of tissue for examination and diagnosis, is, literally, 'a look at life': and when cinemas and picture palaces were introduced they were at first sometimes called 'biographs' – 'living writing/drawing', and are occasionally still called 'bioscopes' (e.g. in South Africa). But see also **ANTIBIOTICS** – which are effective only against microscopic forms of life. See also the **MACRO-** prefix, and under **DIET**.

BIRD-FANCIER'S LUNG An allergic respiratory complaint caused by breathing dust from the feathers or dried droppings of birds. See also **PSITTACOSIS**, **HANGMAN'S FRACTURE** and other occupational/recreational complaints listed under **BREWER'S DROOP**.

BIT Medieval English word for the **UTERUS**, which please see for the connection.

BLADES American medics' slang for surgeons – see also **BUTCHER**. Fortunately such stark nicknames are not used by patients (or, one hopes, in their hearing). Shakespeare comes fairly close to it in *Macbeth*, thanks in part to his arbitrary punctuation, where Duncan's injunction, 'Go get him surgeons', is sometimes spoken by actors as if it were punctuated 'Go get him, surgeons!'

BLASTO-, -BLAST Prefix and suffix derived from the Greek *blastos*, a bud, and denoting a formative or germ cell or embryo. Hence blasto**C(O)ELE**, blastomycosis, etc.

BLEEP CREEP English hospital slang term for a nurse who is alleged to enjoy harassing junior doctors via their pagers.

(A) BLIGHTY A welcome minor wound or sickness suffered – indeed enjoyed – by British infantry soldiers in the First World War to enable them to escape the fighting and gain repatriation to the UK. Some blighties were simulated with an ingenuity that would put a modern **MÜNCHHAUSEN** to shame. Mr Robert Sells reports that 'a useful non-traumatic WW1 blighty used to be a simulation of pulmonary tuberculosis. The recipe was 1) Lose weight by starving. 2) Chew cordite to produce a greenish, sickly complexion. 3) Rub a little barium paste on to the chest below one clavicle to produce a soft opaque shadow on the X-ray, typical of active TB. 4) Prick the back of the tongue just before producing a sputum sample, to simulate haemoptysis, with which TB frequently presents. 5) Mix a little smegma with the bloody spit or, if observed by the MO during the process, chew a little cheese placed in the mouth before entering the examination room. It worked'. Most of the medical words in the foregoing paragraph will be found cross-referenced, but the blighty comes from the Indian subcontinent, modified by British soldiers from the Hindi word *bilayati*, meaning foreign or overseas; but it soon came to mean 'home' – i.e. foreign to native Hindi-speakers. (On balance I think I would rather risk the horrors of the trenches).

BLIND TEST See **PLACEBO**.

BLOOD See **OLD CHARLIE FOSTER**.

BLOOD BANK The term is self-explanatory, but I include it here for the information that the first one was set up by the black New York surgeon Charles Richard Drew in 1940 – when segregation rules prohibited him from donating his own blood.

BLOOD-LETTING The term has an old-fashioned, archaic ring to it, conjuring up the days when removing blood from a patient was considered a cure-all, but the procedure is still carried out in some circumstances, either by **CUPPING** or with **LEECHES**. See also under **PHLEBOTOMY**.

BLUE BABY An infant born with cyanosis caused by a congenital heart lesion, or by incomplete expansion of the lungs. Thanks to two Americans, this condition seldom reaches the news pages now. In 1944, at the Johns Hopkins Children's Hospital in Baltimore, the surgeon Alfred Blalock, working on a premise advanced by his colleague Helen Tausig, developed a surgical technique that allowed blue babies to live, and subsequently live normal – normally coloured – lives.

(THE) BLUES OPENER See **'DOCTOR I WOKE UP THIS MORNING...'**

BOL The Greek word for a ball. See **EMBOLISM**.

BOLUS Latin, via Greek, for a clod, sod or lump of earth, but the word gradually acquired a variety of meanings, often facetious: 'call for the quack with his bolus and glister'. Thus it can be any medicine to be swallowed, perhaps with some reluctance or difficulty; also, 'a medicine of round shape adapted for swallowing, somewhat rounder than an ordinary pill, often used somewhat contemptuously' *(Oxford English Dictionary)*, then 'a small rounded mass of any substance' *(Oxford English Dictionary)*; and, in the *Oxford Concise Medical Dictionary*, 'a soft mass of chewed food that is ready to be swallowed'. In the sense of 'a single dose of a drug, contrast medium, etc. introduced rapidly into a blood-vessel' *(Oxford English Dictionary)* it occurs in the *British Medical Journal* (29 March 1980): 'All treatment was stopped and a bolus of 10 ml of 10% calcium gluconate given'. For the compression of unwieldy boluses into tabloids see under **TABLOID**.

BOMBAY CRUD The same as **DELHI BELLY** and **MONTEZUMA'S REVENGE**, as well as other forms of travellers' diarrhoea.

BOMBUS A humming or buzzing noise in the ears, intestines, etc., that in the ears being presumably audible only to the person who suffers from it, like **TINNITUS**, while the intestinal noise would be **BRUIT**, better audible to an outsider: see also **BORBO-RYGM(US)**. According to an 18th-century edition of

Chambers's Dictionary, bombus can also be 'In music, an artificial motion with the hands, imitating, in cadence and harmony, the buzzing of bees'. What could this mean? But see also **SIBILUS** and **SUSURRUS**.

BORBORYGM(US) From Greek *borboros,* filth. Try saying it under your breath several times (giving due attention to the rolling of the letters r) and you will see why the Greeks chose this word to describe a rumbling in (or from) the bowels, for which a nice old English word is (the) **WOMBLES**. Some early heretics were called Borborites, presumably because of their filthy talk (and who might well have joined with another sect, the Stercoranists – see under **STERCUS**). Trapp's *Commentary on the Epistles* (1649): 'Shunne obscene borborology and filthy talk'. For other echoic terms see **GARGLE**, **SIBILUS** and **RHONCHUS**.

(A) BOTTLE A formerly common request to the family physician: 'Will you give me a bottle, doctor?', meaning a bottle of medicine. It now sounds outdated, as medicines are produced in so many different shapes and kinds – pills, capsules and **TABLOIDS**, etc. In hospital, however, requests for a bottle are usually made to the nurse and produce a bed-bottle, the (now usually disposable) successor to the ceramic and decorative **LIVERPOOL SLIPPER** and other forms, often made by famous potters like Minton, Wedgwood, etc.

BOTULUS Latin for a sausage or small pudding. Hence botulism, food poisoning from bad meat – and also the English word bowel, for bowels and sausages have much in common, physiologically as well as culinarily. Sausages are bowels filled with mixed, minced foodstuff and bowels are sausages filled with digested food. Another relation is *botellus,* the diminutive of *botulus,* and this probably gave us the bottle, which in ancient times was often made from intestines (see also **UTERUS** for a bottle-shape). The British slang expression 'Losing one's bottle' is defined in the *Oxford English Dictionary* as a loss of 'courage, spirits or guts'.

BOVINE SPONGIFORM ENCEPHALOPATHY One of the longest medico-scientific terms ever to be bandied about by laymen and journalists. It began as a veterinary term but was adopted into human medicine when it was found that the animal sickness, also called 'Mad Cow Disease' ('scrapie' in sheep) might be transferred from the meat of cattle to humans who consumed it. The condition was per-

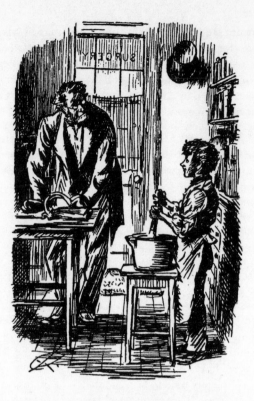

RATIOCINATION

Country Doctor. "DID YOU TAKE THAT BOTTLE OF MEDICINE TO OLD MRS. GAMBIDGE'S? - BECAUSE IT WAS VERY IMPORTANT"
Surgery Boy. "OH, YESSIR. AND I'M PRETTY SURE SHE TOOK IT, SIR!"
Country Doctor (after a pause). "WHAT DO YOU MEAN BY THAT, SIR?"
Surgery Boy. "WELL, I SEE THE SHUTTERS UP AT THE 'OUSE AS I PASSED THIS MORNIN', SIR!"

Punch, May 10, 1879

haps foreseen by Shakespeare, who in *Twelfth Night* makes Sir Andrew Aguecheek say to Sir Toby Belch: 'I am a great eater of beef and I believe that does harm to my wit' (i.3. 90) And in *Henry VI Part II* he has the insult 'Thou mongrel, beef-witted lord!' – but this of course is a reference to a dull bovine brain, not a spongiform one. *Bovine* comes from Latin *bos, bovis,* an ox, *spongiform* explains itself, Greek **ENKEPHALON** means brain, and **PATHOS** is suffering. See also Firkin and Whitworth's *Dictionary of Medical Eponyms (Parthenon Publishing)* for the related Jakob–Creutzfeldt Disease (which, incidentally, is its correct spelling and word-order).

BOW-TIES See under **GREY SUITS**.

BRACHYCEPHALIC Having a short head. See **BRACHYS**, below.

BRACHYS Greek word for short, hence the prefix *brachy-* denoting shortness: brachycephaly, shortness of the skull; brachydactyly, short-fingeredness; brachypenility, shortness of the penis.

BRADYS Greek for slow, prefix *brady-*, e.g. *bradycardia*, a slow heartbeat. See also its opposite, **TACHY-**.

BREWER'S DROOP Temporary male impotence caused by an excess consumption of alcohol, usually beer, which brewers, public-house landlords and their barmen drink in large quantities for professional reasons and saloon-bar drinkers take socially, though the outcome is much the same (see also **ALE GUT** and **BEER BELLY**). A related condition known as 'Derbyshire Droop' was so named after it was found that miners in that county of England were rendered impotent by substances to which they were exposed in their work. For other **'PROFESSIONAL' DISEASES/ SYNDROMES** see **DERBYSHIRE DROOP, CELLIST'S NIPPLE, COFFEE WASHER'S LUNG, DRUMMER'S THUMB, FARMER'S LUNG, FIDDLER'S NECK, FLAUTIST'S CHIN, GAMEKEEPER'S THUMB, GOLFER'S SHOULDER, HANGMAN'S FRACTURE, HOUSEMAID'S KNEE, JEEP-DRIVER'S BOTTOM, MINER'S ELBOW,** etc. Also **RSI**, or **PLOMBOSCILLOSIS** if 'lead-swinging' is suspected. The lungs seem to be the most commonly affected organs, and numerous **PULMONARY** conditions in addition to that mentioned above are listed in the textbooks, e.g. **BIRD-FANCIER'S LUNG**, Pigeon-Breeder's Lung, Airconditioner Lung, Mushroom Worker's Lung, Malt Worker's Lung, Cheese Washer's Lung, etc., and – recreationally rather than occupationally – Snuff-Taker's Lung. **MILKMAN'S SYNDROME** unfortunately does not qualify, and **JOGGER'S NIPPLE** is caused by recreation, not work.

BROMIDE From Greek *bromos*, a stink: bromide of potassium was formerly given as a medicine to calm and sedate patients and – hopefully but usually in vain – to reduce men's sex drive. During the First World War it was added to soldiers' tea in the belief that they would be less likely to rape enemy womenfolk or resort to intercourse with prostitutes (with its attendant risk of the soldiers' incapacitation by **VENEREAL** disease). Anecdote: Two ancient pensioner-soldiers on park bench; one says to the other: 'You know those bromide pills they put in our tea in 1914 to keep down the old how's-yer-father? Well, I think they're beginning to work'.

BRONCH(O)- The breathing-related chest prefix, from Greek *bronchos*, windpipe.

BROTH Also sometimes **SOUP**: two kinds enter the reckoning here. One is the broth prepared by bacteriologists as a medium for the growth of cultures (see also under **AGAR** and **IMMUNISATION**), the other is described under **JEWISH PENICILLIN**.

BRUIT The French word for a noise in the human body which is perceivable through a stethoscope by a second party, not, or not merely, by the person suffering from it. The word is also used for some murmurs. A **TINNITUS** can be heard only by the sufferer. See also **SUSURRUS** and **BOMBUS**.

BTWN GPs' abbreviation for Back-To-Work-Note.

BUBAR Code acronym for 'Buggered Up Beyond Any Repair'. The more outspoken (especially Americans, who seldom use 'bugger'), prefer **FUBAR**.

BUBONIC As in the famous plague. It is a word of somewhat confusing origin: *bubo* is the name for a swollen, inflamed lymph node in places where these are near the surface, especially the armpit or groin. Latin *bubo* also means the groin, but *bubo, bubonis* is a screech owl. Zoologists ignore the medical meaning: for them 'bubonic' means 'owl-like'.

BUCCINATOR The cheek muscle (from Latin *bucina*, a trumpet) – a reference to the trumpet and the way its players puff out their cheeks, as indeed they do in many old paintings and sculptures. Trumpeters who play classical music are, however, taught that this is mimical to a good technique as it wastes breath and diminishes lip control . They therefore leave it to angels (see **CHERUBISM**) and Dizzy Gillespie.

BUCCO Latin word for the cheek.

BUGGERY 'Now mainly used as a technical term in criminal law', says the *Oxford English Dictionary*, perhaps somewhat innocently. Doctors called upon to give evidence in such cases know the legal definitions of this and related activities. The *Oxford Companion to Law* says it is 'The crime of man having intercourse *per anum* with a man or a woman (sodomy), or of a person of either sex having intercourse *per anum* or *per vaginam* with an animal (bestiality). Consent is no defence [especially when the partner is an animal – FS] and both participants are guilty. Since 1967 it has not been an offence in England for a man to commit buggery or gross indecency with another male, if it is done in private, both parties are aged 21 [this was lowered to 18 in 1994], and both consent, but in other circumstances it continues to be a crime'. As for the origin of the word, when things get really vulgar blame the foreigner (see the **FRENCH POX** and cross-references). The French are said to have given the word to the English, from *bougre*, which they in turn derived from the Latin *Bulgaricus*, a Bulgarian, 'a name given to a sect of heretics who came from Bulgaria in the 11th century, afterwards to other 'heretics', to whom abominable practices were ascribed...' says the *Oxford English Dictionary*; and 'bougre' or 'bouger' were earlier English spellings. So much for *le vice Anglais* (and for more about that vice see **FLAGELLATION**). Heresy and buggery – or a combination of both – were in the past thought of as mainly ecclesiastical proclivities: certainly it was what clerics and other high personages liked to accuse each other of. According to a chronicle of 1330 'The king said and did crie, the pape was heretike... and lyued in bugerie'. *Chambers's Cyclopaedia* in 1753 had an interesting sidelight: 'The Buggers are mentioned by Matthew Paris... under the name of Bugares... They were strenuously refuted by Fr. Robert, a dominican, surnamed the Bugger, as having formerly made profession of this heresy'. In some cultures buggery is also the customary form of birth-control, especially in Africa, which is said to be the reason why **AIDS** is a heterosexual disease on that continent.

BULIMIA (NERVOSA) *The Oxford English Dictionary* defines this as 'an emotional disorder occurring chiefly in young women in which "binges" of extreme overeating alternate with depression and self-induced vomiting, purging or fasting [usually combined with] a persistent overconcern with body shape or weight'. That definition strictly applies only to bulimia *nervosa*. Bulimia itself simply means a very hearty appetite, 'a morbid hunger, chiefly occurring in idiots and maniacs, the so-called "canine hunger"...' or, as a quotation from 1398 reveals, 'Bolismus is immoderate and unmeasurable as it were an houndes appetite'. Etymologically, however, bulimia means something like the appetite of an ox, combining a form of the Greek word *bous* with *limos*, hunger, hence perhaps 'eating like an ox'. The bulimics' alternation of guzzling and fasting was known as early as 1598: 'One while the boulime, then the anorexie... rage with monstrous ryot'. See also **ANOREXIA**, as well as various cross-references concerning feasting and fasting, from **BANTING** and **CELLULITE** onwards. There has long been a perfectly good English word for the condition, *bulimy*.

BUNION The name of this unsightly, abnormal enlargement of the joint at the base of the big toe comes from Greek *bounion*, a turnip.

BURSA (MUCOSA) *Bursa* is Greek and Latin for a bag, or wine-skin, hence a 'synovial sac of discoidal form interposed between muscles, tendons or skin, and bony prominences, for the purpose of lessening friction', as the specialist reference books explain. From the same source springs the humble purse as well as the grand *bourse*, where the French transact financial business. See also **HOUSEMAID'S KNEE**.

BUTCHER Medics' facetious slang-word for a surgeon: but not necessarily in criticism of his technique.

Cc

CAC(O)- Prefix from Greek *kakos* meaning bad, evil, excremental, etc., and also sometimes deformity. Cacophony, bad sound; cacogalactia, a condition producing bad milk; cacosmia, whose sufferers perceive normally good smells as bad; and numerous other useful formations. Latin *cacare* means to void excrement. The English slang word cackhanded for lefthanded probably refers to the habit of some Asians and Middle-easterners to reserve their left hand for anal hygiene (making it an insult to offer a lefthanded handshake). It can also refer to anything smeared or daubed – and Joseph Haydn (1732–1809) wrote a little song against the modern (!) painters of his day (or perhaps specifically against the Eszterházy court painter Ludwig Guttenbrunn, who was having an affair with his wife): *Beherzigt doch das Diktum / Cacatum non est pictum* (Remember thou the dictum – but readers will by now be able to translate the rest...) For supposedly good smells see under **AROMA-THERAPY**.

CADAVER The Latin for a dead body, usually an anonymous one as found in the dissecting-room. It literally means 'one who fell over', from Latin *cadere*, to fall – and in Roman times often was applied to the corpses of common soldiers or **PROLES** as well as of criminals (but see also **PAFO**). For the gruesome story of the dissection of living bodies see under **DUODENUM**.

CAECUM A blind-ended pouch in the intestines, to the lower end of which the appendix is attached, from the Latin *caecus*, blind. The Germans say *Blinddarm*, literally, 'blind gut'; and American practitioners prefer the simplified spelling 'cecum'. Until well into the 20th century many people believed that those who swallowed a cherry stone could develop appendicitis, on the assumption that the stone could be trapped in the blind gut and would be unable to get out. Was such a thing ever found during **APPEND(IC)ECTOMY**? And could this superstition have suggested one of the far-fetched adventures of Baron **MÜNCHHAUSEN**? The Greek word for blind is *typhlos*, hence **TYPHLITIS** or perityphlitis, a now almost forgotten word for appendicitis, at any rate a form of it.

C(A)ESAR Familiar abbreviation to describe a Caesarean section, or a baby born by one: a doctor might say that he was about to 'do a Caesar'; and I once overheard a couple of housewives talking in a supermarket, one of whom pointed at her snotty-nosed, very unpatrician-looking child and said: 'He's a Caesar, you know'. Although 'cesar' is a casual abbreviation it is not a modern one. A 1540 translation from the German, of a treatise by Roesslin, has: 'They that are borne after this fashion be called cesares, for because they be cut out of theyr mothers belly, whervpon also the noble Romane cesar the [first] of that name in Rome toke his name'.

CAFÉ-AU-LAIT SPOTS A pale tan **MACULE** whose colour is indicated by its name. One of numerous **MENU CONDITIONS**.

CALCULUS Latin *calx*, a stone, *calculus*, a little stone, e.g. one formed in the body from various deposits (compare also *calcium*). Small stones were used for simple mathematics in the manner of an abacus, hence calculation. See also **LITH-**. The *-culus / -culum* ending always denotes a diminutive.

CALEFACIENT A warming-agent – anything from a good rub-down with a rough towel or the application of a hot-water bottle to the full treatment of clinical **HYPOTHERMIA**. From Latin *calefacere*, to make warm (i.e. *calere*, to be warm + *facere*, to make). As **GALEN** said (paraphrased by Lord Bramwell in 1885): 'Old age is cold and dry, and is to be corrected by calefacients'.

CALLI- The 'beauty' prefix – see below.

CALLIPYGIAN A combination of the Greek word for beauty, *kallos*, and the Latin (via Greek) *pygidium*, the buttock or rump, beautifully buttocked (possibly **APOGLUTIC**): a word which has little if any medical use but is added for light relief. See also **CALLISTHENICS**, below, which are perhaps a little more useful; and **GLUT(A)EUS** as well as **NATES**. Also **STEATOPYGIA** and under **GASTROCNEMIUS**.

CALLISTHENICS From the beauty prefix, above, plus *sthenos*, strength. The Callisthenic Movement was started in the mid-19th century to encourage the parallel development of health and beauty in women through exercise, a most praiseworthy effort (though it is difficult to understand how beauty could be *developed* if not present in the first place). It would have been a kind of precursor of **AEROBICS**, though gentler and not so noisy. Later manifestations of it took the form of mass gymnastics and led to another movement, Health and Beauty.

CALLOMANIA An abnormal condition found, usually but not necessarily, among women, characterised by delusions of personal beauty. But why should it not also apply to men who are particularly taken by the sight or presence of beautiful women?

CALLUS Latin for hardened skin. The word is used in precisely that sense; also for the bony material thrown out around and between the two ends of fractured bone during the process of healing. The spelling 'callous' for these applications is erroneous. That word comes from *callosus*, hardened, related to callus but more usually applied to a state of mind.

CALOR Latin for heat, which gave us – by a somewhat unscientific route – calories. See also **THERM**.

CANDIDA Usually *candida albicans* (surely a tautology – see **ALBUS**: perhaps the clinical equivalent of blanc de blancs?): one of the 'beautiful girls' names' group of diseases, like **AMELIA**, **MYRINGA** or **PRUNELLA**, and a cousin (better not a kissing cousin) to **CHLAMYDIA**. Candida, or candidiasis (see also below) come from Latin *candidus*, white, shining-white, has the same meaning as the Greek-based leukorrhea (English spelling leukorrhoea, from the Greek *leukos*, white + *rhein*, flow), a white vaginal discharge, colloquially known as 'the Whites' or 'Women's Whites'. The French use *les fleurs blanches* as a euphemism for leukorrhoea (see **FLOWERS**). If that were not picturesque enough, there is another name for it, with songbird associations, **THRUSH**. And not only Candida (at present a favourite name among English upper-class families) but Celia, too, unwittingly provided a sickness suffix – see **-CELE**.

CANDIDIASIS The only thing this condition (see above) has in common with candidates, whether for jobs or examinations, is whiteness: because in ancient Rome candidates for office were required to wear a white toga – well-washed, one hopes, and even better rinsed. And why? See under **LOTIUM**.

CANNULA The name for this, a tubular probe inserted into a cavity or tumour to allow the escape of fluid, comes from Latin *canna*, a reed or reed-pipe (diminutive *cannula*). See also **TROCAR**.

CANNULAR In the shape of a tube, also grooved or channelled in form.

CANTHARIDES From the Greek *cantharis*, blister-fly, also known as the Spanish Fly. The dried and

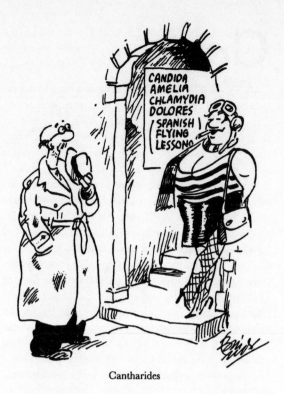

Cantharides

ground insects have been used externally as a rubefacient and vesicant and internally as a diuretic and stimulant to the genito-urinary system, hence the centuries-old belief that it is an **APHRODISIAC**.

CAPIL- Latin *capillus* – the prefix relating to hair or hairlike/hair-thin things, for example fine, thin blood vessels.

CAP(IT)- The head prefix, from *caput*, *capitis*, a head, as in *capitulum*, and *capitellum*, literally 'little head'. The British **GP's** capitation fee denotes payment per head from the **NHS**.

CAPOTE ANGLAISE The French name for a 'French letter', or **CONDOM**, also sometimes given as *capot anglais* (*capot* being the diminutive of *cape*, a cape). *Capote* is 'a long shaggy cloak or overcoat with a hood, worn by soldiers, sailors, travellers, etc.' It is a favourite area for nations to abuse each other. See also the **FRENCH POX** and **DUTCH CAP**.

CAPOTEMENT The sloshing noise made by fluid moving about in a distended stomach. See under **CONDOM**.

CARBUNCLE From Latin *carbunculus*, meaning a small piece of coal. From this it came to mean a

28

precious stone of bright, reddish colour (with reference to a 'burning' effect) and only later an angrily inflamed boil (for the 'boiling' connection see **ECZEMA**). The German word for both the precious stone and the skin eruption is *Garfunkel* (*funkeln*, to glitter). See also **ANTHRAX**, which is the Greek for coal (compare anthracite) and has similar associations with both the precious stone and the virulent, eruptive boils of the infectious disease now specifically known as *anthrax*. Not to be confused with a **CARUNCLE**.

CARCINOMA From the Greek *karkinos*, a crab + the **-OMA** swelling or tumour suffix, later also the Latin word for cancer. The rather questionable, transferred, non-medical use, e.g. 'a cancer on the body politic' was used in classical writings, too, e.g. by Suetonius, who (putting the words into Augustus's mouth) described as 'cancerous' Julia and her son Agrippa 'on account of their incorrigible wickedness'. See also under **ONCOLOGY**.

CARD(I)- The heart prefix, from Greek *kardia*, heart, hence cardiac, of the heart. The upper part of the stomach, nearest the heart, is also called the cardia. Not to be confused with *carn-*, which is the flesh (or fleshy and fleshly things) prefix, as in carnal sin, and which comes from Latin *carn-*, *carno-*, meat or flesh.

CARE IN THE COMMUNITY A clever euphemism coined in the 1990s by ministerial **GREY SUITS** which in practice meant removing mentally ill people from hospitals and sending them home; or, if they had no home, turning them out into the streets, where they were not happy and occasionally murdered fellow-citizens (but see also **DROMOMANIA** for those who like an open-air existence). **COMMUNITY** is one of the indispensable shibboleth words of the **WELFARE STATE**.

CARIES The Latin for decay or rot (compare with 'carrion') now mainly applied to the teeth, sometimes bones. The English word is rhymed with 'Mary's' but the Latin should have three syllables – like 'Marysez'. See also **VIRUS**.

CARINA Latin for a keel, hence any keel-shaped structure: for example, the **TRACHEA** has one. Like **CANDIDA** and other euphonious words it has been appropriated as a girls' name (for which see **AMELIA**). Not to be confused with **KELOID**, even though a keloid scar may be raised.

CARING As in 'the caring professions', etc., a word which came into fashionable use in Britain after the end of the Second World War, with the founding of the National Health Service, or **NHS**. See also **ABUSE**, **GREY SUITS** and **PRIMARY HEALTH CARE**.

CARIOCAS 'A form of lateral movement in a gait cycle in which the sidestepping leg is brought successively behind and then in front of the stance leg' (Mosby). Presumably named after the carioca, a Brazilian dance related to the samba (and a long way removed from **ST. VITUS'S DANCE**. *Cariocas* are natives of Rio de Janeiro, as Londoners are cockneys.

CARMINATIVE An old-fashioned word for a medicine that helps against the wind, that is, alleviates **FLATULENCE**. The origin of the word is far-fetched, from Latin *carminare*, to card (as in wool) and goes back to the theory of humours, by which those humours thought to be responsible for wind were 'combed out like knots in wool'.

CARNAL Fleshly, from the Latin *carnalis*, flesh – as opposed to fleshy, for which the Greek *sarx*, prefix **SARC(O)-** , seems to be preferred.

CAROS/CARUS One of many words for sleep or unconsciousness – see also **COMA**, **HYPNOS**, **LETHARGY**, **SOMNUS**, **SOPOR** and **TORPOR**. From *caros* comes the carotid artery, so named by Galen because he recommended that pressure be put upon it to produce *caros*, unconsciousness: in reality he probably garrotted them – and this word, too, comes from *caros*. Mr Michael Reilly assures me that 'accurate pressure on both carotid bodies at the same time can lead to fainting. Tumours of the carotid body can grow to a large size, and are hard and knobbly: hence 'potato tumour'.

CARPENTER Medics' slang for orthopaedic surgeons (orthopods). For other playful descriptions see **BLADES**, **GIBLET MERCHANTS**, **PLUMBERS** and **BUTCHERS**.

CARPO- The wrist prefix (see below) – but beware of confusions: Greek *karpos* means fruit.

CARPUS/CARPAL Latin *carpus*, the wrist.

CARTILAGE from Latin *cartilago*, gristle. See also **CHRONDROS** and **HYPOCHONDRIA**.

CARUNCLE Not a misprint for a **CARBUNCLE** but a small piece of flesh, from Latin *caruncula*, diminutive of *caro, carnem*, flesh: see above.

CASCARA In Spanish-speaking parts of South America, a canoe made from a tree whose bark yields an extract which for more than a century has given us a powerful **APERIENT**. Its full name is *Cascara sagrada*, or sacred bark, and the Spanish stress the first a, not the second. (A similar mis-stressing affects the substance women paint round their eyes and call 'mascara'. It comes from *mascara*, a mask – and here, in turn, please turn to **ALCOHOL**).

CASTRATION Latin *castrare* meant *any* kind of 'pruning' or 'snipping away', for example, beekeepers called the partial removal of honey from the hives *castrare alvearia*. The name for the removal of the testes (orchidectomy) was therefore originally a facetious usage. Up to the late 19th century this ordeal was inflicted on small boys in order to preserve their treble voices (to satisfy St. Paul's aversion to hearing women in church) and turn them into *castrati*; but the operation had to be performed in early youth. At such an age their musicality might not have become evident, and those who failed to profit from a musical education received the consolation-prize of entry into the priesthood, which must have been brimming with tone-deaf eunuchs. Because ordinands of the Catholic church had to be 'in full possession of their manhood' – the failed male sopranos' livelihood was safeguarded by a clever scheme. When the testes were removed from the little boys they were not thrown away but preserved in a bottle – a kind of insurance policy in case musical promise was not fulfilled. Thus, if ordination had to take place as an alternative to a glittering career in the opera house (or failing that, the church choir), the candidates kept the jar in the pocket during the ceremony – and were thus technically 'in full possession of their manhood'. It makes a good story but Anthony Milner, in his article Sacred Capons (in *The Musical Times*, April 1973) gives a more plausible account of the gruesome things that went on (and which included the crushing of the boys' testes so as to bruise them and inhibit testicular growth). Although the Church piously maintained that amputation of any part of the human body was against its laws unless the body was thereby preserved, it turned a blind eye to castration, presumably because it preserved the voice. See also **CRYPTORCH(ID)ISM**. And having read about beehives at the beginning of this entry, you may wish to turn to **ALVEUS** – and to **HIVES** unrelated to bees.

CAT Computer-Assisted Tomography, also 'CAT Scan'.

CATA- Greek *kata*, down, hence *catarrh*, down-flow; catheter, a tube passed down into the body.

CATACHRESIS Latin (adapted from the Greek) for an improper use of words or the abuse of words. 'The Figure of Abuse if for lacke of naturall and proper terme or worde we take another, neither naturall nor proper, and do vntruly applie to the thing which we would seeme to expresse' (Puttenham, 1589). For the currently fashionable abuse of 'abuse' see under **ABUSE**.

CATARACT Why is this word shared by a violent waterfall *and* the gradual process of advancing opacity of the lens of the eye, leading to impairment of sight? The answer appears to be that in Latin the word denotes not only a waterfall or torrent but also the grating, or portcullis placed in front of it to impair its force. Early English doctors then adopted the Latin word to describe what they called 'a web in front of the eye'. So it was perhaps appropriate that the British Parliament adopted the portcullis as its heraldic symbol, as it might indicate either a torrent of political clichés or a general lack of vision. On the other hand, since the Houses of Parliament have always been situated on the bank of the River Thames, there may be some aquatic connection. For an appropriate quotation see **WEB**.

CATARRHUS Latin word for a flowing-down, a flux from an orifice, the rheum – or catarrh.

CATHARSIS A cleansing. The word is fashionable in television and radio discussions about literary and artistic matters ('Has writing this book been if-you-like a cathartic experience for you?') because of Aristotelean associations – though they might think twice about it if they knew it is also the old-fashioned medical term for a laxative or **APERIENT**, or any flowing-down – see below:

CATHETER Another variation on the above: a tube 'sent down' into the body.

CAUDA Latin for a tail. See also **COCCYX**, or 'cuckoo bone'. The Greek is *cercos*.

CAUSIS A burning, from *kausein*, to burn. Hence *causalgia*, a burning pain: see the suffix **-ALGIA**. See also **KAUSTIKOS, PYREXIA**.

CAVALIER See **ROUNDHEAD**.

CDH Congenital Dislocation of the Hip.

CECUM See **CAECUM**, above.

CELE Greek suffix indicating a swelling, lump, hernia or tumour. As in hydrocele, a swelling caused by accumulation of liquid. Also *-coele* in some formations or spellings, the *o* being as spurious as that in '**FOETUS**', which should always be **FETUS**. Not to be confused with the **COEL(O)-** prefix: this is another instance where spelling-simplifications may spell danger of confusion.

CELLA Latin for 'cell': Greek *cutos*.

CELLIST'S NIPPLE An occupational hazard that may affect some female cellists, and which the medical press occasionally reports, largely for its entertainment value (as it has described **JOGGER'S NIPPLE**). One article suggested the purchase of a padded bra for a cure – though in reality female cellists have always been aware of the threat of irritation to their left **MAMMILLA** and can guard against it even when playing bra-less. All they need do is adjust the moveable spike at the bottom of the instrument, so that the rear top edge of the cello rests against some other bit of their chest. Female cymbal players also have a hard time of it, as there is only one place in their anatomy where they can quickly damp the vibrations of hand-held cymbals between rapidly-damped clashes (watch one of them coping with the last movement of Tchaikovsky's Symphony No. 4 in F minor). Pianists can get *glissando thumb* (and if you need further explanation ask the nearest pianist), brass-players are prone to emphysema and **PILES**, the last-named condition also affecting wind-players (though probably no more than bank managers and their clerks). See also **FIDDLER'S NECK, FLAUTIST'S CHIN, CLARINETTIST'S LIP, HOUSE-MAID'S KNEE,** etc. and many more serious occupational health-risks.

CELLULITE A pseudo-scientific word for body fat, especially the dimply, undulating sort sometimes found on women's bodies. The word was pounced upon in the late 1960s by the slimming industry as a euphemism for fat. For the male equivalent see **ALE GUT** and **BEER BELLY**.

CENTESIS A piercing, from Latin *centeo*, I pierce. Thus the suffix *-centesis* indicates the piercing, puncturing or perforation of whatever it is added to, e.g. *amniocentesis*, puncturing the **AMNION**. The Greek word is *kentron*, a prick or point, from *kenteo*, to puncture (also related to 'centre', i.e. the centre established by pricking a point prior to describing a circle with a pair of compasses), not, as has sometimes been suggested, with 'centesimal', which has been pressed into service to suggest 'taking a hundredth part', e.g. of fluid. See also **ACU-**.

-CEPHAL(O)-/-KEPHALO- Word-element indicating the head; from Greek *kephalos*, head. The English pronunciation varies between 'see-phal', 'sephal' and 'ke-phal'. *Enkephalo-* denotes something that is in the head, hence enkephalon, brain.

CEREBR- Prefix for the brain, from Latin *cerebrum* – usually the front and larger part (the hinder and lower being the *cerebellum*, a diminutive thereof). Gourmets may like to note the fact (and reflect on it) that *cervelat*, that delicious German or French smoked sausage, was formerly made with the finely-minced brains of pigs or cattle: Italian *cervello*, brain. For another gastronomic connection see **INFARCT(ION)** and the various **MENU CONDITIONS**.

CERUMEN A waxy substance secreted by certain glands in the external ear canal: from Latin *cera*, wax.

CERVIX The *cervic-* prefix denotes the neck, which is what *cervix* means in Latin. This sometimes proves confusing for the layman, especially the male, who is likely to have heard only of the female cervix (the neck of the **UTERUS**) and is surprised to find that he also has one. Perhaps the Greek neck-word, *trachelos*, might make things easier. Even more confusingly, men (and only men) can suffer from vaginalitis, inflammation of the vaginal coat or tunic of the testicles. See **VAGINA**. See also **HYSTER-/HUSTER**.

CHALLENGED Until recently this word would have suggested a 'halt-who-goes-there?' kind of challenge, but Political Correctness (**PC**) now dictates that we use 'challenged' instead of 'disabled' – in combination with an adverb indicating *how* a person is disabled (an earlier euphemism, also discarded) or disadvantaged (which is *another*). For example, anyone with a bodily handicap who might formerly have been called or called himself **CRIPPLED** should be described as **PHYSICALLY CHALLENGED**. And if it makes one unfortunate person feel better, so be it.

CHAMBER-POT The familiar domestic receptacle, now largely made obsolete by en-suite bathrooms, formerly played a big part in medical practice, especially for the preliminary examination of urine, etc. Those who placed too much reliance on this form of diagnosis were in the 19th/early 20th century called 'chamber-pot practitioners' (see below). One of the first instructions the medical student was given was 'Do not kick the chamber-pot under the patient's bed'. See **BOTTLE, LIVERPOOL SLIPPER** and **MATULA**.

CHAMBER-POT PRACTICE Wadd's *Nugae Chirurgicae* (1824) describe the practice of Richardus Morton, MD as a 'Chamber-pot practice' – presumably because Morton set disproportionate store by the examination of his patients' urine. Wadd adds, in Latin, '*Alter matulas inspicit, et ubi morbum non invenit, facit*'. See also **STERCORARIAN**.

CHARLATAN Now means an empty pretender to knowledge which he does not possess; this word was originally applied to itinerant vendors of medicines, especially those **QUACKS** who cried up their wares and skills in streets and market-places: see also **MEDICASTER** and **STERCORARIAN**. Some of the most celebrated international pharmaceutical companies can trace their origins to a single charlatan peddling a **PATENT MEDICINE**.

CHASTITY-BELT A lockable belt (also called Girdle of Chastity), usually made of iron and fitted to the pelvic region of a woman to prevent her indulging in (or being subjected to) penetrative sexual activity (at any rate with a partner). According to popular tradition they were fitted to wives of medieval crusaders while their husbands were serving abroad, to ensure that the women remained chaste, produced no bastard offspring and remained free from the **POX** (and their existence may partly account for the frequency of the English name Smith, as silversmiths, tinsmiths, goldsmiths and blacksmiths possessed the skill and equipment to circumvent them). During the 19th century chastity-belts were made for males, and recommended by both doctors and priests, especially in remote American goldmining and prospecting communities in which both homosexuality and prostitution were threats to health and morality. Michael McCormick applied for (and obtained) Patent No. 587,994 from the US Patent Office. His specification was filed on 27 November 1896 in San Francisco, a place where respectable females were at

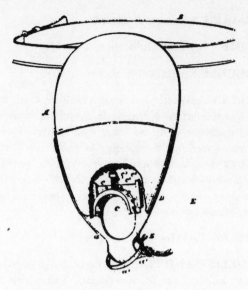

The American Way of Sex, San Francisco 1896

that time in short supply: the Wild West was considered no place for women. 'The objects of my invention (he stated) are ... to prevent involuntary nocturnal seminal emissions; to control waking thoughts and to prevent self-abuse'. To this end he used painful means – what he described as 'pricking-points' – but he maintained that the pain would be momentary and that its prevention was within the control of the wearer, if he diverted his thoughts from 'running in lascivious channels'. 'The device is adjusted to the person by fitting plate A over the abdomen and securing it by belt B. The organ [not shown] is passed through the aperture a, which fits close up around the base...' etc. 'Now, when from any cause expansion in this organ begins it will come in contact with the pricking-points, and the necessary pain and warning sensation will result...' In 1969 an English court ruled that chastity-belts made by a Dorset firm (chiefly for the tourist trade) should carry purchase-tax, while the makers' lawyers argued that as 'safety equipment' they were exempt.

CHD Coronary Heart Disease.

CHEIL- The lip or lips prefix, as in cheilo**PLASTY**, plastic surgery of the lip or lips.

CHEIR Greek for hand. Its associated prefix is *cheiro-*. Cheirognomy and cheiromancy mean reading the hands, i.e. palmistry; cheiralgia is a pain in the hand. In simplified spelling also **CHIR-** as in chiropractor, (*cheir* + *praktikos* = a course of action, *prattein*, to do) a manipulator or masseur. A chirurgeon, which only later became **SURGEON**, is a doctor who works with his hands. The chiropodist (see below) treats only the feet – though with his hands (see **POD-**). See also the Latin hand-word, **MANUS**.

CHERRY ANGIOMA Angioma comes from the Greek *aggeion*, blood vessel + *oma*, the tumour suffix. Cherry, if anyone wonders, from Latin *cerasus*. See also some of the other **MENU CONDITIONS** under their separate headings. In this condition, as well as Cherry Red Spot, the red colour and round shape are the significant signs. Also known as De Morgan's Spots.

CHERUBISM In Old Testament Hebrew *k'rub* (plural *k'rubim*) means an angel. Cherubism is an abnormal hereditary condition showing bilateral swelling of the cheeks – just like cherubs blowing the wind or the **BUCCINA**.

CHICKEN-POX The popular name for *varicella*, a mild eruptive illness which chiefly attacks children. The name is thought to refer to the mildness of the disease – but consider my theory about speckled hens, under **VARIOLA**.

CHIEF/PRINCIPAL NURSING OFFICER The title of the highest-ranking nurse in British hospitals, a position which formerly carried the friendly and respected appellation of Matron. All this was swept away by demands for terminological sex-equality – and in truth 'Matron' (from Latin *matrone*, literally 'big mother' or, in English usage, 'a married woman usually with the accessory idea of moral or social dignity' – *Oxford English Dictionary*) sits uneasily on the shoulders of a male nursing-boss. The change was brought about not for semantic reasons but as part of the headlong rush for reallocating old jobs by giving their holders **PC** or grandiose titles. A glance through the Health Appointments columns of the daily newspapers will be found instructive: one day's crop in a single paper included a Primary Care Strategy Development Officer, a Joint Planning and Development Worker Substance Misuse, a Reprovision Consultant, a Mentoring Project Co-ordinator, an Evaluation Manager, a Human Resources Health Management Advisor [sic], a Motion Analysis Scientist and numerous Clinical Studies Co-ordinators, Audit Facilitators, Counsellors, Field Workers, Cost Containment Managers, Case Workers and Operations Directors (administrative, not surgical operations). Soon

afterwards, Stockport Healthcare NHS Trust offered a £21,000 p.a. post to a Reward Manager, Richmond Healthcare Trust advertised for a Joint [sic] Implementation Manager [soft-drug abuse?]; Hillingdon Health Agency had £45,000 to spare for a Director of Acute Commissioning; Haringey wanted a Member's Support Manager; and in NW London there was a demand for Drop-In Workers. One doctor reports that in his hospital the number of offices occupied by hospital administrators increased in five years from 3 to 26, all with their own secretaries. Administrative hospital workers are collectively (and disrespectfully) called **GREY SUITS**. For a relic of the more human past see **ALMONER**.

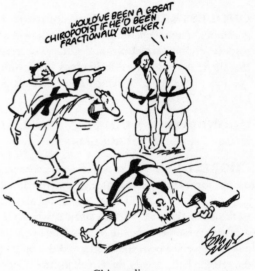

WOULD'VE BEEN A GREAT CHIROPODIST IF HE'D BEEN FRACTIONALLY QUICKER!

Chiropodist

CHIROPODIST Originally the preferred word for a medical auxiliary or **PARAMEDIC** who treated ailments of both the hands and the feet, from Greek *cheir* + *podos*, foot (see **PED-/POD**) but now usually and more accurately described as a **PODIATRIST**.

CHLAMYDIA From Greek *clamys*, a cloak: a microparasite which comes in various forms and can live in the conjunctiva of the eye (*chlamydia trachomatis*), in birds (*chlamydia psittaci*) and the private parts of both men and women. See **CANDIDA** and its cross-references for other pretty names suitable for girls.

CHLOR(O)- Prefix denoting light-green or yellowish colours – though, just to confuse matters, chloroform is a colourless and volatile liquid. Chlorine gas is yellow, though mustard gas (or dichloro-diethylsulphide), which one would expect to be of a mustardy-yellow colour, is a colourless, oily liquid and a powerful poison and vesicant. It was first used in warfare in 1917 by the Germans at Ypres.

CHLOROSIS From Greek *chloros*, the colour green. See also **GREEN SICKNESS**, or the 'virgins' disease' (1681), below.

CHOL(E)- The prefix indicating bile, from Greek *chole*, bile (hence cholera). Also cholemesis, the vomiting of bile; cholelithiasis, gallstones; cholecystectomy, the removal of the gallbladder: see **CYST-** and **-TOM**. Also **MELANCHOLIA** and **EMESIS**.

CHOLECYST- Prefix denoting anything related to the gallbladder. See also **CYST-**.

CHOLESTERIN The chief constituent of gallstones, a term consisting of the Greek words for, respectively, bile (see above) and stiffness or solidity. But there are other word-formations, each with its specialised meaning, of which cholesterol is best-known to the layman.

CHONDROS Greek for gristle. The Latin is *cartilago*. See also **HYPOCHONDRIA**.

CHOREIA Greek for the dance; hence chorea, the name for rapid, involuntary, spasmodic and purposeless body movements, or grimacing, also called *Chorea Sancti Viti* or **ST. VITUS'S DANCE**, which please see for its presumed religious origins. The word *choreia* has also given us both the chorus and the orchestra, though the latter was in the Greek theatre a kind of singing-and-dancing *place*, not a collection of musicians. For another doctoral dance-step see **CARIOCAS**.

CHRISTMAS DISEASE Not a 'Seasonally Affective Disorder' caused by over-indulgence – see **SAD** – but a mild form of h(a)emophilia found in a family with the surname Christmas and described by R. Briggs *et al.* in the *British Medical Journal* of 27 December 1952: 'If this definition of haemophilia is accepted then the seven cases recorded in this paper are ... a newly recognised condition which we propose to call "Christmas Disease", after the name of the first patient examined in detail'. Later (1961) the serum factor which is different in this form of haemophilia was named 'the Christmas factor'.

CHROM- The prefix denoting pigmentation, from Greek *chroma*, colour. Hence chromatopsia, abnormal colour-vision, etc.

CHROMOSOMES For a definition see a proper dictionary: the word literally means 'colour body': and see **SOMA**.

CHRONIC Said of a disease that persists for a long time: from the Greek *chronos*, time, and the opposite of **ACUTE**. The word is frequently misused in popular speech to mean bad, severe or objectionable (**HYSTERICAL** is often used when the speaker means 'funny'). Patients asked, 'Is your pain acute?', often reply, 'Yes, doctor, chronic'.

C/I Pharmacist's abbreviation for contra-indication, that is, the conditions under which a certain drug should not be prescribed or taken. See **CONTRA-**.

-CID(E) The 'killing' suffix, from Latin *cidere*, to kill (also to cut, presumably because most felonious killings in ancient times were carried out by the knife). Derivations range from spermicide to germicide, fungicide, infanticide, regicide – even circumcision – or, as a last resort, suicide. Cider (even its roughest form) has a quite different origin.

CIRCU(M)- The 'around' prefix. *Circum* is the Latin for round, hence circulation (i.e. the going-round of the blood); circumcision, cutting round; circumanal, around the **ANUS**; circumoral, around the mouth; etc. See also **RADIO-**.

CIRCUMCISION The surgical removal of the **PREPUCE** of the **PENIS** (and, among certain primitive, woman-hating peoples, of the **CLITORIS** – see **FEMALE CIRCUMCISION**). When carried out on Jewish boys for religious reasons the operation is performed by a *mohel*, a specialist circumciser who is neither necessarily a rabbi nor a doctor, though these two offices may be also held, incidentally. Most parents are now happy to entrust the procedure to a paediatrician, who does it under clinical rather than clerical conditions. But rabbis and mohels were said to acquire remarkable skills in the procedure, and some, it was claimed, were so quick at the job that the child had no time to cry out. In the Jews' Cemetery of Bridgetown, Barbados, a graveyard inscription dated 15th March 1782 commemorates Benjamin Massiah, who was 'Reader of the Jews' Synagogue for many years without Fee or Reward and performed the Office of Circumciser with Great Applause and Dexterity' (see my *Dead Funny: Another Book of Grave Humour*, Pan Books, 1982). Circumcision used to be common among the British and American middle-classes and its alleged advantages and drawbacks are under constant and often heated debate. One notable American doctor feels so strongly that it is a form of mutilation that he not only had his own prepuce restored but offers an ingenious form of plastic surgery he has devised: as the Germans might say, '*Foreskin durch Technik*'. Female circumcision, as mentioned earlier, is practised only by savages; but as some of these are very rich and live in (or have free access to) Western countries they often try to prevail upon respectable, qualified surgeons to carry out this gruesome and illegal operation on the womenfolk under their subjection. See also **INFIBULATION**.

CIRRHOSIS A disease of the liver, from the Greek *kirrhos*, orange-tawny-coloured – though it should be added that the ancient Greeks neither grew nor knew this far-eastern fruit.

CISVESTISM Truly there is a word for almost every condition, however unusual. The word means 'the practice of wearing attire appropriate to the sex of the individual involved but not suitable to the age, occupation or status of the wearer' *(Mosby)*. The word comes from *cis*, this side + *vestis*, garment (though surely the intention is to indicate not *this* side but 'the far side'?) In the way cisvestism most commonly asserts itself it is more often called Mutton Dressed As Lamb.

(THE) CLAP The popular name for venereal infections – especially **GONORRH(O)EA** (which, according to the old student joke, is derived from the fact that 'You don't know whether it's gone or here'). The *Oxford English Dictionary* says 'of uncertain origin' but quotes the old French *clapoir*. After all, the French have traditionally – if unfairly – been blamed for spreading venereal infections. See **(THE) (FRENCH) POX** and, for a dubious 'cure', **ANIMAL BATHS**.

CLARINETTIST'S LIP A painful affliction often suffered by players of that instrument, caused by pressure between reed and lower teeth which is taken by the lower lip in between. See also **CELLIST'S NIPPLE** and cross-references.

-CLAST, -CLASIS The 'breakage' or 'fracture' suffixes.

CLAUDICATION From Latin *claudicare*, to limp, though specialist textbooks offer different shades of meaning. Latin *claudere* means to shut, close (see

CLAUSTRUM below), and *claudus* means lame. The Emperor Claudius was born with a deformed foot and a consequent limp, but although various suggestions have been made, no precise connection has been established.

CLAUSTROPHOBIA A morbid fear of being shut, locked or trapped in enclosed spaces. For the opposite of this condition see **AGORAPHOBIA**. *Clostrum* is Latin for a bolt or lock, claudere to close, shut or lock (see also **CLAUDICATION**, above); and from this were named enclosures, closed place, cloisters, etc. The **GREY MATTER** of the brain also has a claustrum.

CLAUSTRUM For this and other architectural terms used by doctors see **ATRIUM** and follow the cross-references; see also the previous entry.

CLAVICLE The collarbone, from Latin *clavicula*, a small key, bar or bolt of a door... 'because the collarbone was compared to the key of a vault ... or because its form is that of the ancient bolt, (Littré, quoted by the *Oxford English Dictionary*). In ancient times it was called the **FURCULUM**, or 'merrythought', but this is now reserved for the wishbone of birds, especially those consumed at table. As two persons each hold on to one end of the wishbone they make a wish (or think a merry thought), and break the bone in two: the one who retains the bigger part of the fracture gets his wish.

CLEAVAGE LINE I know what most males reading this book will *think* this means, but in fact it is a dermatological term indicating a striation in the skin at a place where tension of the subcutaneous tissue, or a fold, usually occurs, e.g. on the palms. The name for the other kind of cleavage dates from only about 1945 and American film censorship, and is more interestingly defined by the *Oxford English Dictionary* as 'the cleft between a woman's breasts as revealed by a low-cut décolletage'; and (more delicately) by the American censor's office of the time as 'the shadowed depression dividing an actress's bosom into two distinct sections'.

CLEFT LIP The more appropriate name for what is often insensitively called a 'hare lip': a usually reparable congenital anomaly in the upper lip.

CLEVER DICK LOOKS SILLY CLOT Mnemonic for the vertebral bones of the spinal column: Cervical, Dorsal, Lumbar, Sacrum, Coccyx.

CLIMACTERIC Usually applied specifically to the female **MENOPAUSE**, more rarely to the loss of sex drive in males; but Latin *climacter* means *any* critical period or epoch in human life, from *clima*, a slope, or staircase (another **ARCHITECTURAL TERM**). In other words, it's downhill all the way.

CLINGONS Strictly 'cling-ons'. See under **FARTLEBERRIES**.

CLINIC From Greek *klinicos*, one who reclines on a bed *(klino)*, i.e. as a patient. Clinic orginally therefore described the patient himself (compare cleric) but the meaning was later transferred to the place where patients lay, or were treated. Martial uses *clinicus* in the sense of a doctor (i.e. clinician) as well that of a pall-bearer/gravedigger – what Americans call one-stop shopping. See also **AMBUL-**.

CLINICAL ASSOCIATES An attempt by **GREY SUITS** to rename the ancient and honourable calling of nurses. See also **CHIEF/PRINCIPAL NURSING OFFICER** and **ODA**.

CLITORIS The female homologue of the male penis. The name is said to be derived from the Greek word for 'to shut', from which the medical-Greek *klitoreis* was constructed. Other languages refer to the little organ as 'the tickling-spot', e.g. *Kitzler* in German (*kitzeln* = tickling), so it might be reasonable to assume that the clitoris related to the old English word tickle or tickling, which the *Oxford English Dictionary* defines as 'To be affected or excited by a pleasantly tingling or thrilling sensation; to be stirred or moved with a thrill of pleasure...' There are numerous slang expressions for the little organ, e.g. *button, man in a boat and peeping sentinel,* all no doubt invented by men, which surely gives the lie to the now common assertion by militant women that 'most men don't know of its existence; or, if they do, where to find it and what to do with it'. But to say that it was 'discovered' by early medieval anatomists must be disputed. Their owners would have found theirs first, without necessarily publishing their discovery (see also under **BARTHOLIN'S GLANDS**). A writer of 1650 names, and accurately describes the aspect of, the clitoris, as like 'a little **YARD**'; but classical literature appears not to use the word at all, although the authors were full of enthusiasm for the part (especially when writing about **TRIBADES**). The Romans called it *landica* – when they dared, for this was considered so indecent a word that it was usually euphemised or described rather

than named: Cicero only referred to it as 'a bad word' *(cacemphaton)*; and *Lewis and Short* include *landica* but refuse to give a definition – merely advising the reader to consult another dictionary! It survives in old French as *landie* and was used by Dr Francois Rabelais when he specifically meant the clitoris. *Clitor, Clitoris, Clitorium* are mentioned by Livy and Pliny – but as pertaining to a town in Arcadia, a mountainous region – doubtless a tourist spot today.

CLOACA Latin for the hind-gut. Originally from *cluere*, to purge but there may be a connection with an artificial conduit or canal constructed in Rome by Tarquinius Friscus by which the city's filth was carried from the streets into the Tiber; and therefore also the Roman name for a sewer or drain in general. See also under **COPRO(S)**, **F(A)ECES**, **STERCUS** and, immediately below, **CLOACINA** the goddess who watched over it all.

CLOACINA The Goddess of the Sewers, though this particular role may have been fancifully ascribed to her later. She was still considered to be active in Victorian Britain, though no longer regarded as a goddess. Before the nature of infection was fully understood, the drains were considered to be an essential part of both public and private health. *Cassell's Book of the Household* (c. 1880) in the chapter about *Operations in the Home*, states, 'Much will depend on the condition of the drains, for if they are defective, convalescence will be prolonged, and the patient's chances of recovery materially diminished'. According to Pliny, quoted in *Lewis and Short*, the Cluacina [sic] Venus was so called 'because the Romans, after the end of the Sabine war, purified themselves in the vicinity of her statue with myrtle branches'. They probably had to. John Gay (1685–1732), the author of *The Beggar's Opera*, wrote in his *Trivia, or the Art of Walking the Streets of London* (1716):

> *Then Cloacina, goddess of the tide*
> *Whose sable streams beneath the city glide,*
> *Indulged the modish flame: the town she roved,*
> *A mortal scavenger she saw, she loved...*

...and, more to the point of her specialty, a verse I copied from a lavatory (cloakroom/toilet) wall in an institution much frequented by learned persons. The author is unknown to me – maybe he was the graffitist himself.

> *O Cloacina, goddess of this place,*
> *Look on thy suppliants with a smiling face.*
> *Soft yet cohesive let their off'rings flow*
> *Not rudely swift, nor obstinately slow.*

Perhaps Cloacina (who might have been a distant and grubbier relation of **HYGIEIA**) could legitimise for us the word 'cloakroom' as used for the much-euphemised place for which no satisfactory modern term has yet been found that is both factual and polite (although in fact a cloakroom was literally a place where cloaks were kept, Latin *clocca* or *cloca*, a cape, the same word as the French *cloche*, a bell, from its shape). Because drains were so important in the health of the people their construction was welcomed with many a flourish, and the poets of the day sang their praises. Samuel Carter, who flourished in the first half of the 19th century, thus extolled the London sewerage network:

> *Magnificent, too, is the system of drains,*
> *Exceeding the far-spoken wonders of old:*
> *So lengthen'd and vast in its branches and chains,*
> *That labyrinths pass like a tale that is told:*
> *The sewers gigantic, like multiplied veins,*
> *Beneath the whole city their windings unfold,*
> *Disgorging the source of plagues, scourges and pains*
> *Which visit those cities, to cleanliness cold.*
>
> *Well did the ancient proverb lay down this vital text:*
> *'Cleanliness for human weal to godliness is next'.*

CLONIC See **TONIC**.

CLYSTER From a Greek word *clusis*, a drenching, to drench, rinse or wash out. The clyster, administered by injection into the **RECTUM**, was considered to be a remedy for anything from costiveness to poisoning. The pipe or syringe used for the purpose became the basis for many medical jokes and also a derisive or abusive name for doctors themselves: *'You powder'd pigs-bones, rubarbe glisters!'* (Fletcher, 1621); and its musical possibilities were not overlooked: Beaumont and Fletcher also jocularly describe it as a 'hoboy' (in *Knight of Malta*, c. 1616). Nor was its likeness to a **DILDO** ignored. See also **ENEMA**.

-COCCUS The 'germ' suffix. From the Greek *kokkos*, a seed, berry or grain (Latin *coccum*), i.e. something very small, hence the association with bacteria. See **STREPT(O)-** and **STAPHYLO-** for descriptions of their shape.

COCCYX/COKKYX The Latin word for a cuckoo as well as for the vestigial 'tail' at the bottom of man's spine, also known as the 'cuckoo bone' (Galen's *os coccygis*) – because it was thought to look like that bird's beak. See also **COXA**.

COCHLEA Latin for a shell (snail or cockle), hence also for the snail-like spiral part of the inner ear – a typical example of an everyday Latin word used as a scientific term. The Latin *cochlea* comes from the similar Greek word for a spiral staircase, Archimedes' water-screw and indeed anything spiriform or screw-like. It is also thought to be the origin of the expression 'warming the cockles of the heart', from the heart's supposed resemblance to a large cockle-shell. The *Oxford English Dictionary* gives a Latin version of the expression in a quotation from an anatomical treatise on the heart, dated 1669.

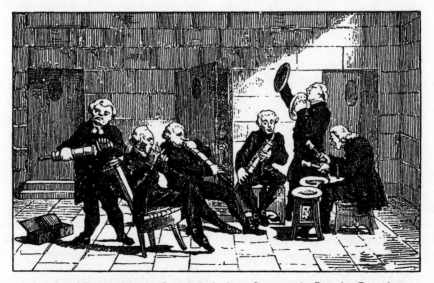

A group of French doctors of ca 1808 playing a Courante (or Running Dance) on Clysters and Enemas, with Close-stool drum accompaniment

COCKTAIL 'We don't serve cocktails', the GP might say to a patient (possibly a **DOORHANDLE**) who demands a prescription for several drugs for different conditions he thinks he suffers from ('Oh and while I'm here, doctor...'). Newspapers reporting suicides or suicide attempts often claim that the victim had taken 'a (lethal) cocktail of drugs'.

C(O)ELIAC Adjective referring to the belly or intestines, from Greek *koilia*, belly, *koilos*, hollow. See also **ENTERON**.

COEL(O)- The 'hollow' and 'empty' prefix, from Greek *koilos*, hollow. The coelom is the body cavity of the developing embryo; coelosomy, a congenital anomaly characterised by the protrusion of the viscera from the body cavity (*coel-* + soma, body). Not to be confused, e.g. by possible spelling-simplification, with **-CELE**.

COFFEE GROUNDS VOMITUS One of the unappetising **MENU CONDITIONS**: blood from the stomach having turned dark-brown or black, usually because of a bleeding peptic ulcer, and having the colour and consistency of ground coffee.

COFFEE-WASHER'S / COFFEE-WORKER'S LUNG A pulmonary occupational affliction: see also **BREWER'S DROOP**.

COITUS The medical word for sexual intercourse (also 'coition') comes from the Latin *coitio, coitionem*, which literally means 'a uniting, a banding or going together'. *Coming* together would be *convenire* (a fact of which the organisers of medical *conventions* should be aware). In other words, as in the biblical phrase 'the ram went with the ewe' and numerous rustic expressions, 'going together' was what ordinary people said. Today, a girl who confides to her doctor that she is 'going out' with her boyfriend usually means she is 'going' with him in the above sense. The English verb 'to coit' is bad English made out of good Latin, and also an accidental contraction of 'co-habit', which means living, not necessarily sleeping, together – though then again, sleeping is not necessarily involved in coition. The whole business of sex is hedged-about with careless euphemisms and careful circumlocutions. The meaning of **COITUS INTERRUPTUS** is self-evident. For this see also **APOSIOPESIS**.

COITUS INTERRUPTUS Needs neither translation nor definition: the act of withdrawal by the man before **ORGASM** just before the end of man–woman sexual **CONGRESS** so that the **SEMEN** is discharged outside, not inside, the woman. You will find more about it under **ONAN**, who paid for it with his life. See also **PULSUS ALTERNANS**.

COLIC From Greek *kolikos*, relating to the colon; hence the 'severe paroxysmal griping pains in the belly', as the *Oxford English Dictionary* puts it, although colics can happen in other places as well, e.g. the kidney or the gallbladder.

COLON The greater portion of the lower intestine, but the word was also used for the gut in general, as well as for the stomach; but then the ancients got their digestive processes rather confused. The word comes from the Greek *kolon* meaning food (*colostomy* combines that word with Greek stoma, meaning the mouth – in this case, of course, an artificial 'mouth', or opening). Further confusion is caused by the fact that the explorer and navigator English-speakers know as Christopher Columbus was called, in Spanish, Cristobal Colon, so that many places named after him have a curious ring to English ears, e.g. the Teatro Colon, the famous opera-house in Buenos Aires. The colon is also a punctuation-mark stronger than a semicolon but weaker than a full stop; in old English, from Latin *colere*, to till: a colon is a husbandman or gardener – hence the colonies and, a back-formation via French, 'colon' for a colonial.

COLPOS The Greek *kolpos* has the same connotation as the Latin *vagina*, or fold (i.e. in the skin) though *kolpos* originally also meant 'the bosom', or 'the womb' in a slightly poetic way, as we speak of 'the breast' as a seat of the emotions. It suggests that the Greek doctors preferred the euphemism (in the same way as some people still say 'stomach' when they mean the belly) to the Romans' vernacular: *vagina* was a sheath or scabbard, *uterus*, a bottle, *penis* a tail. Even today few laymen know the meaning of any of the *colpo-* formations (colposcope, colpitis, colpocele, colpotomy, etc.), whereas they would know at once what a vaginoscope is for.

COMA In Greek, *koma* meant a deep sleep or lethargy. Now, unnatural and prolonged sleep or deep unconsciousness. See also **HYPNOS, SOMNUS, SOPOR, STUPOR** and **TORPOR**.

COME TO TERMS WITH... One does not wish to be unsympathetic to human pain, grief or disaster, but must nevertheless be aware that clichés soon lose their force and meaning; and without these four words **COUNSELLORS** would be out of a job.

COMMINUTION   Of bone: the fracturing or crushing into several pieces: not to be confused with 'commination', which is the threat of punishment or divine retribution.

COMMON COLD   This has so far defeated the best medical and scientific brains, but according to Sir Robert Bruce Lockhart (1886–1970), 'As a cure for the cold, take your toddy to bed, put one bowler hat at the foot, and drink until you see two'. For a Scotsman like Lockhart, toddy, or hot toddy, would have been a mixture of whisky, hot water, and sugar or honey – in proportionate quantities according to taste.

COMMUNITY   A word over-used by politicians, theorists and workers in the British **WELFARE STATE**. Any term, word or concept to which it is attached is thought to gain a glow of benevolence and **CARING**, e.g. Community Health Centre, Community Care, Community Immunisation, Community Action, Community Dog Warden, etc. It is nearly always either redundant or meaningless, especially when applied to secular or **ETHNIC** minority groups, e.g. 'the homosexual community'. 'Community leaders' are usually unelected, self-appointed and highly vocal spokesmen for their particular group.

CONCUPISCENCE   Almost the same as **LIBIDO** but less popular with the general public: no-one has ever sued anyone for alleged 'loss of concupiscence'. Like *libido* it originally had general, not merely sexual, meanings; from Latin *concupere*, to have a great longing – for *anything*, perhaps a glass of beer or a smoked salmon bagel.

CONDOM   There is no evidence that the contraceptive sheath was invented by and named after 'an 18th-century physician, Dr Condom' (possibly Cundum or Cundom), as is often alleged in popular journalism. Dr Condom, whoever he was, is said to have recommended the use of a pig's bladder or fish membrane, and such was indeed used by the self-styled great lover Giacomo Casanova de Seingalt (1725–98). Dr Samuel Johnson's biographer James Boswell (1740–1817) used a sheep's **CAECUM** – but caught the **CLAP** all the same; and Dr Stephen Lock says, 'I was taught at Cambridge that Roman soldiers excised the planta(ris) muscle of dead opponents to use for the purpose' (but Mr Stephen Reilly questions this: 'It is a miserable, narrow strip of vestigial muscle lying below the **GASTROCNEMIUS**; by no stretch of the imagination could it ever have been used to protect even the most minuscule penis: its only claim to fame is that it sometimes ruptures during athletic activity'). It should, of course, be pointed out that these early sheaths were not intended to protect the women against unwanted pregnancy but the men from possible infection by women ('the Condum being the best, if not the only, Preservative our Libertines have found out at present' – *Turner on Syphilis*, 1717). As an anonymous English poet of 1744 wrote: 'Let not the Joy she proffers be Essay'd/ Without the well-try'd Cundum's friendly Aid'. No Doctor Condum, Cundum or Cundom has ever been found in London street-directories, not even in the London Telephone Directory, where the most curious old English family names survive; and in any case, the first recorded mention of a 'condum' is dated c. 1706, so he would have been a very precocious '18th-century physician' indeed. The nearest English name is Condon, but this spelling has not been recorded for the sheath. There is a French town called Condom (you can't miss it – it is a few miles south-east of Bordeaux near a place called Sore) and this provides the most likely provenance for a 'Dr Condom'; but the place was never noted for a rubber industry – which would have made the 'French letter' really French. On the contrary, someone recently discovered that during the 18th century hundreds of condoms were exported from England to France for the personal use of Louis XV; so the boot is, so to speak, on the other foot, and it would make the French term for the condom, *capote anglaise*, more seminal than counter-abusive. (But see also the **DUTCH CAP**). Since the **AIDS** scare the Americans have also taken the word 'condom' to their hearts, whereas they would previously have called it a 'rubber' (causing frequent confusion with an English eraser). But international mix-ups are common in this matter: the 3M company at one time marketed a form of self-adhesive 'sellotape' called *Durex*; and there is an American brand of contraceptive sheath called Cello, pronounced 'sello' but written like the musical instrument, much to the dismay of cellists. The advent of **AIDS** elevated the condom to the status of a late-20th-century icon and the word is on everyone's lips, whether in church or at dinner-parties. Even children who know nothing of the urges that may lead to its use are familiar with the object ('Hey, Johnny, I found a condom on the patio!' – 'What's a patio?'). Commerce has tried to make the product 'attractive to the end-user' (as the advertisements inappropriately put it) by producing condoms in different colours and flavours – though this is not a new idea either: the *Oxford English Dictionary* gives a quotation from Pattison's *Cupid's Metamorphosis* of 1728: 'Happy the Man, who in his Pocket keeps/ Whether with Green or Scarlet Ribband bound/ A well made Condum'. The latest development is the 'female' condom, a sheath 'worn' by the woman which looks (and probably feels) like one of those plastic bags dispensed in tear-off rolls at the vegetable counter of Safeways (and is probably about as safe). Its trade-name takes the first two syllables of 'feminine' and the last of 'condom' to produce Femidom. (*'Femicon'* was doubtless considered but rejected in anticipation of difficulties with French-speaking purchasers). See also under **PROPHYLACTIC** and **MENARCHE**. In the late 1980s a French international footballer called Jean Condom gave much pleasure to his supporters – unfortunately not as a goalkeeper but as a rugby star. His family probably hailed from the town mentioned earlier.

CONFERENCE From Latin *conferre*, to bring together, consult together, or gather together for joint examination and comparison of material. Conferences are an important element in the dissemination and exchange of specialist knowledge – although many a conference has turned into a **SYMPOSIUM**. Francis Bacon (1561–1626), English lawyer, writer and philosopher, Lord Chancellor and Adviser to Queen Elizabeth I, wrote 'Reading maketh a Full man; Conference a Ready Man; and Writing an Exact man'. Also **DROMOMANIA** and **SEMINAR**.

CONFINEMENT A strangely archaic-sounding word for childbirth, delivery and accouchement, still current in everyday English speech ('she had a difficult confinement...'). It really means being shut up, kept in one place or imprisoned – but then, the aspect of pregnant women used to be considered distasteful to some. Until comparatively recently a pregnancy in the British royal family would be announced in a circumlocutory statement such as, 'Her Royal Highness will be fulfilling no public engagements until further notice'. From then onwards her growing belly would be kept decently hidden from the public. The expression 'confined to a wheelchair' is rightly now considered politically incorrect, as it usually is.

CONGRESS Latin *congressus*, a coming-together, and hence an old-fashioned euphemism for **COITUS** – 'sexual congress' in full (just as the word 'sexual' before it, as it is usually omitted before 'intercourse'). In this sense it is not often used in the United States of America, understandably, as their Congress is part of the legislature. Smaller congresses or **CONFERENCES** are convened by professional bodies in their various disciplines: see under **SYMPOSIUM** and **DROMOMANIA**.

CONIUGARE Latin, to unite. Hence the conjunctiva, which 'unites' the eyelid with the ball of the eye; and conjunctivitis, an inflammation of it, or 'pink eye'. And see **PHLYCTEN**.

CONSULTANT Formerly the noun lacked the *-ant* ending and was 'consult', from Latin *consultus*, a skilled adviser. Dr Samuel Johnson (1709–84) is quoted by his amanuensis James Boswell, 'So, we have a Juris consultus, a consult in law'. The modern title of Consultant (Medical Officer/Physician/Surgeon) is no older than the late/middle Victorian age. The *Oxford English Dictionary* noted its first known occurrence in De Styrap's *Medical Ethics* (1878): 'In Consultation it is customary for the family doctor to precede the Consultant into the sick-room...' – but as De Styrap gives the position a capital C it seems likely that by then the word 'consultant' already commanded respect. See under **GREY SUITS** and its various cross-references for the dress favoured by consultants and other toilers in the medical field.

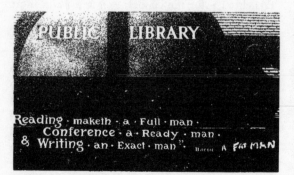

Francis Bacon's dictum, improved by a health conscious graffitist, over the entrance to Kensington Library, Livepool (Photo: Reg Cox)

CONSUMPTION See **PHTHISIS** and **TB**.

CONTAGIOUS/INFECTIOUS See **INFECTIOUS/CONTAGIOUS**.

CONTRA- The 'against' or 'opposite' prefix. See **C/I**.

CONTRECOUP The effect of a blow, an injury or a fracture, which is produced exactly opposite, or at some distance from, the part actually struck. Those familiar with the English board-game shove-ha'penny or the toy known as 'Newton's Balls' will have observed this effect of transmitted energy. Contrecoup is one of the few French words used in medicine (**MENARCHE** and **TOURNIQUET** are others): the English 'counterblow' is not really appropriate.

CONVALESCE(NT) From the Latin words *con* (together) + *valescere*, to gain strength (see also **-ESCENT**). We would now unhesitatingly say 'recuperate', but this was once considered an intolerable Americanism which no respectable English doctor would have used. Here is the English satirical magazine *Punch* on the subject in 1864: 'Another Yankeeism nearly as illiterate as "reliable" [!] has just been imported by the *Etna* [a famous early steamship] in one of Reuter's telegrams. This communication, one of those evil ones which corrupt good language, informs us that General Grant is very ill, and that, "as the army is about to settle into winter quarters, it is urged by General Grant's physicians that he should go home to recuperate". Some years ago Mr Buckstone, in a farce, acted a Yankee's part, in which he had to say. "If I live from July till eternity, I shall never obliviate this..." The formation of "recuperate" from *recupero*

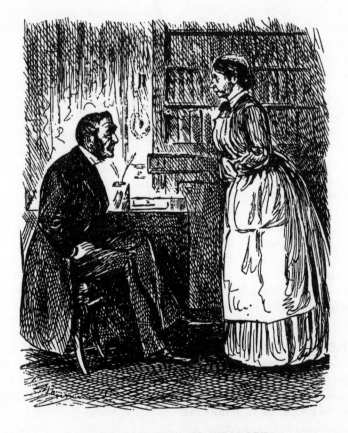

"NO ONE IS A HERO TO HIS VALET."
Sir Arthur Pillson, Bart., M.D, F.R.C.P., &c., &c., &c. "AND ARE YOU BETTER, SIMPSON, AFTER THAT MEDICINE I GAVE YOU LAST NIGHT?"
Cook. "WELL, I CAN'T SAY AS I HAM, SIR HARTHUR; AND TO TELL YOU THE TRUTH, IF YOU'VE NO OBJECTION, SIR HARTHUR, I SHOULD LIKE TO CONSULT A REGULAR MEDICAL MAN."

Punch, November 11, 1882

may be more defensible than that of "obliviate" from *obliviscor*, but still "recuperate" is a needless corruption of Latin. Why not stick to "recover"? Besides the French word *recuperer* has a distinct meaning and signifies to retrieve. An American might, without any impropriety beyond that of affectation, talk about action to recuperate his dollars, but how can people who call themselves members of the Anglo-Saxon family use such language? As for you who owe allegiance to Her Majesty, and are in duty bound to maintain the purity of the Queen's English, consider "recuperate" President's English, spurious, base, villainous; pray you, avoid it'. Thus wrote the English satirical magazine *Punch* in the middle of the 19th century. Both 'recuperate' and 'reliable' have become respected words: but 'obliviate', which came so naturally to *Punch*, was current only between 1660 and 1850, then to be all-but forgotten. No-one can stop language from changing, and once a neologism catches on it will not wither until the wheel of fashion turns again. As for *recover*, we can no longer use it as a synonym for 'recuperate', as each word acquired a separate connotation during the 20th century.

COPRO- Greek *kopros*, dung, the prefix for excrement or filth. The Latin is *faex, faecis*; also *stercus*. Copro- usually indicates human excrement, hence copro**PHILIA**, a love of excreta (coprolagnia when taking a sexual form), which in some persons induces sexual excitement – to the disbelief and astonishment of the rest of the population, most of whom are repelled by stercorous matter and its **FAECAL** smells. An even more extreme abnormality (which hardly bears thinking about) is coprophagia, for the meaning of which see under the **-PHAG(E)-** prefix/suffix. The implications of copro- should make hyphen-shy writers think twice before spelling co-production 'coproduction', for this drastically alters its meaning. See also **FAEX, FAECIS**. See also **AROMATHERAPY**.

COPROLALIA 'Talking dirty'. Most people who do it do it because they want to, and some use foul language because they lack the word-power and intelligence to do otherwise; but it is also one of several symptoms indicating the **GILLES DE LA TOURETTE SYNDROME**, whose often perfectly respectable sufferers cannot help themselves and utter obscenities without realising it – though one might ask, if they are so respectable how do they know the words?

COPULATION From Latin *copula*, a link; which is also the name of an organ-stop.

CORN See **KERATIN**.

CORN FLAKES This familiar breakfast food has a medical origin. We owe many of their various and ingenious forms to the American surgeon John Harvey Kellogg, a Seventh Day Adventist by religion who, in 1866 at the age of 24, managed the Western Health Reform Institute at Battle Creek, Michigan. As a confirmed vegetarian he would ask audiences in his lectures, 'How can you eat anything that looks out of eyes?', and developed certain vegetarian foods, such as a form of peanut butter and numerous dried cereals.

CORNEA The horn-hard circular part in the front of the eyeball, from the Latin *cornea tela*, horny tissue, later *hornea tunica*, horny coating. See also **KERAT(O-)**.

CORNED BEEF RASH A rash with a self-explanatory name; and one of the **MENU CONDITIONS** – perhaps related to the **SPAMMIE**.

CORONARY Short for coronary thrombosis or **INFARCT(ION)**: an obstruction of the blood-vessels of the heart 'which encircle parts like a crown' and are therefore described as 'coronary', crown-like – in popular parlance a heart attack (which if sudden and fatal is almost invariably prefaced in the press by the obligatory description of 'massive'). Other linguistic origins of stoppages will be found under **EMBOLISM** and **THROMBOS(IS)**.

CORPULENCE From Latin *corpus*, a body (living or dead, e.g. corpse), thence *corpulentia*, grossness or fleshiness of body, mentioned by Pliny and others: in old English it often appears as corpulency. See **BANTING, BULIMIA, CELLULITE, OBESITY, OREXIS, PINGUESCENCE** and **PYKNIC**.

CORTEX Latin for bark, rind or shell, hence the outer **GREY MATTER** of the brain.

CORTISONE From half the above word + the -one suffix of **HORMONE**: a steroid hormone found in the **ADRENAL** cortex and also produced synthetically as a drug.

(SAINTS) COSMAS AND DAMIAN The patron saints of physicians, called 'The Moneyless Ones', who were canonised for charging no fees. Whether for this or other reasons, doubts have been expressed that they really existed: some say they were merely a christianised concept of the twin sons of Zeus. This theory is supported by the fact that no dates of birth or canonisation have ever been put forward. The twins were martyred at Cyrrhus in Syria, allegedly for their Christian faith but perhaps – who knows – by disappointed patients.

COSTA Latin for a rib.

COSTIVENESS A contraction, via the old French *costevé*, of the Latin *constipatus*. It is often used as a polite alternative for 'constipated' – but is NOT a posh way of saying 'costly', contrary to the view of many journalists, councillors and others, e.g. 'The government is embarking on yet another costive road-closure scheme' (traffic blockages?). This is the appropriate place to mention that in early medicine **FLAGELLATION** was thought to be a cure for costiveness; also that this may be the reason why the British public-school system, which encouraged regular bowel movement and for centuries used flogging to enforce discipline, perhaps invented it as *le vice Anglais* (but see also under **BUGGERY**). Of the renaissance prince, composer and murderer, Carlo Gesualdo of Venosa, his doctors said, *Princeps Venusiae musica clarissimus cacare non poterat, nisi verberatus a servo ad id adscito* ('the Prince of Venosa, most illustrious musician of his age, was unable to shit without having first been flogged by a servant...') – though the information that Gesualdo wore 'a beatific smile' during the treatment suggests that the Prince may have enjoyed it for a different reason. See also **FLATULENCE**.

COUNSELLING During the two closing decades of the 20th century social workers of the **NHS** and **GREY SUITS** swelled in numbers with the creation of well-paid posts whose incumbents administer a kind of verbal **PLACEBO** to patients and/or their relatives. They may enlighten them about the nature of the condition, break bad news and console them, and gently try to make them feel better. This was formerly done by the family doctor or priest, by friends, or by the victims' own relatives (who may now, however, be too busy seeing their compensation lawyers – see **AMBULANCE CHASERS** – or giving TV interviews). British counsellors soon formed their own trades union, the British Association of Counselling, and subdivided themselves into various **SPECIALTIES**, such as Grief Counsellors, Rape Counsellors and Crime Victim Support Counsellors, etc. Municipal counselling services work in close co-operation with police and rescue workers: a day after we reported the theft of some garden furniture (by thieves who never got nearer to the house than 50 yards) we received a telephone call from a counsellor kindly offering her services to help us **COME TO TERMS WITH** the loss of a couple of antique cast-iron urns. Some British universities offer degree courses in Counselling.

COWORKER One who works together with another, a co-operator, e.g. in a research project: 'We are co-workers with God' (J. Shute, *Judgement and Mercy*, 1643). The necessary hyphen, is now often modishly omitted – suggesting not the work of doctors but veterinarians.

COWPOX A mild infectious disease characterised by a pustular rash which pointed the way to **IMMUNISATION** by **VACCINATION**. In 1721 London suffered a smallpox epidemic which took many lives. Lady Mary Wortley Montagu – with great faith and courage (or ignorance) – had her 5-year-old daughter inoculated in the presence of leading physicians, and the child developed only a mild visitation of the disease. The physicians were so impressed that George I had two of his grandchildren inoculated – but only after the procedure had been tested on 11 charity school children, and on six inmates of Newgate Prison, who volunteered in return for having their death sentences commuted (see under **DUODENUM** for a classical example of dissection carried out on volunteer criminals by Erasistratus). But in 1713 the London physician John Woodward had received a letter from a Greek physician, Emanuel Timoni of Constantinople, describing a method of preventing smallpox by what was quite clearly an earlier form of immunisation. Timoni reported that another Greek physician, Giacomo Pylarini of Smyrna, had removed some of the thick liquid from a smallpox pustule, rubbed it into a small scratch made with a needle on the skin of a healthy person, and thus protected that person, who developed a mild case of smallpox but nothing worse.

COXA Latin for the hip or haunch, hence coxalgia, coxarthritis, etc. The Greek is **ISCHION**. See also **COCCYX**.

COXENDIX Pliny's word for the hip-bone (see above) which has not gained much currency in English-speaking countries.

CRANBERRY JELLY STOOLS The same as **REDCURRANT JELLY STOOLS** – one of the unappetising **MENU CONDITIONS**; and for mulberries, see under **MOON MOLARS**.

CRANIUM From the Greek word *kranion* for a skull; but strictly the brain-case or brain-pan.

CRASH TEAM In British hospitals, a team of doctors and nurses on standby for the resuscitation of patients who have suffered cardiac arrest.

CREMASTER The Greek for a suspender, as might have been used for socks or trousers had they worn such garments. Now the word is applied to the muscles of the spermatic cord by which the **TESTES** or **GONADS** are suspended.

-CRET- Part of the Latin *cerno, (crevi, cretum)*, to separate into different parts. Hence such words as discerning, discrete, secret, secretion, excretion, and of course secretary – one who is privy to secrets.

CRETIN Originally this meant the same as Christian (Swiss patois, *crestin, creitin*): one of a class of dwarfed, deformed and mentally impaired people found in certain Alpine valleys from the middle of the 18th century, thence applied to a certain form of impairment. The 'Christian' connection arose from the fact that they were distinguished from the brutes as 'human creatures', though so deformed mentally and physically. See also **MORON**.

CRIBRIFORM With lots of holes, from Latin *cribrum*, a sieve, *cribrare*, to sift.

CRINATE Hairy, from Latin *crinis*, hair. And incidentally, *crin* is the name of the horse-hair-stiffened fabric from which crinolines (in old colloquial English 'arse-coolers') were made. See also **PIL(US)** and the Greek **TRICHOS**.

CRIPPLE(D) This word is no longer acceptable in polite speech, and is usually replaced by gentler expressions like 'disabled' or 'wheelchair-bound' and (the latest **PC** favourite, **CHALLENGED**. The Bible uses it only once, in *Acts* XIV, 8, and brings an interesting alternative to 'lame': 'And at Lystra there sat a certain man, impotent in his feet, a cripple from his mother's womb'. The *Good News Bible* changes this (rather lamely) to 'lame from birth and had never been able to walk'. Shakespeare, in *Timon of Athens*, has the chilling lines, 'Thou cold sciatica, cripple our senators, so that their limbs may halt as lamely as their manners'. But in spite of the fact that the disabled are sometimes heard to say it of themselves, and even use the lighthearted abbreviation 'crips', it remains a most insensitive word: proponents of **PC** have a point. See **SCIATICA**.

CROTCH The 'fork' of the human body, where the legs join the trunk, better than the alternative, crutch, which is more usefully reserved for an auxiliary or substitute leg to help the lame, one-legged or legless to walk. Both are probably related to Latin *crus, cruris*, a leg, and there is a Nordic word that sounds like a relation. Old-time physicians used to speak politely of the bit between the legs as the 'intercrural area' – the place where one may get the **DHOBI ITCH**, or **TINEA** *cruris*.

CROTOS In Greek a form of castanet or rattle used to beat out the rhythm in music, hence the **DICROTIC** or double, beat of the heart.

CROUP 'To cry hoarsely, to croak as a raven, frog, crane, etc.', says the *Oxford English Dictionary*, giving an example of 1513 of 'byrdis crouping in the sky...' – an echoic word imitating a sound from nature. The dictionary also describes croup as 'An inflammatory disease of the larynx and trachea of children, marked by a peculiar sharp ringing cough...' Croup, we are also told, was the popular name for this condition among the people of south-east Scotland and 'was introduced into medical use by Professor Francis Home of Edinburgh in 1765'.

CRUMBLIES Junior doctors' slang for old and frail people.

CRYPTOGENIC (DISEASE) Literally a disease of *secret* origin, but this is in fact a code term: e.g. 'cryptogenic cirrhosis' would be another way of saying 'I don't know what the hell is causing this **CIRRHOSIS**' (my informant adds 'But the term is impressive enough to send a bill' for). See also **GOK** and **IDIOPATHIC**.

CRYPTORCH(ID)ISM Undescended testicles, from *kryptos*, Greek for hidden, secret + **ORCHIS**, testicle. The congenital absence of one or both is *anorchism*. The text-books say that this, unlike **CASTRATION**, does not affect hormonal development. But cases have been known of boys who kept their treble voice and prolonged their work in church choirs into adulthood, with the constant risk of its sudden loss. The German writer J. W. von Archenholz, who chronicled his adventures on *A Trip to Italy* (published in an English translation by Joseph Trapp in London in 1791) relates a 'musical disaster' which he claims befell a castrato singer in Naples in about 1765, although it was really a case of *cryptorchidism* (also seen

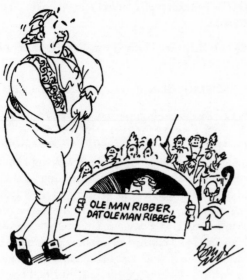

Cryptorch(id)ism

more meticulously spelt *crypto-orchidism* and contracted as *cryptorchism*): 'A very peculiar accident happened a few years ago to a singer of the name of Balani. This man was born without any visible signs of those parts which are taken out in castration. He was, therefore, looked upon as a true-born castrato; an opinion, which was even confirmed by his voice. He learned music, and sung for several years upon the theatre with great applause. One day, he exerted himself so uncommonly in singing an arietta, that all of a sudden those parts, which had so long been concealed by nature, dropped into their proper place. The singer from this very instant lost his voice . . . and with it lost every prospect of a future subsistence'. (Quoted in *The Castrati in Opera*, by Angus Heriot, published by Calder, 1960). See **CASTRATION** and **TESTES**.

CTD American doctors' secret code abbreviation for Circling The Drain, said of a patient who is thought to be dying. Also **PBAB**.

CUBITUS The elbow, hence the *cubito-* prefix in conjunction with various anatomical terms. The word has an interesting history, coming from *cubare-*, *cumbere*, to lie down, to recline, which the Romans did even at mealtimes, supporting themselves on the propped-up elbow and eating in a semi-*recumbent* position, probably to the detriment of their digestion. Like most lying-down words *cubare* became a euphemism for sexual intercourse and Tacitus uses it in that sense: a *concubi*ne is someone to lie *with*. Like the foot, the

cubit was an 'anatomical' measurement, the distance from the elbow to the fingertips. The word also gave us **INCUBATION**, the period in which a disease 'lies' dormant (not to mention the hatching of eggs after the mother-bird has lain upon them) and the incubus, which in nightmares lies heavily on a sleeper (who is either dreaming of sex or troubled by indigestion – his supper *lying* heavily in his stomach). See also **DECUBITUS**.

CULTURE From Latin *cultura*, cultivation, growth. In biology, the maintenance of organisms under artificial conditions and in a suitable nutrient medium so that they can multiply. See also **GREY SUITS**.

-CULUS, -CULUM, -CULA These Latin endings always denote a diminutive, e.g. *calculus*, a little stone, *vasculum*, a little vessel, etc.

CUNEIFORM Wedge-shaped.

CUNNUS, CUNNI Another Latin word for the **VAGINA**, though it was already obscene in classical Latin and, like the related English 'cunt', was used offensively by the Romans, too, in a transferred sense, of a person, usually female. *Cunnus* appeared to play no part in polite medical or scientific terminology, apart from *cunnilingus*, which, however (like **FELLARE**), is not a medical condition. In old English, especially of the 17th and 18th centuries, 'cunny' was used for the same organ (also a pet name for a rabbit or coney, a furry thing, but derived – perhaps punningly from the Latin *cuniculus*, a rabbit or coney). *Cunnus* may also be related to *cuneus*, a wedge and/or a similar word meaning a ditch – which was another word facetiously or picturesquely used by the Romans for the female sex organ; as was **FOSSA**, another word for a ditch. See also **COLPOS**, **FICA**, **LANDICA** and **VULVA**.

CUPIDITY Another word for lust or **LIBIDO**, and named after Cupid, the Romans' counterpart of **EROS**. See also **LAGNEIA**.

CUPOLA The small dome-shaped summit of the **COCHLEA**. From Latin *cupula*, a little cask or small vault (barrel vault?). One of the **ARCHITECTURAL TERMS** scattered about these pages.

CUPPING An old-fashioned remedy akin to bleeding (for which see **LEECH**). Dry cupping was done by applying a heated cup or glass to the skin which, as it cooled, caused a swelling and increased the circulation or drew blood to the surface of the skin. With wet cupping a small incision was first made in the skin, so that the blood would be drawn out and flow into the cup. Cupping and Vibrating is something different – procedure to remove fluid and mucus from the lungs, carried out not with a cup but the cupped hands.

CURE/REMEDY An important distinction in the – now carefully-formulated – rules for the advertising of medicines.

CURETTE One of the rare French words, from *curer*, to clear or cleanse: a surgical cleansing, scraping or scooping instrument for the purpose of *curettage* in various parts of the body (see also **D&C**). The word is now also applied to a suction instrument used for the same purpose. But a curate of the church does not cleanse souls. He is merely in charge of them, a curator – from Latin *curatus*.

CURRY ANUS An inflammation of the anus and surrounding area, accompanied by a burning sensation, observed in young English persons (almost invariably males) addicted to takeaway curries (usually eaten **AMBULANT** and with fried potatoes). As they like their curry hot, it burns them on both entering and leaving them. Dr Peter Dangerfield recommends the simple and cheap cure of keeping a roll of toilet-tissue in the deep-freeze before using it on the affected part.

CUT- The skin prefix, from Latin *cutis*, skin. See also **DERMA**.

CUTICLE See above: from Latin *cuticula*, a little skin.

CYANOSIS Blueish discoloration of the skin.

CYESIS An old-fashioned name for pregnancy, like the French *enceinte* for 'pregnant', which was used in England at a time when such a condition was not mentioned in polite circles except by euphemisms, e.g. 'In a certain ('delicate' or 'interesting') condition, in happy anticipation, in the family way, a lady-in-waiting', etc., or else disguised by foreign words. In British royal circles announcements that 'Her Royal Highness has cancelled all public engagements until further notice', would let the world know as clearly as saying, in Nelson's words, that 'England Expects'. Under **PSEUDOCYESIS** you will find a limerick.

CYST(O)- The bladder (or hollow sac) prefix, from the Greek *cystis*, (or *kystis*), bladder. Hence all manner of combination terms like cystalgia, cystectomy, cystitis, and, of course (in a non-urinary sense), a *cyst*, an abnormal, hollow sac filled with liquid or semi-liquid matter.

CYTO- The 'cell' prefix, as in *cytopathic, cytochemistry*, etc. *Cytos* is Greek for a cell – Latin *cella*. Also the anglicised suffix *-cyte*, e.g. cystocyte, leukocyte, etc.

D*d*

Δ The Greek Letter D, or *delta*: shorthand for 'diagnosis, e.g. 'Δ influenza'.

D&C Sounds like a do-it-yourself store but in fact stands for dilatation and **CURETTAGE**, a gynaecological procedure (also facetiously referred to as Dusting and Cleaning). Experts say it is now usually done by a different method which should be abbreviated to D&S – Dilatation and Suction.

-DACTYL- Prefix/suffix element from the Greek for fingers or toes. The Greek word in full is *dactylos*, the Latin, *digitus*, which please see, below, for futher information.

DAY TRIPPER Casualty officers' code for a presumed or likely cause of certain accident injuries. Victims are often pedestrians who claim to have 'tripped and fallen over a paving-stone'. In English urban areas, where **AMBULANCE CHASERS** are not the only seekers after compensation, such persons are usually **PAFO**s who wish to turn their minor accidents to lucrative account. In municipalities or hospitals where claims for injury compensation are kept on a database, computer searches have shown that tripping runs in families: once a member of the family has tripped over a paving-stone all his relations manage to trip over the same obstruction. 'Victims' themselves now use the term – as they cash yet another insurance check. See also **PLOMBOSCILLOSIS**, **RSI** and **WHIPLASH**.

DE- A useful but double-edged prefix. In its most frequently used sense it means to take away, remove or lessen, like depilate for removing hair; desensitise, to lessen or remove sensitivity; dehydrate, to remove water, dementia, the separation of a person from his mind – and in extreme cases, decapitation, the removal of the head. But another form of *de-* intensifies the word element it precedes, like depression, which is not a removal of pressure but an increase; defiling, to dirty or to soil, not a negation of it (an ancient modification of the word meaning 'to foul'); and denigration, to blacken, not unblacken. The difference can be (but often is not) emphasised by the pronunciation: 'dee' for reversal of meaning, 'deh' for intensification. The last-named example should therefore be pronounced 'deh-nigg-rate', not 'dee-nigh-grate'.

DEAD HAND SYNDROME See **VWF**.

DEAF-AND-DUMB People who are totally deaf from birth cannot *hear* others speak, and are therefore unable to imitate them. Thus they cannot learn normal speech and remain *dumb*, an Old Norse, Gothic and Old English word meaning speechless, mute. Unfortunately the German word *dumm* (as in *Dummkopf*) was erroneously assumed by German immigrants (mostly in the USA) to mean the same as the English 'dumb', and so they started to use 'dumb' in the sense of 'stupid' (e.g. 'dumb blonde') – which deaf people obviously are not. As a result of this misunderstanding, deaf-and-dumb is now a politically-incorrect term (except to the deaf-and-dumb, who usually have no such qualms). In recommended **PC** usage, the correct word is 'a non-verbal person' or some formation containing the word 'challenged', though 'mute' is surely acceptable. Even the innocuous 'deaf-mute' is disapproved of by some. For the record, the German word for 'dumb' in its correct sense is *stumm*, which has also been naturalised into American English as 'shtum', meaning 'to remain silent'.

DÉBRIDEMENT An old French term, literally 'un-bridling' a horse, but meaning in practice the removal from a wound of damaged tissue or foreign matter – indeed *débris*.

DECIBEL One-tenth of a bel, and the bel is named after Alexander Graham Bell (1847–1922), the electrical engineer and aptly-surnamed inventor of the telephone: to have called a unit a 'bell' would presumably have been too confusing. Abbreviated *db* or *dB*, decibels are used in hearing-tests and when checking dangerous noise-levels. The rustling of leaves or pages of a Bible can register approximately 10 dB; a jet-plane taking off and heard from 200 yards' distance about 140 dB, causing physical pain and, on continuous exposure, permanent deafness. A rock-and-roll or 'heavy metal' band (featuring a 'lead' guitarist?) can register 110 dB, 'ameliorated' to 90 dB by an average-volume walkman – both splendid ways of increasing the already vast profits of the hearing-aid industry. A sound-level increase by 10 dB roughly doubles subjective loudness, so that 120 dB is twice as loud as 110 dB.

DECUBITUS The recumbent position, the manner or posture of lying in bed: Latin *decumbere*, to lie down. Decubitus ulcers are more usually called bed-sores. See **CUBITUS**, **INCUBUS** and **SUCCUBUS**.

DEF(A)ECATION From *defaecare*, to cleanse of dregs or residue, to purify: *de* + *faeces*, dregs. The purification meaning (often spiritual or religious) came before, and for some time existed side-by-side with, the now universal one of emptying the bowels.

DELHI BELLY Popular name for any form of **DIARRH(O)E(I)A** contracted by British forces, colonists or travellers in the Indian subcontinent (also **BOMBAY CRUD**): **GIPPY TUMMY** in Egypt, **MONTEZUMA'S REVENGE** in Mexico and the **TURKEY TROTS** in Turkey.

DELIRIUM The Latin word for madness, although in modern medical use it generally denotes not so much dementia but incoherent speech, hallucinations, restlessness, etc., resulting from disturbances in the functions of the brain, perhaps during high fever. People sometimes absurdly declare themselves 'deliriously happy', often abbreviated to 'I was delirious!' **FATUOUS(NESS)** has similarly lost its force. See also **HYSTER(ICAL)**.

DEMENTIA From Latin *demens, dementum*, out of (one's) mind. See **MENS, MENTIS** There used to be a good English word, now disused, demency.

DE MORGAN'S SPOTS See **CHERRY ANGIOMA**.

DENGUE FEVER This mosquito-borne infectious and eruptive fever, which is epidemic and sporadic in East Africa, has a false etymology. It is usually said to be named from the Spanish word *dengue* meaning fastidiousness, prudery or a short veil – which, in the the context of the condition, is meaningless. In fact it is a Swahili word, better written *denga, dinga*, or *dyenga* (in full, *ka dinga pepo*), which means 'cramp *(dinga)* caused by an evil spirit' *(dengo)*.

DERBYSHIRE DROOP A form of temporary male impotence – see under **BREWER'S DROOP** – and cross-references, from **CELLIST'S NIPPLE** to **FARMER'S LUNG, FLAUTIST'S CHIN, FIDDLER'S NECK, GAMEKEEPER'S THUMB, HANGMAN'S FRACTURE** and **HOUSEMAID'S KNEE**, etc. – but also **RSI, PLOMBOSCILLOSIS** for possible 'lead-swinging' conditions.

DERBYSHIRE NECK Endemic thyroid **GOITRE** caused by a low intake of iodine, e.g. in limestone environments such as are found in parts of Derbyshire.

DERMA Greek for skin producing numerous words (mostly via the genitive *dermatos*): dermatology, dermatoplasty, dermographia, dermatitis, etc. See also **EPI-**; also under **CUT-**, for the Latin equivalent is *cutis*. See also **EXCORIATE**.

DEXTER Latin for 'right' – the right-hand side, also right-handed (and dextrous, as left-handed people were once thought to be 'clumsy' – as well as sinister!). Dextrocardia: a rare congenital condition in which the heart is on the right, i.e. the wrong, side. The Greek is *dexios* – both in the right/correct and the right-handed sense. Another Latin word for the left is *laevus*.

DHOBI ITCH Popular name for **TINEA** *cruris*, or **RINGWORM** of the crotch – a name evocative of British colonial medicine, especially military. Hindi *dhob* means washing, and a *dhobi* the servant engaged to wash clothes. The poor man was blamed for a condition which doubtless arose from either an infestation or, more likely, from soldiers' aversion to soap and water: when in doubt – blame a foreigner, as with the **FRENCH POX** and other international misattributions.

DI- The 'double' or 'pair' prefix – see below.

DIA- (DYA-) Prefix of separation, from the Greek word meaning through, throughout, complete – but also asunder and to separate, as in dialysis, separation, from *dia* + *luein*, to lose.

DIABETES The Latin word for a syphon, from a similar-sounding Greek word meaning 'a passing-through', because the condition (whether *diabetes insipidus* or *diabetes mellitus*) is characterised by an immoderate passing of urine: 'Diabethe, the pyssyng euill' (1565). See also **BANTING**.

DIACLASIA Literally 'breaking across', e.g. a fracture made deliberately by a surgeon to correct a deformity or previous, but badly-set, fracture. The suffixes -clast and -clasis denote 'breaking' or 'crushing' – remember the iconoclast who breaks images.

DIAGNOSIS See **GNOSIS**.

DIAPEDESIS The Greek word for 'oozing through', in medical use of blood cells through the unruptured walls of blood-vessels.

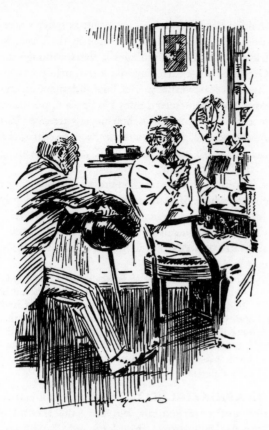

Patient. "I HEAR THEY'RE SAYING THAT JONES, THE MAN
YOU'VE BEEN TREATING FOR LIVER COMPLAINT,
HAS DIED OF HEART TROUBLE."
Doctor (acidly). "WHEN I TREAT A MAN FOR LIVER TROUBLE
HE DIES OF LIVER TROUBLE."

Punch, September 27, 1911

DIAPHRAGM See **PHRAGMA**.

DIARRH(O)E(I)A Greek **DIA-** (see above) + *rheein*,
a flow: a 'flowing-through'. In medical language it
means an uncomfortably or even pathologically
copious flow from the bowels; and as such the word
is so well established that one can no longer use it as
a general term, for example to describe free-flowing
road-traffic. In about 1894, when *The Times* reported
that 'Mr Gladstone has had a smart attack of
diarrhoea and will not be attending the House [of
Commons] for a few days', the word was still
considered to be outside the vocabulary of ordinary
people.

DIASTOLE A 'placing apart', e.g. the dilatation of
the heart walls, which is a normal part of the cardiac
cycle. See **SYSTOLE**.

DICROTIC The double beat of the heart or pulse.
For an explanation of the origin of this word see
CROTOS.

DIDYMI The testicles, and the Greek for twins,
doubtless used by the ancient Greeks in exactly the
same slightly facetious way as a modern man might
speak about his 'pair' (of balls). (In fact the twins are,
in this instance, invariably non-identical). *Di-* is the
'double' prefix, e.g. diplegia, paralysis of both legs –
see **-PLEGIA**. *Epididymis*, the part above and adjacent
to the **TESTES**, i.e. the tube for storage and transmission of **SPERM** to the **VAS DEFERENS**.

DIET Food and drink considered with regard to
their nutritional qualities, from Greek *diaita*, though
this had a wider meaning than alimentary consumption: the course of life, the way of living and thinking
– hence also the parallel meaning of the word, for a
parliamentary assembly. Perhaps this is why, whenever the Israeli cabinet is shown in session, plates,
cutlery and fruit are seen on the table. See also under **BANTING, PRIMARY HEALTH CARE, REGIMEN,
VITAMINS,** etc.

DIGITUS Latin for finger. The five are
distinguished by various ancient names alluding to
their functions. There are two for the thumb, **HALLUX**
and **POLLEX** (sometimes interchangeable with the big
toe). The first finger is the *index* finger (in German
Zeigefinger, or pointing finger), also *digitus salutarius*, the
greeting finger. Today it has acquired other
connotations: in round-ball football, when held aloft,
it is the 'I've-just-scored-a-goal' finger, and when
jabbed by massed spectators, the 'send-'im-off'
finger). To the Romans it was the finger 'accompanying the singing' (i.e. the conducting-finger)
as well as *liceri digito*, the 'auction finger', for indicating
bids. Today it would also be the 'Ranting Politician's
Finger', each syllable marked by a jab in time to the
speech; also the Angry Finger, jabbed in the direction
of a quarrelling-partner (or even into his chest, when
it probably leads to a fist-fight). The first two fingers
played a recognised part in ancient oratory and
rhetoric*. The fourth is the *digitus annularis* (also
anularis) in English the annular, or ring finger, also
the **LEECH** finger, medical or physic finger, in Latin
digitus medicus or *digitus medicinalis*, because it was used
by ancient doctors for **PALPATION**. In ancient times
the ring finger was thought to contain an artery that
led straight to the heart, hence its use for wedding

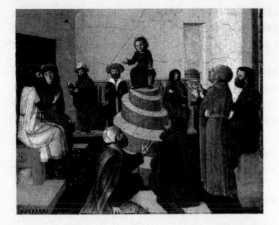

Bernardino Butinone's The Christ Child disputing with the doctors – who respond with some unusual finger signals. (National Gallery of Scotland).

and engagement rings. Urquhart's translation of **RABELAIS** (1653) has, 'Upon the medical finger of the same hand he had a ring.' In modern terms it might also be the 'show-business vanity finger', because male television personalities traditionally use it for scratching their head without disturbing their coiffure – a practice not as modern as might be thought: both Juvenal and Seneca observed and described the habit: *scalpere caput digito* – '... of effeminate men fearful of disarranging their hair' (Lewis and Short's *Latin Dictionary*) – a habit for which Pompey was ridiculed. Next to it, the little finger, *digitus minimus*, often used for relieving an itch in the ear or extracting wax from it, was therefore called even by the ancients the *digitus auricularius* – in English ear finger, in German *Ohrfinglein* – and thus described even in old fingering-charts for wind instruments; while the middle finger (again in popular as well as musical-instrument use) was described as the *digitus infamis, digitus impudicus, digitus lascivus or digitus* **TRIBADIS**, the lewd, wanton, impudent or rubbing finger: old English country-folk called it the 'courting finger'; (*tribadis* in fact suggests either lesbian, or female auto-erotic, associations – the classical writers thought of *everything*). Southern European people – and increasingly also Anglo-Saxons – jab their impudent finger upwards (palm facing up) to the same purpose and (in the same manner as English still jab two, meaning 'F... you!'). The original meaning of *lascivus* was sportive but was soon widened to include amorous sports. The ancients spoke of the left hand as the *amica manus*, because it was (and still is in some cultures) reserved for sexual and excretory purposes; thus to use it for

shaking hands is taken as an insult: in other words, *amica manus* means more user-friendly than friends-friendly. The Greek for finger is *dactylos*, though the Greeks do not seem to have made so much sport with theirs, at least verbally. But final judgment on this point must be deferred until I have an opportunity to examine a copy of Echtermeyer's treatise, *Über Namen und symbolische Bedeutung der Finger bei den Griechen und Römern* – 'On the Names and Symbolic Meaning of the Fingers among Greeks and Romans' (1835). It is, however, unlikely to explain the bunched five-finger gesture which African motorists and others angrily jab at each other. It means, '*Five* men took part when your mother conceived you'. See also **WHITLOW** – and **TRIGGER-FINGER**, unknown to the Romans as they had no firearms.

*The National Gallery of Scotland has a painting by Bernardino Butinone (fl. 1484–1507) entitled 'The Christ Child disputing with the Doctors', showing both Christ and the Doctors employing various finger-signals that were recognised aids to philosophical discussion, the doctor in the foreground giving Him a full, palm-upward, splayed two-finger sign which is now interpreted quite differently.

DILATION/DILATATION Both mean expansion and enlargement, but only the second is etymologically correct, from Latin *latus*, broad, says the *Oxford English Dictionary*. See also **D&C**.

DILDO An ancient device which sometimes combined female sexual pleasuring with what was until recently delicately called 'feminine hygiene'. The *Oxford English Dictionary* says it is 'A word of obscure origin ... also the name of the penis or phallus, or a figure thereof, (or) an artificial penis used for female gratification; the *lingam* of Hindu worship; formerly, also, a contemptuous or reviling appellation of a man or lad; and applied to a cylindrical or "sausage" curl'. Until the advent of oral contraception such a device was found in many households, fitted with a rubber bulb that could be filled with warm water (and possibly a spermicidal agent) and 'legitimately' used by women for post-coital douching as well as simulating a male ejaculation – 'Ingram's Whirling Spray' being the most widely advertised. Some of the dildoes (battery-powered 'vibrators') now sold in sex shops as 'sex aids' also have such an additional facility, in the shape of a water-fillable imitation **SCROTUM**. The word is thought by some to be a corruption of Italian *diletto*, delight, and figures in the works of numerous English writers and dramatists, e.g. Thomas Nashe, Ben Jonson and William Shakespeare. In his play *The Chaste Maid*,

Thomas Middleton (?1570–1627) mentions a dildo manufacturer (who has a **TINNITUS** – any connection?): 'What, has he got a singing in his head now? Now's out of work he falls to making dildoes'. A song by the English composer Thomas Morley (?1557–1602) has a street seller of household goods repeatedly offering among the wares from his tray, by way of refrain, '... and a dildo, dildo, diddle-diddle dildo'. The *Oxford English Dictionary* says that test-tubes, because of their long, cylindrical shape, were once called 'dildo-glasses' – officially, and not just by dirty-minded medical students. In classical literature it was called *fascinum*, and was – among other things – worn as an amulet to ward off the evil eye (see under **PRIAPUS**): for some of the 'other things' see Gaius Petronius (d. c. AD 65): *'profert Oenothea scorteum fascinum, quod ... paulatim coepit inserere ano meo'*. See also **TRIBADE**. In French literature the dildo goes under the name *godemichet* or *godemiché*, in Italian *diletto* (see above) or *passatempo*.

DIPHTHERIA So named in the 19th century (also diphtheritis) via the French *diphthérie* after the Greek word for skin, hide or leather; from the appearance of the mucous membrane of the throat and air passages. See also **CROUP**.

DIPSA Greek for thirst, so dipsomania is literally 'a madness for drink' (see **MANIA**), though originally such a craving was not necessarily for alcoholic drink. See also **ALCOHOL**.

DISCRETE From Latin *discretus*, separate, distinct. In medicine, discrete spots are separate, scattered about, not coalescent or confluent ones, as in discrete smallpox (from French *variole discrète*). Although the dictionaries tell us that the spellings 'discreet' (wise, considerate, circumspect, e.g. the soul of discretion, like your family physician) and 'discrete' (meaning separate, as above) are often taken as interchangeable, it is surely worth differentiating between them. Both have the same Latin origin, but the two meanings parted company in Late Latin.

DISSECTION From Latin *dissecare*, to cut apart, i.e. into pieces, usually a human cadaver, an essential part of every doctor's training. The now common pronunciation 'die-sect' shows how much the loss of Latin has compromised the use of words, for it suggests the spelling 'di-sect', a recognised word meaning to cut asunder, like 'bi-sect'. For the gruesome story of dissection of a living body see under **DUODENUM**. The first dissection of human bodies – presumably of **CADAVERS** – took place in 1235 at the School of Medicine at Salerno, Italy. During the Greek periods such experiments were carried out on 'volunteers' – criminals who were promised their

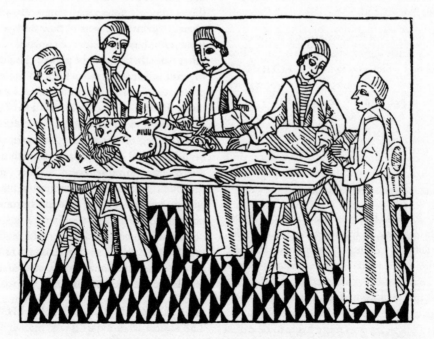

A dissection, from a book published in Lyons in 1482

'freedom' if they agreed to help anatomists with their enquires.

DISTAL From Latin *distans*, further from, apart, beyond; as opposed to *proximus*, producing proximal, near, intimate.

DIURETIC From Greek *diouretikos*, promoting urine.

DIVERTICULUM In Latin, a byway, deviation or diversion – also a wayside shelter or refuge, e.g. such as can still be seen on old road-bridges to offer temporary refuge to pedestrians as they shelter from passing vehicles. Hence, in medicine, a pouch or sac (plural diverticula) at a weak point or points in the alimentary tract. The word was used facetiously in ancient Rome also for a place where diversions are on offer, e.g. a brothel.

DIZYGOTIC Of twins, those derived from two separate ova and therefore not 'identical'.

DNA Abbreviation of deoxyribonucleic acid, a biochemical term relating to **CHROMOSOMES** (nuclear material containing the genetic code which 'instructs' cellular elements to make proteins). DNA has entered popular consciousness as 'genetic fingerprinting' in **FORENSIC** medicine.

DNA Used in outpatient clinics for 'no-shows', meaning Did Not Attend.

DNR Code for Do Not Resuscitate (e.g. in the event of a patient's suffering cardiac arrest): an abbreviated instruction which gets as close to **EUTHANASIA** as is at present legally possible. The direction is seldom seen on paper and the request usually comes from the patient himself. *Suscitare* is the Latin for to raise or raise up, related to resurrection, which has acquired a more specialised meaning and is later, post-biblical, Latin.

DOA Dead on Arrival. See also **BBA**.

DOCTOR In Latin this word means a teacher, an instructor, from *docere*, to teach (to teach the docile, i.e. those willing to be taught); also *doctus*, learned, with provision for a female teacher being called a 'doctoress' (Latin *doctrissa*); while in German-speaking countries some middle-to-high-ranking medical practitioners in hospitals are still called *Dozent*. To the Romans a physician was more likely to be called a *medicus*. Doctorates may be gained in many faculties

– which is why the world is teeming with non-medical doctors – engineers, scientists, philosophers, politicians, etc. (some doctorates can be purchased from certain institutions and even well-known politicians flaunt them). Medical doctors, by comparison, are comparatively rare: practitioners in medicine are usually addressed as 'doctor' merely out of courtesy. While fully qualified to practise they are more likely to possess a bachelor's or licentiate's degree but no doctorate, which requires a separate examination. British surgeons are traditionally addressed as 'Mister', however many doctorates they have earned – a long-established practice going back to the days when surgeons doubled as barbers (or vice versa): both trades needed sharp knives and the barbers already had them (though France banned barbers from performing surgery as early as 1731). Female surgeons of today are content to be called 'Mrs' or 'Miss' (but not, it seems, 'Ms'). Thus a male physician married to a female surgeon would be addressed as 'Dr and Mrs', two surgeons as 'Mr and Mrs', a male surgeon and a female physician as 'Mr and Dr' (while in Germany a completely non-medical *Hausfrau* who happens to be the wife of a doctor enjoys the honorific title *'Frau Doktor'*). It is also traditional in Britain for doctors (of any sort) modestly to refrain from prefacing their signature with their doctorate (unless in parentheses), just as people with the honorific prefix 'Sir', 'Lord' or 'Dame' do not sign theirs (though newspaper letter-editors annoyingly often do print names as if they had). On the other hand, continental doctors not only do so but add any other titles they may have picked up: a *Herr Doktor* of my acquaintance who had also been given a professorship and an honorary doctorate signed himself 'Professor Dr Dr ...'. The *Oxford English Dictionary,* incidentally, includes a doctor-fish and surgeon-fish, of the genus *Acanthurus*; and it should be added that in colloquial English the verb 'to doctor' has unhappy connotations: 'to castrate – usually an animal' – and 'to disguise, falsify, tamper with or adulterate', perhaps appropriate for many a political doctor (or the latest fad, for the political 'spin doctor' whom you will find, suitably enough, next to **SPHINCTER**). (See also **(TO) HOSPITALISE**). It should also be noted that in America veterinarians as well as dentists are also addressed as 'doctor'.

'DOCTOR, I WOKE UP THIS MORNING...'
The almost traditional 'Blues' opener for consultations with the **GP**.

DOCTORS' COMMONS A term often misused (e.g. in the press) as though it referred to medical doctors. It was, from 1509, the common table and dining-hall of the Association or College of Doctors of Civil Law in London.

DOCTOR'S COUPÉ The motorised successor of the horse-drawn Doctor's Buggy, the traditional two-seater form of transport used by UK doctors. With the advent of the motor-car the concept was applied to a small two-seater car, having room for passengers only in a small 'dickey' seat at the back which was open to all weathers, thus discouraging the vehicle's use as an informal **AMBULANCE**. American family physicians of the early decades of the 20th century preferred a Model-T Ford, whereas the English doctor's favourite was the Bullnose Morris two-seater with dickey. A special issue of the magazine *The Light Car* of 8th July 1914 carried the heading *Aesculapius and the Light Car* and was aimed at 'doctors who are contemplating the purchase of a motor-car'. The Lagonda Light Car was advertised as 'An ideal doctor's coupé'.

DOLICHOCEPHALIC Having a long, narrow head, from Greek *dolichos*, long + *kephale*, head. As opposed to **BRACHYCEPHALIC**.

DONOR From Latin *donator*, a giver, *donare*, to give, to present – of one's own free will. In 1994 it was reported that China had no shortage of 'donor' organs for transplantation – because useful organs were removed from executed criminals; also that executions were sometimes carried out in such a way that victims were still alive when their organs were removed, so as to ensure maximum freshness. If the story is true it is reasonable to assume that condemned prisoners would be killed in the operating-theatre, with the intended recipient ready and anaesthetised, to save refrigerated transport. Stories of human rights abuses are nothing new from China, but are Chinese doctors – shades of the notorious Nazi mutilator Dr Mengele – really willing to lend themselves to such practices? If so it would reduce transplantation to a while-you-wait, Chinese takeaway business. But the mutilation of living persons in the interest of science is nothing new: see **DUODENUM** for a tale of 'living' dissection.

DOOLALLY An unbalanced state of mind, named after a place called Deolali in Marashtra, India. It was originally British services slang but is now in general use and is, informally, heard in both general and hospital practice. According to Fraser and Gibbons, *Soldier and Sailor Words* (1925) the term in full is Delolali tap, 'mad, off one's head'. It was an Army camp in Deolali which was said to have been the cause of many men 'doing queer things' – possibly as a result of some local condition not suspected or understood.

DOORHANDLES Patients who 'remember' another complaint just as they are about to leave the GP's surgery. In reality it may have been the main purpose of their visit, but they lacked the courage to mention the problem during the interview; and even then they may explain that the enquiry is only **FOR A FRIEND**. See also **HEARTSINKS**.

DORSUM Latin for the back or posterior, adjective dorsal. Also the upper aspect, e.g. of the penis.

DOSE/DOSAGE A simple derivation – from Latin *dosis*, a giving (originally Greek *didonai*, to give) and distantly related to the **DONOR**. It does, however, depend whether the word is used by the doctor or, colloquially, by the patient: 'I seem to have got a dose, doctor' has nothing to do with a pharmacist's prescription. Perhaps this is why the unnecessary elongation 'dosage' has come into use (compare 'bag and baggage' – though not 'cab and cabbage'). For other doses, given or caught, see under **POX**.

DOUBLE BLIND TEST See **PLACEBO**.

DOUBLE DIPPER Someone who defrauds the Social Services by making two claims for the same thing – both probably false anyway.

DOWAGER'S HUMP For the benefit of those unfamiliar with the conventions of the hereditary British aristocracy it should be explained that a dowager is a widowed titled lady who, after losing her husband, retains the title and rank she acquired on marriage to him. For example, Countess Birdbrain, wife of Admiral Earl Birdbrain, retains her title after the Admiral's death (divorce does not count, or the system would be overloaded) and becomes the Dowager Lady Birdbrain when their married son, his heir, succeeds on his father's death to the hereditary earldom. At this point the son's wife becomes the Countess Birdbrain, and his mother the Dowager Countess. The same applies to other hereditary British titles like dukedoms, baronies (i.e. lords) and baronetcies. And after all that, the explanation:

Dowager's Hump is the popular English name for a form of **KYPHOSIS**, a curvature of the spine brought on by old age. This is perhaps all the more noticeable among aristocratic ladies, who are customarily taught ramrod-straight deportment by their governesses and finishing-schools. There is also 'Dowager's Bottom', but this, alas, is more suitable for inclusion in a gazetteer than this book, being a small village in the South of England. Bottom in this sense means, of course, a piece of low-lying land, more common in the USA than Britain. See **LORDOSIS**, which, however, is not related to the peerage; also **LEMON-ON-TOOTHPICKS**.

DOWN'S SYNDROME The now normal name for **MONGOL(ISM)** (also Langdon–Down Anomaly), which did not come into use until 1961, when it was accepted that to call people with this kind of chromosomal abnormality 'Mongols' was demeaning both to the sufferers and the people of Mongolia. The term 'Leper' is also now disapproved of.

DPI/DPT Code abbreviations used by some **GPs** in their practice-notes about female patients who complain of various unspecified and vague symptoms. 'This lady is in need of Deep Protein Input (or Treatment)' means she could do with more sex.

DRIP Universal abbreviated term for an intravenous infusion. Also nurses' term for a new doctor who has to be shown everything.

-DROM(O)- The prefix/suffix denoting movement or speed, e.g. a **HIPPO**drome, which for the Greeks meant a racecourse. See also **PRODROMAL**.

DROMOMANIA Compulsive vagabondage, or a pathological impulse to travel – which the Germans translate (but use in a more light-hearted form) as *Wanderlust*. In some vagrants it may sometimes be combined with **CLAUSTROPHOBIA** and/or the **GILLES DE LA TOURETTE SYNDROME**: some apparently homeless street-dwellers in big cities are doubtless claustrophobic dromomaniacs who cannot bear to remain in an enclosed space such as a house or apartment. However, inveterate attenders of conferences may also be prone to it, although this might be better named dromo**PHILIA**. The condition is often observed among British Members of Parliament, who join numerous Anglo-foreign 'Friendship Groups' and which provide them with free travel and lavish hospitality (all of which must be declared). Local-government officials, too, benefit from such arrangements, especially those whose towns or cities are 'twinned' with foreign ones, enabling them to combine official business with private pleasure. See also under **SEMINAR** and **SYMPOSIUM**.

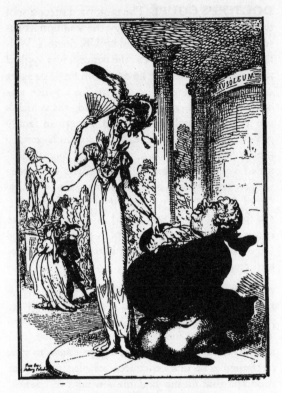

Dropsy courting Consumption
Thomas Rowlandson

DROPSY Usually 'the dropsy'. First so called in the 13th century, written dropesie or dropecy, it referred to an excessive accumulation of fluid in the body, or parts of it; but early diagnosis would often have confused it with obesity. The word dropsy seems to have gone out of use – certainly out of fashion – and been replaced with more scientific terms, e.g. **(O)EDEMA**. Women who experience an uncomfortable fulness at some part of their menstrual cycle speak of 'fluid retention'. See also **ANASARCA**.

DRUM BEAT A type or classification of rectal wind. See under **FLATULENCE**.

DRUMMER'S THUMB A form of **TENOSYNOVITIS**, perhaps a genuine form of **REPETITIVE STRAIN INJURY**; possibly related to, or synonymous with, **GAMEKEEPER'S THUMB**. For other 'professional' illnesses see under **BREWER'S DROOP** and numerous cross-references.

DUCK-BILL See **SPECULUM**.

DULA? DOOLA? DHULA? This word was recently bandied about without further explanation on a BBC family programme, and clearly referred to a female birth-helper who is not a trained midwife but comforts the birthing mother, wipes her brow, etc.

DUODENUM In full, *duodenum digitorum*, or twelve fingers' breadth: the first portion of the small intestine (in the literal German language it is called *Zwölf-fingerdarm*, literally, 'twelvefingergut'): for the second portion, see **JEJUNUM**; also **DIGITUS**. The duodenum was named by the physician, Herophilus of Chalcedon, who flourished around 270 BC. With another doctor, Erasistratus of Ceos, he procured criminals who were released from prison on condition that they submitted to medical 'experiments'. The two doctors then proceeded to dissect them 'while they were still breathing [and] observed parts which nature had formerly concealed, and examined their position, colour, shape, size, arrangement, hardness, softness, smoothness, connection...'. They maintained that 'it is not cruel, as most people allege, to cause pain to guilty men – and only a few at that – so as to seek out remedies for innocent people of every age'. After the experiments the criminals were presumably returned to prison – as **CADAVERS**. The quotation above comes from an unidentified ancient source cited in the *Oxford History of the Classical World*. Stories like that of Erasistratus may be responsible for many a Christian martyrdom. That of St. Erasmus, for example, who had his intestines wound out of his living body with the help of a windlass (whose resemblance to a capstan meant that he also doubled as the patron saint of sailors); and that of St. Agatha, who was martyred by mastectomy. During the delirium of her torture St. Peter appeared to her and alleviated her pain, but she eventually died from her suffering. She is usually depicted carrying her severed breasts on a platter – and their resemblance to bells and cottage loaves, respectively, made her the patron saint of both bell-founders and bakers.

DUTCH CAP A thin rubber or plastic contraceptive cap with a 'rolled' flexible rim that fits over the **CERVIX**. The original Dutch cap was a lace bonnet, which also has a rolled rim. other terms of interna-

tional insult include the **FRENCH LETTER** (under **CONDOM**) and the analogously named French **CAPOTE ANGLAISE**.

-DYNIA A pain suffix, rarer than **-ALGIA**. For example proctodynia, pain in the rectum; (also proctalgia). See **PROCTOS**.

DYS- Greek prefix denoting abnormality, difficulty or impairment in or of whatever follows: hence dyslexia, bad reading; dysmenorrhoea; bad menstruation, dyspepsia, bad digestion; dyspnoea, difficulty in breathing (not 'bad breath', for which see **HALITUS**); dysuria, difficulty in urinating, etc.

DYSARTHRIA A speech disorder, says the *Concise Oxford Medical Dictionary*, in which linguistic content and meaning are normal but pronunciation is unclear. This perfectly describes the delivery of many radio and television reporters. See also **LERESIS**.

DYSENTERY Literally, 'bad guts': see **ENTERON** and the **DYS-** 'dysfunction' prefix.

DYSFUNCTION A popular catch-all word, half Greek (from the *dys-* prefix) and half Latin-based English (from *functio*, a performance, a functioning). For some reason the all-Latin malfunction is less popular and associated more with badly working machinery than the human body.

DYSGRAPHIA Strictly this means the inability to write coherently, as a manifestation of brain damage – but also it is used to describe atrocious handwriting, e.g. that sometimes seen on doctors' prescriptions which the **PHARMACIST** was obliged to decipher before the advent of computer print-out prescriptions. **DYSLEXIA** (below), may also be loosely applied.

DYSLEXIA Combined from two Greek elements meaning, together, 'bad reading' (see **DYS-**, above): a developmental disorder affecting the ability to acquire reading and writing skills. The *Merck Manual of Diagnosis and Practice* says the **(A)ETIOLOGY** of this condition is 'unknown' – indeed in some cultures the condition itself is unknown: for example, the Japanese have no word for it, though their young are obliged to learn an infinitely more complex language than do English children. Japanese children spend between one-and-a-half to twice as much time each week in the classroom as English or American children. Dare a layman suggest that in otherwise normal children (i.e. those having no perceived neurophysiological disorder) dyslexia may simply be a lack of familiarity with the *look* of letters and words, or that some learning disabilities may in fact be teaching disabilities (but see also **ALEXIA**)? Show me a healthy child who cannot distinguish between the look of his teddybear and his stuffed rabbit, his brother and his cousin. Many misuse the word, saying 'I'm afraid I'm rather dyslexic' when they mean 'I'm a poor speller'. The now almost universally used adjective and noun 'dyslexic' – and worse, the ugly-sounding plural noun 'dyslexics' – are strictly erroneous formations. Would you call those who suffer from **DYSPEPSIA** 'dyspepsics? No, they are dyspeptics. Therefore the 'correct' adjective/noun is 'dyslectic' – plural noun 'dyslectics' (and the same applies to **ANOREXIA** and its sufferers). The *Oxford English Dictionary* gives the *-tic* forms first, adding the *-xic* only in deference to common usage (for dictionaries record – they do not prescribe). There is no sanction against getting things *right*, and those who care might as well use 'dyslectic/ dyslectics' and – at the risk of being 'corrected' by sub-editors, bystanders and others – fly a small, defiant flag of rectitude.

DYSPAREUNIA When doctors use this word they mean difficult or painful coitus – painful for the woman, that is; but the term comes from **DYS-** the Greek prefix of malfunction + **PAREUNOS**, 'lying together in bed': so it should really be applicable to both sexes experiencing such difficulties.

DYSPEPSIA Indigestion. It comes from **DYS** + peptos, cooked, so it more accurately means 'badly cooked' – the bad digestion being assumed to be the result of bad cooking.

DYSPHEMIA Literally, 'bad language', but in doctors' language it means stammering, and presumably other speech defects.

DYSPRAXIA From Greek **DYS-** + prassein, to do. An inability of, or difficulty in, performing skilled, coordinated movements or tasks. Even the merry **SPOONERISM** has been classed as a medical problem, and may not be simple **LERESIS** but a combination of dyspraxia and **DYSARTHRIA**. See also under **ALBINO**.

DYSTROPHIA/DYSTROPHY Literally 'defective nourishment', now used in the sense of defective growth.

DZ Short for **DIZYGOTIC**, meaning unalike twins derived from two separate **OVA**, as opposed to those who are **MONOZYGOTIC**. And **ZYGOTE**.

E*e*

ECT Electro-Convulsive Therapy. See also **ZAP**.

ECT(O)- From Greek *ectos*, outside. Hence *ecto-parasites*, living outside the body; ectodermic, outside the skin (see **DERM**), etc. See also under **PARA-**. The corresponding 'inside' prefix is **ENDO-**.

-ECTOMY The cutting-out suffix. See **-TOM**. See also the 'within' prefix **ENDO-**.

ECTOPIC Out of place, outside the proper place. From Greek *ektos*, outside + **TOPOS**, place.

ECZEMA From the Greek *ek*, out, over + *zeein*, to boil, i.e. to 'boil over', though eczema is now a more general and usually allergic skin condition, not one that normally produces a raised skin temperature or boils, let alone boils over. The English word boil is not related, and is derived from an Old English/Teutonic root. See also **ANTHRAX** and **CARBUNCLE**; and **ZEEIN**.

EDEMA The American-preferred spelling of **OEDEMA**, a swelling, from Greek *oidema*.

ELECTUARY A medicinal conserve or paste consisting of a powder or other medicine mixed with honey, preserve or syrup of some kind to make it more palatable; or one that melts in the mouth. Since the advent of soluble capsules which the patient can swallow without tasting the drug or drugs contained therein, little has been heard of electuaries, and the vehicle (or bulk) enclosing the active ingredients is now more often called the **EXCIPIENT**. Medieval doctors called it an *electuarium*, from Latin (via Greek) *lingere*, to lick (out); and this has nothing to do with elections, or with politicians' desire to make their policies appear more palatable. But the adjacent entry in *Lewis and Short* is *electio, electionis*, a choice, selection, etc., and also gives *vitiatarum electiones*: 'the option given to a violated maiden whether her ravisher should be put to death or shall marry her...' (Tacitus). See also **ELIXIR**, below.

ELIXIR A medicine or other preparation alleged to possess powerful or even magical qualities in curing disease. Many a **PATENT MEDICINE** was sold under this name until the law began to insist on more factual and accurate descriptions. Its origin may be found in ancient Egypt, where Arabs claimed to possess a magical powder called *al-iksir* which enabled them to turn common substances into gold (a feat they accomplished many centuries later with a substance called oil). A Roman Latin word, *elixare*, meant to stew or extract by boiling, but may be unrelated; and the likeness to lingere (see under **ELECTUARY**, above) should also be noted.

EMBOLISM The presence in an artery of an obstruction, an embolus, which is usually but not necessarily a blood clot. From Greek *embolos*, a plug (*bol* is the Greek word for a ball), Latin *embolus*, the plunger of a pump, i.e. something inserted. In non-medical use, in the study of time, an embolism is the intercalation of a day in the calendar to correct the difference between the civil and the solar year (or the occasional addition of an extra, seventh, 'pip' in the British Greenwich Time Signal); and in the Roman Mass an embolism denotes the prayer after the Canon, beginning 'deliver us', which is inserted between the Lord's Prayer and the Prayer for Peace. It also gave us, via Latin *emblema*, the word emblem.

EMBRYO The Greek-based word for the Latin **FETUS**.

EMERITUS The Latin description of one who has been retired or discharged from active service or occupation. To the Romans it meant primarily a soldier who had served his time and was then sent packing. Today only the 'merit' element of the word is acknowledged in the creation of Emeritus Professorships, though some say that they heard a snatch of the song, 'We don't want to lose you but we think you ought to go'. This seems to apply also to the creation of the artificial but grand-sounding post of Conductor Emeritus of an orchestra. See under **FETUS** for 'effete'.

EMESIS From the Greek *emeein*, for the action of vomiting, possibly related to Latin *emittere*, to send out, expel – or indeed emit. The equivalent Latin word *vomere* means to throw up, hence **VOMIT**. Haematemesis (see the **H(A)EM(O)-** prefix) is vomiting blood. See also **REMISSION**.

EMETIC A substance that causes vomiting, voiding something which has been swallowed. From Greek *emeein*, to vomit, *emetikos*, something that has the power to induce it. The suffix is *-emesis* – see above. *Emetikos* originally meant greed for food.

-EMIA See **-AEMIA**.

EMPHUSAEIN/EMPHYSAEIN Greek, 'to inflate', to blow into, or up (with air), hence emphysema, etc. It also means to play the flute – though it is more often the players of brass, not woodwind instruments who are sometimes subject to this illness.

EMPIRICUS Latin, from Greek *empirikos*, for a physician who for his diagnoses relies on experience, with an element of intuition: Greek *empeiria*, experience. The word empirical is now more often used in a general, not necessarily medical, sense. See **SALTUS EMPIRICUS**.

ENCEPHALITIS Literally, inflammation of the brain, from Greek *enkephalon*, brain + *-itis*, the inflammation suffix. See also **ME**, and **ENKEPHALON**, below.

ENDEMIC From Greek *en*, in + *demos* the people: something, usually an illness or **SYNDROME** which is constantly or frequently found in certain communities or places, e.g. **THALASSEMIA** in Mediterranean countries. But see also **ENDO-** below. See also **EPIDEMIC** and **SPORADIC**.

ENDO- From the Greek *endon*, within. Numerous composite terms are constructed with it, e.g. endocardium, inside the heart, endocrine (+ *krinein*, separate) secreting internally, etc. Endoscopy means 'looking within'.

ENDOMETRIUM The lining of the womb; but endometry means the internal measurement of *any* part. See **METRA**.

ENEMA From the Greek *enhienai*, 'to send in'. A liquid or gaseous substance introduced ('sent into') the rectum. The older (but less correct) pronunciation used to be 'en*ee*ma', and the meticulous plural was enemata. See also **CLYSIS** for an old English name for the enema, the stock joke-instrument of ancient doctors, the clyster.

ENKEPHALON Greek for the brain, from *en*, in + *kephalos*, head – literally 'that which is in the head', hence the numerous *encephal(o)-* formations (*encephal-* and *enkephal-* are legitimate alternatives). The Latin equivalent is *cerebrum*, producing *cerebr-* words.

ENO'S A well-known British **LAXATIVE** 'fruit salt'. Like **KRUSCHEN SALTS** it is almost part of popular folklore (certainly popular parlance) but is still with us. Eno's was first produced in Newcastle upon Tyne in the late 19th century by J.C. Eno, a pharmacist. By 1880 Eno had set up subsidiary firms in London as well as North and South America. See also **ANDREWS LIVER SALTS**.

ENTERON Greek for gut or intestine (Latin *intestinus*). Hence the adjectives enteric (and intestinal) concerning the guts, and dysentery, literally 'bad guts', gastro-enteritis, etc. (see each of the elements of the last-named under its own heading).

ENURESIS From Greek *enurein*, to pass urine. Usually applied to involuntary bed-wetting, but strictly describes any kind of urinary incontinence.

ENVIRONMENT From Greek *en*, in + *viron*, circle. Although an old word, known to the classically educated since the 17th century, it lay dormant until the late 20th, when it was woken with a kiss-of-death from sociologists and dragged into their vocabulary. Since the 1970s it has been a kind of verbal wildcard, appliable to any situation, combinable with numerous ideas of social medicine: the quality of air ('the environment we breathe') and harmful agents contained in it; water or food and their quality (perhaps containing 'environmental carcinogens'); the disposal of household and industrial waste ('environmental services'), etc. In truth we cannot now do without it, though a little ingenuity would soon produce alternative expressions for some applications.

ENZYME In the Greek Church this is the name for the bread, from *en* + *zume* or *zyme*, to leaven, or ferment, with which the Eucharist is administered. The word was first used in the medical/scientific sense by the German biochemist W. Kühne in 1877, who adapted it into the German Enzym. In 1881 the English scientist W. Roberts suggested '..the desirability of adopting this term into English, with a slight change of orthography, as "enzymes", and also of coining from this root the cognate words... enzymosis and enzymic'.

EPHEBIATRICS A vain attempt by Sir Douglas Hubble (1900–1981) to create a new **SPECIALTY** for those looking after adolescents (writes Dr Stephen Lock) – a kind of intermediate stage between **P(A)EDRIATICS** and **GERIATRICS** or **GERONTICS**. From Greek *ephebos*, Latin *ephebus*, 'a young (male) citizen from eighteen to twenty years of age, during which he was occupied chiefly with garrison duty', and was therefore presumably a **PROLETARIAN** performing his military service. (They are also the years in which Israeli citizens of both sexes carry out compulsory military service, so the practice is kept alive in at least one Mediterranean country). See also **HEBE-**. The 1990 edition of *Mosby's Pocket Dictionary of Medicine* includes the word, so Hubble's effort may not turn out to have been in vain after all.

EPI- Greek *epi*, on, upon, over, on top, etc. Hence epidermis, the (outer) skin (see **DERMA**) – or, as Ambrose Bierce defines it in *A Devil's Dictionary*, 'The thin integument which lies immediately outside the skin and immediately inside the dirt' (see also below for what he has to say about **EPIDEMIC**. The epiglottis means *over* the **GLOTTIS**. See also under **LEPSIS**.

EPIDEMIC If **ENDEMIC**, above, is *among* the people, an epidemic means *all* the people, or a visitation *upon* the people, perhaps by a **PLAGUE** or **PEST**. Ambrose Bierce's *A Devil's Dictionary* calls it 'A disease having a sociable turn and few prejudices'.

EPIDIDYMIS From Greek *epi*, and *didymis* the **TESTES**: the part above and adjacent to them, i.e. the tube for storage and transmission of **SPERM** to the **VAS DEFERENS**.

EPINEPHRINE From Greek *epi*, upon + **NEPHROS**, kidney. An **ADRENAL** hormone.

EPIDERMIS Greek *epi*, and *derma*, skin. The outer, superficial and non-vascular layer of the skin. The old English name for it is scarf skin.

EPISIOTOMY From Greek *episeion*, the **PUBIC** region + the -otomy suffix, from *temnein*, to cut. A surgical procedure often used in childbirth.

EQUALITY OFFICER Most British hospitals employ at least one, though the post (one of the **GREY SUITS**) carries somewhat loosely defined duties and responsibilites. In 1994 the City of Liverpool appointed to the office of Deputy Lord Mayor a convicted prostitute and passport-application forger who also occupied the full-time post of Equality Officer in a local Maternity Unit. Although most citizens knew what the activities of Deputy Lord Mayor, prostitute and passport forger involved, no-one had the slightest idea of what the duties were of an Equality Officer, especially in a Maternity Unit. See also **RIGHTS WORKERS**.

EQUI- The Latin prefix denoting equality – equal to the Greek **ISO-** but less often used. Equipotent, of equal (pharmacological) strength.

EROS The Greek god of love (**CUPID** to the Romans) who gave us eroticism and all things erotic.

ERUCTATION A belch – perhaps the result of a **BORBORYGM(US)**. In Latin it literally means 'throwing up', just as ejaculation is 'throwing out'.

ERYTH(RO-) Prefix for red things, e.g. eryth(r)ema, the abnormal reddening of the skin, even through blushing; erythrocyte, a red blood cell, the antibiotic erythromycin, red-coloured pills. From Greek *eruthros*, red (though Greek colour-words may be confusing because some are multi-descriptive, others narrowly specific). See also **CYT(O)**.

-ESCENT Suffix for forming words meaning 'becoming', as in convalescent, getting better; tumescent, beginning to swell; pubescent, showing signs of sexual maturity, etc.

ESOPHAGUS The simplified American spelling of (o)esophagus, which please see for the connection.

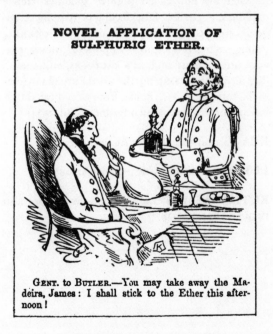

NOVEL APPLICATION OF SULPHURIC ETHER.

GENT. to BUTLER.—You may take away the Madeira, James: I shall stick to the Ether this afternoon!

Cartoon in *The Liverpool Lion*, 1848

ETHER From Greek *aither*, air. A volatile liquid used as an early anaesthetic which, like **LAUGHING-GAS**, was sometimes taken recreationally.

ETHNIC In its ancient meaning the Greek word *ethnikos* is defined as 'national, heathen, neither Christian nor Jewish'. Today the meaning has been widened and usually relates to people belonging to a minority 'ethnic' group whose members retain their customs or social views. For certain apparently 'racist' diseases prevalent among 'ethnic' groups see **COMMUNITY, ENDEMIC, FAVISM, KURU, TAY-SACHS DISEASE** and **THALASS(ANA)EMIA**.

ETIOLATED Pale, sickly or colourless, e.g. like celery that is grown without light. From French *étioler*, which comes from Old Norman *(s')étieuler*, to turn into straw. (See also under **SKELETON** for dried-out bones.) The name Estelle originally denoted a transparently fair-skinned girl. Not to be confused – though Americans do, because of their simplified spelling – with:–

ETIOLOGY Nothing to do with the preceding entry: just the American way of writing **AETIOLOGY** – one of several instances of spelling-reforms that are potentially confusing.

EU- The Greek prefix of goodness, well-being, or for what are now called 'positive' qualities. Hence euphoria, a (possibly false) feeling of happiness, eugenics (see **-GEN**, below) producing good offspring (though often propounded as political movements with sinister aims) and, as a last resort, euthanasia. (See also **THANATOS**). But the word Eustachian (medulla, tube, valve, etc.) comes from a celebrated Italian anatomist, Bartolomeo Eustachius (d. 1574).

EUA Examination Under Anaesthetic.

EURUS Greek for 'wide' – hence aneurysm.

EUTHANASIA Literally 'a good death'. See also **DNR** and **THANATOS**.

EXCIMER LASER Used in **PRK**. Its scientific definition is beyond the scope of this book, but the *Oxford English Dictionary* quotes the *New Scientist* (13 November 1986): 'The excimer laser ... emits ultraviolet light that cuts and marks materials without damaging them with heat... They are gas lasers that emit light when a halogen atom and a rare gas combine temporarily'.

EXCIPIENT From Latin *excipere*, to take up, to receive: the **ELECTUARY** or bulking-agent containing a medicine.

EXCORIATE From Latin *excoriare*, to flay, to strip off the skin (in botany, the bark), though fortunately this is used mostly in a figurative way (e.g. 'excoriating abuse') – and perhaps as the ultimate description of scratching an itch. See also **SARCO-** for (flesh-) biting sarcasm.

EXCRETION See **-CRET-**. For a mnemonic about it see under **SKILL**.

EXQUISITE When describing pain this meant acute, intense, keen – and probably highly localised. But as the word is now more often used to describe pleasure, excellence, or well-finished workmanship, 'exquisite pain' is found chiefly in older writings on medicine. See also **AGONY**.

EXTRA- Not 'additional', as in modern use, but 'outside', used as a prefix.

EXTROVERT Psychologists' term for a sociable person with an outgoing personality. Classical scholars say it should be extravert. The opposite is intravert.

EXUDE To ooze out, originally applied only to sweat, from Latin *ex* + *sudor* ('sweat out') but now anything that oozes from the pores, a wound or an incision, etc., may be said to exude.

F*f*

F *See* **FT**.

F(A)ECAL *See below.*

FAECES From Latin *faex, faecis*, dregs, left-overs, etc. and hence also waste matter voided at the end of the digestive process. See also **STERCUS** and the Greek **COPRO-**.

FAF See under **(IT'S) FOR A FRIEND** – a request for advice, usually made of a **GP** by a patient, and allegedly on behalf of a third party.

FALLOPIAN TUBES These two slender ducts (through which ova pass from the ovaries to the uterus) are named after their discoverer, the Italian anatomist Gabriele Fallopio (1523–62).

FANNY Traditional acronymic nickname for a member of the First Aid Nursing Yeomanry, a British voluntary nursing-service founded by upper-class ladies who wanted to help the wounded during World War I. They also gave brave and sterling service at the front during World War II, when 'Joining the Fannys' was the aim of many society ladies, who could 'do their bit' in the company of other women of their social class. Their name may subconsciously have been inspired by the memory of Miss Fanny Keyser, who with her sister Agnes founded **KING EDWARD VII'S HOSPITAL FOR OFFICERS**. 'Fanny' is also a mild dysphemism with anatomical associations (see under **GLUT(A)EUS** and **PUDENDA**) which is worth mentioning only because British and American definitions differ as to its precise location. According to that prolific wartime historian Ben Trovato, General Eisenhower asked an English woman who had a daughter named Fanny serving as a F.A.N.Y. nurse, 'How long has your Fanny been at the front?' – and received a reply which is not suitable for this book.

FARMER'S LUNG An occupational lung disease, allergic alveolitis (see **ALVEUS**) caused, under certain conditions, by exposure to hay. For other occupational conditions see under **BREWER'S DROOP**.

FARTLEBERRIES Doctors unfortunately encounter these more often than the fastidious reader might suspect, especially in casualty rooms and on people who failed to heed their mothers' injunction always to have clean underwear and observe anal hygiene, 'in case you get run over'. Fartleberries (alternatively called 'cling-ons') are **F(A)ECAL** fragments clinging to the anal hair, also known (especially in the Tyneside area of England, says Dr George Cook) as 'winnets', while in Derbyshire, according to Dr Stuart Marshall-Clarke, they are 'cleg nuts'. Grose's *Dictionary of the Vulgar Tongue* had the word in its first edition (1785), but unaccountably dropped it in subsequent ones. The *Oxford English Dictionary* shuns it, too. It appears in Partridge's *Dictionary of Slang and Unconventional English*. Dr Erich Geiringer reports a precise Austro/German equivalent, *Farzenbeeren* (or *Furzenbeeren*) – *Farz* or *Furz*, fart. *Médecins sans frontières* indeed. See also under **FLATULENCE**.

FASCIA Fibrous connective tissue of various kinds (for which see a medical dictionary) or bundles of it. The word is derived from the same source as the Roman emblem of magisterial power, the *fasces*, an axe tied into a bundle of sticks, which Italian fascists annexed as theirs. In anatomy the *fasci* are thin sheaths of fibrous tissue investing a muscle or other tissue; and for **FASCINUS** see below. Mr Louis J. Beddall recalls a limerick dating from the time of his student-days and the Italian fascist movement:

> *A medical student named Long,*
> *Whose spelling was not very strong –*
> *When writing his thesis*
> *Wrote 'fasces', not 'faeces'–*
> *But was he so very far wrong?*

FASCIITIS An affliction of the above. See also **NECROTISING FASCIITIS**.

FASCINUS Vulgar classical – presumably not medical – Latin for the penis, in other words, a man's 'whole bundle of tricks', also facetiously called his '(wedding) tackle', meaning the penis and testicles together.

FASTIGIUM Another **ARCHITECTURAL TERM**: Latin for a summit or peak, e.g. the ridge or highest point of a house; hence the name for the acme or greatest intensity of an illness or the highest point of a fever.

FATFOLDER A patient who sees his family doctor frequently and therefore accumulates many case-notes: a phenomenon overtaken by conversion of patients' notes into computer files. 'Fatfilers'?

FATUOUS(NESS) From Latin *fatuus*, foolish. Now a mildly derogatory term of reproof, but formerly a recognised form of **DEMENTIA** or imbecility. As Erskine's Scottish Law cruelly defined it in 1773: 'Fatuous persons, called also idiots…who are entirely deprived of the faculty of reason and have an uniform stupidity and inattention in their manner and childishness in their speech'.

FAUCES The upper part of the throat. Originally, in a Roman building, a passage. Other Greek/ Roman architectural terms adopted into medical/ anatomical use include **ATRIUM**, central chamber; **CLAUSTRUM**, an enclosed room; **FOCUS**, fireplace; **FORNIX**, an arch; **PORTA**, an entrance; **TRABECU-LUM**, from *trabs*, a little beam or bar; **PHRAGMA**, a dividing partition or wall; **VESTIBULUM**; ante-chamber; and **THALAMOS**, inner chamber.

FAVISM A hereditary form of anaemia which, like **THALASS(ANA)EMIA**, mainly affects Mediterranean people: the name is derived from the broad bean, *Vicia fava*, which is supposed to be the cause of it. See also **SICKLE-CELL AN(A)EMIA** affecting mostly Africans and Afro-Caribbeans.

FEBRIS Latin for fever, hence febrile. Also **PYREXIA**.

FEEBLE-MINDED Now a politically incorrect term – see under **MORON**.

FELDSHER Since the mass exodus of doctors from the former Soviet Union, most of them Jewish, this word is now occasionally heard in English. In Russian it means a kind of **PARAMEDIC**, not unlike the 'barefoot doctor' of China – a person who has received some rudimentary training in medicine and emergency surgery but is without formal professional qualifications; medical orderlies in the British armed forces are therefore feldshers of a kind. The word has a slightly Jewish ring to it but it does not appear in Yiddish dictionaries ('My son the feldsher' would not sound very impressive). It is Old German, originally *Feldscher*, an army field-surgeon, and a corruption/contraction of *Feldscherer*, 'field-shearer' (i.e. hair-cutter): in other words, a military barber–surgeon. In the (now rapidly shrinking) ranks of the British army the bandsmen have always been trained as Medical Orderlies and Stretcher-bearers – the traditional secondary role of military musicians, a sensible arrangement, as most musicians would probably not know what to do with a rifle. As there are now even more Russian Jewish emigré musicians than doctors there need be no shortage of musical feldshers in any future war. Their favourite prescription would doubtless be for **JEWISH PENICILLIN**.

FELLARE Latin for sucking, whether in infantile feeding, for other 'innocent' purposes or sexual gratification (e.g. *fellatio*). Unfortunately the latter use has rather monopolised the word, although there is a perfectly good Latin-based synonym for this kind of sexual intercourse: irrumation, from *irrumare* (perhaps jocularly derived from *ruminare*, chewing the cud). The Romans distinguished these activities with various names, on a who-does-what-with-which-and-to-whom basis, between a female performing the act on a man (for the other-way-round see under **CUNNUS**), in which case she becomes the *fellatrix* or *irrumatrix*, while a male is a *fellator* or *irrumator*. In ancient Rome irrumation was used also as an act of humiliation inflicted on a captured enemy – a practice horrifyingly revived by some sadistic rapists of the present time (and whenever it figures in a court case one must wonder why the victim never makes the obvious counter-attack while having her attacker in his or her power).

FEMALE CIRCUMCISION The surgical and often crude removal of – at the very least – the **PREPUCE** of the **CLITORIS**. This surgical assault is forbidden in civilised countries but is nevertheless secretly performed by some Western practitioners on young girls who are brought to them. Like **INFIBULATION**, the operation is intended to keep a woman faithful to her husband by destroying her sexual pleasure – and allegedly heightening his. Male **CIRCUMCISION**, however, is legally practised on about one-sixth of the world's male population, for both religious and hygienic reasons.

FEMIDOM Trade name of a 'female' **CONDOM**, under which please see for the connection.

FENESTRA Window, in Latin, and therefore any opening – window-shaped or not. Hence fenestration, described by a medical friend as 'an overdressed word for making a hole', e.g. in a sinus or ear-drum – a term, he suggests, that is ripe for defenestration.

FERAMONE See **PHEROMONE**.

FETUS This is the one and only correct spelling, and not an American simplification, of what is in Britain usually written 'foetus'. Latin *fetus*, means offspring, although a result of an etymological misunderstanding the 'wrong' spelling has been around since the middle ages as 'foetus'. The related 'effete' is also often misunderstood, being now often used as if it meant effeminate (a misinterpretation of the *eff-* opening). It means 'worn out by childbirth'. See also **EMERITUS**.

FIBULA The long or splint bone of the outer side of the leg, from the Latin for a buckle or clasp, because of its resemblance to the tongue of the latter. See also **TIBIA** and **INFIBULATION**.

FICA Another colloquial Latin word for the **VAGINA** (which was itself a layman's term facetiously used by the Greek doctors in Rome so as to make themselves understood by the Romans). *Fica* seems to appear only in sexually-facetious texts, adapted from *ficus*, a fig, which was used both for the **ANUS** (in this application a *dried* fig, no doubt) and the vagina. If you cut a fresh fig in two on its vertical axis and inspect the pink, open halves you will better understand the comparison to the aspect of the vagina. (Much the same applies to the aspect of half a **MALUM**, or apple, perhaps more so.) The fig connection may also be related to 'fucking', via the old German *ficken*, which is still the standard vulgar German word applied to that activity. A gentler one is *feigeln* – literally, 'to make the fig, or to fig'. See also **CUNNUS**, **RIMA**, and **VULVA**.

FIDDLER'S NECK An often painful and ugly pressure discoloration found between the neck and chin of violinists, at the place where they grip their instrument. Padding helps a little to alleviate it, but it is every violinist's mark of Cain (at any rate of those who practise assiduously). To the uninitiated it looks just like a love-bite (or rather love-suck), so that female violinists often get an 'I-know-what-*you*-were-doing-last-night' look. See also **CELLIST'S NIPPLE** and other occupational complaints.

FINDO (FIDI, FISSUM) Latin, to cleave, split, divide. Hence the fissure. When the fissure splits something in two it becomes **BIFIDUS**, **BIFIDA**.

FIRM A group of English hospital doctors headed by a consultant and consisting of him or her as 'boss', a registrar, one or more house officers (formerly 'housemen'), and students, who make up the largest number of the firm.

FISTULA Latin for any kind of pipe, whether used in plumbing or music. Its medical application ('a long, narrow, suppurating canal') would in Roman times simply have likened a pathological manifestation to an everyday object. It also gave us the word festering. See also **TIBIA** and **SYRINGE**.

(THE) FIVE Fs MNEMONICS (1) An unexplained swelling in the abdomen could be due to **F**luid, **F**latus, **F**(a)eces, **F**(o)etus or **F**at. (2) The most common predisposing qualifications for gallstones: **F**emale, **F**ortysomething, **F**at, **F**air and **F**ertile. The alliteration 'Fair, fat and forty' occurs in Sir Walter Scott's novel *St Ronan's Well* (chapter 7).

FLAGELLATION Apart from its psycho-sexual aspects, which do not concern us here (and which the French call, with unjustified sanctimony, *le vice Anglais*) a good beating was in ancient times regarded as a recognised treatment for **COSTIVENESS**, or constipation, which please see. See also under **BUGGERY** and **PROCTOS**.

FLATULENCE From Latin *flatus*, wind, *flare*, to blow, which also gave us monetary inflation (and see **VENTUS** for other windy derivations). Flatulence is produced by the air we swallow by aerophagy ('eating wind') and which is mixed with gas created by digesting/decomposing food in the stomach and **COLON**. Together they produce the familiar, uncomfortable distension of the **ABDOMEN** which clamours to be relieved. Not to release them was formerly considered, like costiveness, a threat to health; and as it is the only health problem whose relief may be accompanied by a comic noise, flatulence has since ancient times been the subject of levity. If the wind travels upwards and out through the throat, it is politely called an eructation, Latin *ructare*, to belch, and is seldom involuntary (unless appearing as hiccups). The other kind, moving downwards and released through the **ANUS**, is socially less acceptable but has a more interesting linguistic history. The Greeks called it *perdein*, the Romans *pedo*, the Italians *peto* and the French *péter*; and the *pétard* one is 'hoist' with (as in *Hamlet*) was a minor explosive charge used for blowing small holes in defences, or forcibly opening doors ('hoist' here meaning blown into the air): see also **TREPAN**. It gave the punning French a fruitful source for word-games: when

Princess Margaret decided not to marry Group Capt. Peter Townsend their newspapers printed headlines like **MARGARET RENONCE A PETER**. There is nothing wrong with the old English word *fart*, first seen in written form in about 1250 in the bucolic round *Sumer is icumen in* attributed to John of Fornsete, a Monk of Reading Abbey (*'Bulluc sterteth, bucke verteth'*) but medical persons are reluctant to use it, preferring some of the numerous other polite euphemisms that will be found in this book. Ancient treatises abound on flatulence – though they usually descend into ribaldry. Among them are Thurlow's *Essays on Wind* of 1825 and a French dissertation, *L'art de péter, Essai théori-physique et méthodique...* (Paris, 1776). However, neither Mark Twain's famous privately printed essay, nor songs on the subject by Purcell and Mozart, pretend to have any scientific basis. The 16th edition of the *Merck Manual of Diagnosis and Therapy* (1993), the GPs' Bible used in most surgeries, continues the tradition. After dwelling in great detail on the physiology and chemistry of flatulence it describes various types – and does so in everyday language not used elsewhere in this learned tome (and as close to **COPROLALIA** as such an important reference-book will ever get); and while echoing Thurlow, who in his *Essay* states 'There are five or six different species of fart...', *Merck* is able to classify only four:

'Among those who are flatulent, the quantity and frequency of gas passage shows great variability. As with bowel frequency, persons who complain of flatulence often have a misconception of what is normal. In a study of 8 normal men aged 25 to 35 years, the average number of gas passages was 13 ± 4 in one day, with an upper limit of 21 per day... On the other hand, one study noted a person who expelled gas as often as 141 times daily, including 70 passages in one 4-hour period...This symptom, which can cause great psychosocial distress, is unofficially described according to its salient characteristics: (1) the 'slider' (crowded elevator type), which is released slowly and noiselessly, sometimes with devastating effect; (2) the open sphincter, or 'pooh' type, which is said to be of higher temperature and more aromatic; (3) the staccato or drumbeat type, pleasantly passed in privacy; and (4) the 'bark' type (described in a personal communication) is characterised by a sharp exclamatory eruption that effectively interrupts (and often concludes) conversation. Aromaticity is not a feature. Rarely, this usually distressing symptom has been turned to advantage, as with a Frenchman* referred to as *Le pétomane*, who became affluent as an effluent performer and who played tunes with the gas from his rectum on the Moulin Rouge stage'.

According to some authorities flatulence of type (1) is in Scottish dialect known as a 'feist', defined in dictionaries as 'a noiseless breaking of wind' and also 'a weak person' – lending a different flavour to the currently popular Anglo-American term 'feisty'.

One aspect that has yet to be researched is the impact of human flatulence on the environment. When the Commonwealth Scientific and Industrial Research Organisation studied the methane output of cattle with the help of infra-red and chromatographic sensors, it found that each cow produced 110 gallons of methane a day, and reported that 'cows may be inflicting three times more damage to the atmosphere than previously thought'. (Information from undated newspaper cuttings, c. 1994.)

*He was Louis Baptiste Pujol (1857–1945), and you can read about his life and work in my *Music through the Looking-Glass* (Routledge & Kegan Paul, London, 1984).

FLAUTIST'S CHIN See also **CELLIST'S NIPPLE**, **HOUSEMAID'S KNEE**, etc.

FLOATERS See **STEATORRH(O)EA**.

(THE) FLOWERS English euphemism, current from the 15th century onwards but now all but forgotten, for the **MENSES**.

FLU See **INFLUENZA**.

FOCUS When we say, 'The fireplace makes a nice focus for our living-room' we repeat an age-old idea. *Focus* is the Latin name for a hearth, which in a Roman dwelling was indeed the focus – the centre of warmth and, at night, light. When such a fireplace was a large opening in the middle of a house, a kind of central, open-to-the-sky room, it was an **ATRIUM**. See also **FORNIX**, **THALAMOS** and **VESTIBULUM** – all medical words with **ARCHITECTURAL** origins. Apart from its ophthalmological meaning, the *focus* is the principal site of an infection or disease.

FOETUS See **FETUS**, above, and **PARTURITION**, below.

FOLLICLE Latin *folliculus*, a little bag, which it resembles. It is the diminutive of *follis*, a bellows – which, of course, a follicle also resembles.

FONTANELLE French modification from the Latin word for a small fountain, hence the name for the membranous spaces in the head of a newborn infant. The pulsation observed in these spaces was thought to resemble bubbling.

(IT'S) FOR A FRIEND Commonly said in GPs' surgeries by patients too shy to admit that the complaint is really their own (just as autograph-hunters always say 'It's for my child'). Such patients may be coded as **FAFs** in their Patient's Notes and could also be **DOORHANDLES**.

FORAMEN From the Latin *forare*, to bore (in the physical, not social or conversational, sense): hence an opening or a hole, particularly in a bone, plural *foramina*.

FOREIGN-ACCENT SYNDROME Observed in a 46-year-old American who began speaking in a foreign accent after being involved in a car crash, and reported in *Medical World News* in 1993. Presumably the condition was previously observed also in many psychiatrists of the older, post-Freud generation, though for different reasons.

FORENSIC As in forensic medicine or science: see **FORUM**, below. A curious change in the pronunciation of this word must be recorded: during the 1980s many people, doctors included, abandoned the old pronunciation 'for-en-sick' and started using a buzzing z –'for-en-zick', as they also do in many other English words.

FORMUS Another term for a tumour: *Lewis and Short* says it is Latin for a glow, or warmth. Note also Sanskrit *gharmas*, the English and German words *warm* and Greek *thermos*.

FORNIX Latin for an arch or arch-like structure, e.g. the *fornix cerebri* in the brain. In Roman architecture it is a vault or cellar – and it was in such underground places that brothels were situated. From *this* comes the word *fornication*. Latin *fornicarius* is a fornicator; *fornicaria*, a prostitute (what Lord Macaulay would *not* have called one of 'the lays of ancient Rome'). The presence of three vault-like *fornices* in the **VAGINA** is purely fortuitous. Other **ARCHITECTURAL** terms are cross-referenced.

FORUM The Roman place of assembly, where matters of public interest were debated and judicial

as well as other business performed. This gave its name to **FORENSIC** medicine; and in some American universities the word 'forensic' is traditionally used to describe certain debating practices.

FOSSA Latin for a ditch, hence the *fossae* found in the elbow joint and other places; and also one of the facetious Roman words for the **VULVA**. See also the various cross-references under **CUNNUS**.

FRACTURA Latin for a break, breach, fracture or cleft. The abbreviation/sign used in medical notes or reports is #. This is perhaps related to its use in proof-reading to mean 'extra space': not, surely, in music, where it is a sign indicating the sharpening of a note by a semitone.

FRAENUM Latin for a bridle, diminutive *fr(a)enulum*: a small fold of skin, of which the human body has several.

FRANK SIGN An acquired oblique fissure of the ear-lobe associated with coronary disease, hypertension and diabetes, named after its discoverer, the American physician Dr S. T. Frank. See B. G. Firkin and J. A. Whitworth's Dictionary of Medical Eponyms (Parthenon Publishing). There is also an **O-SIGN** and a **Q-SIGN**.

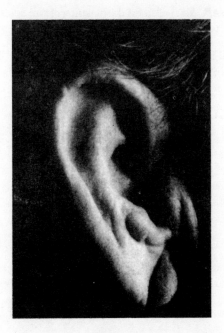

Frank Sign

FREMITUS Latin for a growl. Several kinds of fremitus may be perceived from the chest by **AUSCULTATION**, or sometimes **PALPATION**. See also **RALE**.

FRENCH LETTER See under **CONDOM** and **CAPOTE ANGLAISE**.

FRENCH POX See **POX**.

FRIGHT, FIGHT or FLIGHT The three commonest activities or emotions for which the body produces **ADRENALIN(E)** (epinephrine). Others may be musical, theatrical or sporting performances, oratory, debate – and many things requiring a reserve of energy or stamina, a delay in the onset of fatigue, or the overcoming of stage-fright.

FRINGE MEDICINE A collective term for various systems of treatment that are not regarded by the medical profession as orthodox, and whose efficacy may be disputed. See also **AROMATHERAPY**, **MESMER** and **QUACK**, etc. But some of these treatments have been known, like **ACUPUNCTURE**, to move inwards from the fringes.

FT (also F) Pharmacists' abbreviation for *fiat*, 'let it be done'. Liverpool-trained medics will remember their university's motto, *Fiat Lux*, 'Let there be light'.

FUBAR You will guess the meaning of this acronym after turning to **BUBAR**.

FUGERE Latin, to flee (see also below). The centrifuge, which rotates at great speed and causes matter to 'flee from the middle'.

FUGUE Latin *fuga*, flight. Most people know the word as an English musical term for a composition in two or more voices or parts which enter one after another and are harmonised according to the strict – yet breakable – laws of harmony and counterpoint. To psychiatrists (and increasingly also lay persons and journalists) fugue is a manifestation of neurosis, a flight from one's own identity, often involving panic, a physical removal to another place, usually with some form of amnesia, etc. It may also denote part of an epileptic seizure.

FULMINANT/FLUMINATING Indicative of a rapid and sudden onset of a severe condition, e.g. an infection, fever or **H(A)EMORRHAGE**. From Latin *fulmen, fulminis*, a thunderbolt, especially one which sets on fire, like that which Zeus might have hurled.

FUNCTIONAL OVERLAY One of the newer medical jargon terms, indicating an emotional aspect of an organic disease whose symptoms may continue long after its clinical signs have disappeared.

FUNDHOLDING An administrative–medical innovation of the early 1990s which raises strong views among NHS doctors and patients, in one way or another. I therefore simply record it as an addition to the language. Suffice it to add that 'Market Forces' and **GREY SUITS** (or at any rate 'Grey Suitism') are involved in it.

FUNNYBONE That part of the elbow over which the **ULNAR** nerve passes and which produces a far-from-funny sensation if accidentally struck. Read about the wishbone and merry-thought below.

FURCULUM Formerly the name of the **CLAVICLE**, but now reserved for the wishbone (or 'merry-thought') of birds. And merry thoughts might lead us to the **FUNNYBONE**, above.

Gg

GA (Pronounced in separate letters, G.A.): abbreviation of General Anaesthetic.

GADGET See **PLEDGET**, where you will also find a widget.

(GA)LACT- The milk prefix, from Latin *lac*, milk, itself from Greek *galaxias, gala, galact-*.

GALEN The most celebrated physician of the 2nd century AD and, unlike the health- and medicine-related gods, he was a real person. He was born in Asia Minor and studied medicine in Greece and Egypt. In AD 163 he was appointed physician to the Emperors Marcus Aurelius and Commodus and effectively established Greek-based medicine in Rome. His numerous writings on the art of healing influenced doctors for centuries to come. Andrew Boorde, 'of Physicke Doctour', had a – probably imaginary – portrait woodcut of him published in 1547:

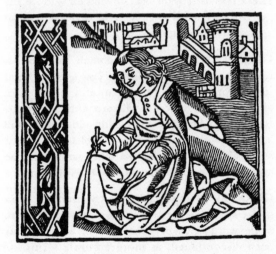

GALVANISM Electricity developed by chemical action, as first described in 1792 by Luigi Galvani (b. 1737). Galvanic cautery (electrocautery), galvanic electric stimulation, etc. are still used, and so is the galvanometer in certain diagnostic instruments, e.g. electrocardiographs (ECGs). See also **MESMERISM**.

GAMEKEEPER'S THUMB Nothing to do with Lady Chatterley, alas, or her friend Mellors, but the name for a dislocation of the thumb, said to be an occupational risk of gamekeepers who dispatch an injured, or imperfectly shot, game-bird by breaking its neck in a single, one-handed movement. See also **HANGMAN'S FRACTURE** and other occupational conditions, real or fanciful, listed under **BREWER'S DROOP**.

GANGLION Greek for a knot, hence the name for a knot-like swelling (a ganglion is found also in the nervous system). The plural is *ganglia* – often erroneously used in the singular, like 'a bacteria' or 'a diverticula' (but see **VERTEBRA**). The effective treatment for some ganglia was said to be a sharp blow with the Family Bible.

GANGRENE From the Greek word for gnawing, *gangraina*, because the affliction is thought to 'eat away' the flesh. See also **NECROSIS**.

GARG. Pharmacists' abbreviation for:–

GARGLE One of the most expressively onomatopoeic words. It comes from the Greek *gargarizo*, to rinse the mouth, from which is derived the Latin *gargarisma*. In German *Gurgel* is a word for the throat; and one of the anatomical names for the **UVULA**, now rare, is *gargareon*, and the (etymologically related) gargoyle water-spout also rinses his mouth. The French word is even more echoic: *gargouiller* – say it with a mouth full of liquid while rolling your *r* in the French manner and you have gargled; and to them *gargouillis* means intestinal rumbling – like **BORBORYGMUS**.

GAS PASSER Medics' slang for an anaesthetist.

GASTR(O)- The stomach (or belly) prefix, from the Greek *gaster*, belly; hence all manner of combination-words such as gastroenterology, gastritis – and indeed, gastronomy – see the various elements of these words under their separate entries.

GASTROCNEMIUS The chief muscle in the back part of the leg, which gives it a protuberant or 'bellying' form, from Greek *gastroknemia*, the calf of the leg, literally 'the belly of the leg'. Ballet-dancers' gastrocnemii are usually especially well-developed. In days gone by, before women revealed so much of their build to passers-by, 'a finely-turned calf', or calligastrocnemia, would have been remarked upon by men as readily as **CALLIPYGIA** still is.

GAY This has been a frivolous euphemism for homosexuality since the mid-1930s, but by the 1970s and 80s it became the accepted **PC** way of describing both male and female homosexuality. However, in this field the vocabulary constantly shifts, and by the early 1990s militant homosexual men and women had declared 'gay' to be patronising and started to call themselves 'queers' (previously regarded as offensive). But 'gay', a useful little word, meaning happy, merry, joyous and cheerful, was an early casualty of sexual innuendo, used of prostitutes and their customers from about 1630, and was a standard word for any dissipated person well into the 20th century, and a specifically homosexual one from about 1930.

(THE) GAY PLAGUE Tabloid newspapers' crude name for **AIDS**.

-GEN- From Greek *genein*, to reproduce: the growth pre- and suffix, and a generally hard-working word-making element which indicates coming-into-being, growth or cause, e.g. carcinogen(ic), something which promotes the growth of cancer. See also **GENESIS**, below, and **PARTHENOGENESIS**.

GENDER REASSIGNMENT Euphemistic description of sex-change operations.

GENE This, the name of a biological unit of genetic material and inheritance, comes (like the Latin **GENESIS**, see below) from the Greek *genein*, to reproduce.

GENERIC DRUGS From Latin *genus*, kind: drugs or medicines sold under the name of their principal contents, not the makers' owned and patented brand-name. Aspirin was originally a proprietary **PATENT MEDICINE** which later entered the public domain (and was only then written with a small initial *a*). See also **PATENT MEDICINE**.

GENESIS The name of the First Book of the Old Testament comes from the Latin (itself derived from Greek) for the act of creation. Thus it refers not only to God's heroic six-day week but also to all the frantic begetting that goes on in the opening book of the Bible so as to generate the characters for the succeeding ones. Indeed an ancient Scottish translation renders the Book of Genesis as 'the Buke of Swiving'. This would not have been as ribald as it seems today: it simply put the title into the vernacular, 'swyving' being the Old English word for sexual congress. Such straightforwardness makes one wonder what that old Scots Bible has to say about Onan.

GENIO- The chin or lower jaw prefix. See also **MAXILLA**.

GENITO- The reproduction/generation prefix: Latin *genitor*, parent or begetter.

GENTLE PERAMBULATORS An aperient medicine prescribed in England from the middle of the 19th century: a cleverly named product, as it suggests that it will make the patient 'go'. Others include(d) **ANDREWS LIVER SALTS**, **CASCARA**, **ENO'S**, **PERISTALTIC PERSUADERS**, **KRUSCHEN SALTS** and more.

GENU Latin for the knee, hence to genuflect, bend the knee, *genu varum*, bow-legged and many *genu*-prefixes, used also for knee-shaped parts. (Roman plumbing had *geniculi*, or 'knee-joints', as modern plumbers call them, or else 'elbows'.) The corresponding Greek word for the knee is *gonu* (and almost all other languages, from Sankrit to Old Norse had similar-sounding words). See also **KNEEJERK**.

GEORGE The traditional name for the articulated **SKELETON** used by medical students for study, at any rate when it is a real skeleton: modern plastic replicas apparently do not qualify for a name.

GERIATRIC Usually a misnomer. The word is constructed from the Greek prefix *ger-* (*geras*, old) and *-iatr-* (from *iatros*, a physician) and is therefore applicable only to people who are both old *and sick*. It should not be applied to healthy old persons (still less, facetiously, to worn-out or obsolete machinery, as in 'This bike is getting positively geriatric'). The appropriate word for the old is **GERONTIC**.

GERM(S) Of impeccable ancestry – from late Latin *germen*, sprout, hence germination – the medical use of the word as, vaguely, the 'seed' of a disease, has been discontinued, as more accurate terms for organisms, infections and infestations have become available.

GERONTIC From Greek *geron*, an old man. The study and science of ageing and old people is gerontology, not geriatrics. See also **EPHEBIATRICS** and **P(A)EDIATRICS**.

GERONTOPHILIA The *geronto-* prefix, from the above, plus the Greek 'love' suffix **-PHILIA**: a special fondness or sexual preference shown by younger people, usually women, for, usually, older men –

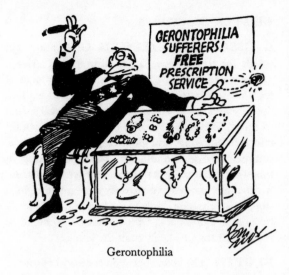

Gerontophilia

especially rich ones, money being the most powerful aphrodisiac known to woman. The opposite condition – young men falling for much older women – has also been observed, but more rarely. Freud's disciple Ernest Jones called it the Grandfather Complex and described it as a psychosexual condition. Older objects of young desire may disagree with him.

GERRY Hospital slang: short for a geriatric patient – and, of course, also for a chamber-pot, though this, being an abbreviation of jeroboam, a large pot, would be written with a j.

GEUSIS Greek for taste – hence *ageusia*, lack of taste sensation. See the Latin equivalent, **GUSTUS** and **ANOSMIA**, which is related to it.

GI Abbreviation of gastro-intestinal; also a member of the American armed forces.

GIBLET MAN/MERCHANT In facetious professional slang, usually among junior doctors, a surgeon.

GIGGLE-INCONTINENCE An inappropriate, involuntary passing of a small quantity of urine, usually on the part of females and caused by excessive laughter. 'Not a dry seat in the house' may be a theatrical exaggeration but something of the sort can really come to pass, so it is advisable when attending comedy shows to inspect one's seat before taking it. It may also occur during the female orgasm – more rarely in combination with laughter. See also **LAUGHING-GAS**.

GILLES DE LA TOURETTE SYNDROME It would be impractical to fill this little book with all discoverers of conditions named after them – and besides, there already exists such a book (*see Bibliography*) – but M. de la Tourette must be an exception. The **SYNDROME** he described shows itself in facial and/or bodily tics, often combined with involuntary **COPROLALIA**, or obscene speech. It has – absurdly – been suggested in one of many posthumous diagnostic theories that Mozart suffered from it, because of his childish liking for dirty talk (mostly excretory, not sexual). But no contemporary of the composer ever mentioned that he had a nervous tic – and if his dirty talk was a 'syndrome', most of his family and friends, and a large part of the Viennese population, suffered from it. Peasants always talked in an earthy manner, but for the middle and upper classes it was a passing fashion, probably started by a novel by Christoph Wieland, which describes an imaginary place called *Abdera*, where even fine ladies used coarse and *disgusting* language: *abdere* is Latin for 'to hide away': see under **ABDOMEN**. Also **GUSTUS**.

GINGIVA Latin for the gum. It appears not to be etymologically related to ginger (Latin *gingiber*), in spite of the powerful effect this deliciously pungent root can have on the mouth.

GIPPY TUMMY Popular name for any form of **DIARRH(O)E(I)A** contracted by British forces, colonists or travellers: 'gippy' at first meaning Egypt but now used as a general term. Also **DELHI BELLY** and **BOMBAY CRUD** in India, **MONTEZUMA'S REVENGE** in Mexico (called **TURISTA** by the natives of South American countries) and the **TURKEY TROTS** in Turkey.

GLABROUS A word that might have been invented by Lewis Carroll. It comes from Latin *glaber*, smooth, bald and is used to describe, hairless skin.

GLADIOLUS Part of the breast-bone: the diminutive of Latin *gladius*, a sword, and named in allusion to its shape, like the name of the flower. A gladiator was a swordsman. See also **XIPHOID**.

GLADSTONE BAG A small, oblong leather portmanteau rounded in shape and opened laterally at the top, named after the English statesman and Prime Minister W.E. Gladstone (1808–98). It was for a long time associated with the visiting physician but has been superseded by more carefully arranged cases with special compartments appropriate for modern drugs and equipment. Gladstone also gave his name to a cheap French claret (after he reduced the excise duty on it) as well as a four-wheeled carriage which was perhaps succeeded by the **DOCTOR'S COUPÉ**.

GLANS The Latin word for a gland, hence words like glandular. It is also the medical name for the rounded bit at the end of the penis and of the corresponding part of the **CLITORIS**. In both medical and colloquial German that part is called *Eichel*, acorn (but literally 'little oak'), but then, *glans* was the normal, everyday Latin word for an acorn ('tall oaks from little acorns grow', as the saying goes). This is another example of a medical term now in polite and scientific use which for the ancient Romans was the popular, sometimes even facetious, word. The Greek word for an acorn is *balanos*, hence balanitis, inflammation of the end of the penis. It seems that whenever people spoke of the procreative or digestive parts of the body, or parts considered 'shameful' (see **PUDENDA**) there has always been a wider choice of euphemisms.

GLASGOW COMA SCALE Devised to give a reliable and objective way of describing the conscious state of a patient and often used for the prediction of the final outcome. (Teasdale, *The Lancet*, ii 81, 1974). For other 'geographical' namings see the **MANCHESTER OPERATION/REPAIR** and the **LIVERPOOL SLIPPER**.

GLAUCOMA The assertion that the Eskimo (or Inuit) have 30 words for snow is probably a fancy, but the Greeks certainly had a wider range of words than most languages for colours. *Glaukos* stood for a blueish, greyish green, hence glaucoma.

GLAXO The name of this international pharmaceutical group is based on the Greek *gala*, *galaxias*, milk, and Latin *lac*, with the prefix (**GA**)**LACT-**. The company name was chosen by the founder of the Glaxo Group, Joseph Nathan, a Londoner who in 1853 emigrated to Wellington, New Zealand and in about 1900 bought a milk-drying process. He tried at first to register the name 'Lacto', but this had already been taken. Glaxo was therefore the second choice − but ultimately it matters not what you christen your baby: when he grows up and makes his mark the name will prevail. (The Company recently merged with Burroughs Wellcome and is now known as Glaxo Wellcome.)

GLISTER See **CLYSTER**.

GLOSSA/GLOTTA/LINGUA Greek and Latin words for the tongue, hence also speech. Also a glossary, like this book, trading in a simple form of *linguistics* and attempting to list words and explore their meaning. Various other formations will spring to mind, like glossitis − one of the many harmful effects of smoking; and glossectomy, cutting off the tongue. Also glossolalia, St. Paul's 'speaking in tongues' (and usually in nonsense speech): see **LALIA**, which may cross-refer you to dirty talk − and the glo'al stop, by which some English-speakers (e.g. Londoners, Scots and Tynesiders), who cannot be bothered to move their tongue, lazily omit the letter *t*.

GLOTTIS The space between the vocal cords.

GLUCAGON From Greek *gleukos*, sweet wine + *agon* (from *agein*, to lead, to bring): a hormone produced by the **PANCREAS**.

GLUCUS Latinised from the Greek *gleukos*, see above, and meaning sweetness. Hence glucose, glycogen, etc. Doctors and chemists seem to prefer this, the Greek-based form, to the pure Latin equivalent *dulcis*.

GLUT(A)EUS Maximus, medius and minimus − the three muscles which form the buttock and move the thigh. The Latin word comes from the Greek *gloutos*, the rump. *Gluteus* is now the favoured spelling, in English as well as American. See also **FANNY**.

GNATHOS Greek for the jaw; *maxilla*, *mandibulum* in Latin. Is it mere coincidence that many English words concerned with things we do with the jaw start with *gn-* : gnashing and gnashers, gnaw, gnap ('to bite in a snapping fashion' - *Oxford English Dictionary*), gnar, gnare, gnarring ..? See also the numerous 'wetness' words starting with sp-.

GNOSIS Greek for knowing, recognising (and both these words are derived from that root): hence also diagnosis, determining, recognising or identifying a condition by observing its symptoms; and prognosis − knowing, or more likely guessing, how a condition is likely to develop (but see **GOK** below). Agnosia means the failure to recognise somebody or something.

GOITRE The word for a morbid enlargement of the thyroid gland of the neck is French, and comes from the Latin *guttur*, the throat. See also **DERBYSHIRE NECK**.

GOK Short for 'God Only Knows', i.e. the doctor's coded admission, perhaps in a person's case-notes, of an inability to diagnose his condition: or as the Greeks would have called it, *agnosis*. See **CRYPTOGENIC**, **GNOSIS**, above **IDOPATHIC** above; and **WOOS**, below.

GOLDEN HOUR The first hour after an accident, when the victim stands the best chance of being successfully treated. The following 60 minutes have been described as the 'Silver Hour', depending on the seriousness of the injuries.

GOLFER'S SHOULDER One of the professional or activity-based conditions recounted under **BREWER'S DROOP**.

GOMER Doctors' code term imported from America: it means 'get (him/her) out of my emergency room', usually said by a casualty-officer if he thinks the patient has a trivial complaint.

GONAD One of the primary sex glands, e.g. the **TESTES** or **OVARIES**, adapted from *gonos*, the Greek word for seed, generation or reproduction.

GONORRH(O)EA From Greek *gone*, seed and *rheein*, flow: the infectious discharge was originally thought to be **SEMEN**. See also **(THE) CLAP** and **GONAD**. Also **ANIMAL BATHS**.

GOUT From the Latin *gutta*, a drop of fluid, a drip – see also **GUTTAE**. The name is derived, says the *Oxford English Dictionary*, from the notion of the 'dropping' of a morbid material from the blood in and around the joints. It is also related to the Old French *égout*, a sewer. The big toe is most commonly affected, usually one belonging to a man. Shakespeare's *II Henry V, i* has 'A pox of this gout! or, a gout of this pox! for the one or the other plays the rogue with my great toe'.

GP The British General Practitioner, or family physician.

GPI General Paralysis of the Insane, the last stages of **SYPHILIS**.

-GRAM The that-which-is-written suffix, from Greek *gramma*, a record. Sometimes interchangeable with the *-graph* suffix, below. There are, for example, cardiograms as well as cardiographs, mammograms and mammographs, though the accepted interpretation is often that the 'gram' is the examination and the 'graph' the written result.

GRAN- From the Latin *granum*, grain. As in conditions such as granulation, granuloma, etc.

GRANNY-DUMPING Usually happens on the Friday before a holiday period, when relatives try to avoid leaving elderly relatives at home alone, so they have them admitted to hospital. Often accompanied by pleas of **SMBD(D)**. See also **PATIENT-DUMPING**.

-GRAPH(O)/(IA) Suffix, from Greek *graphein*, writing, used in combination with many other elements, often used in connection with a recording-instrument, e.g. electrocardiograph, audiograph: also dermographia, a sensitivity of the skin which results in marks, e.g. slight scratches or even pressure, producing temporary weals – literally, 'writing on the skin'. See also **-GRAM**, above.

GREEN PYJAMAS Informal name for the clothes worn in operating-theatres. See also **GREY SUITS**.

GREEN SICKNESS The old English name for chlorosis, an an(a)emic disease which mostly affects girls about the age of puberty and lends a pale or greenish tinge to their complexion. Shakespeare mentioned it several times: 'And making many fish-meals, that they fall into a kind of male green-sickness'; (*Henry IV, Part II*). John Dryden speaks of 'Languishing maids in the green-sickness'; and like **BULIMIA** it seems sometimes to to have been accompanied by eating-disorders: 'The mischief that young Girls do themselves, who are inclined to the green Sickness, by taking great Quantities of Chalk, Lime and other Absorbents...' (*James, 1746*) – cases of **PICA**, perhaps. English writers and poets of the 17th and 18th centuries often referred to the Green Sickness in a facetious, sexually-suggestive manner; indeed the song about *My Lady Greensleeves* is all about 'giving a girl a green gown'; for in the days when most illicit amatory activity was carried on out-of-doors young women often returned home with the sleeves of their garments stained at the elbows (perhaps there is somewhere a song about My Lord Greenknees). In England the Feast of May (May 1st) used to be considered the appropriate day for a girl to lose her virginity. As Robert Herrick (1591–1674) wrote, in his poem, *Corinna's Going a-Maying*,

> *There's not a budding Boy or Girle this day,*
> *But is got up, and gone to bring in May...*
> *Many a green gown has been given;*
> *Many a kiss, both odd and even.*

GREY MATTER Not only a facetious way of describing 'braininess' (or otherwise, as in 'he is lacking in grey matter') but a proper, scientific description of a part of the brain and nervous system.

GREY SUITS Also abbreviated to 'Suits', in British hospitals, the name given to administrators who, in a factory, would be called 'white-collar workers'. In the British National Health Service the Grey Suit **CULTURE** has proliferated to such a degree that books have been issued explaining simple medical terminology to the administrators (*see Bibliography*), although so far no book has appeared which explains the administrators' complex jargon to the doctors. It should be added, however, that the 'health workers' (as the unlovely term now describes all who toil in that field) who are most likely to come into conflict with Grey Suits are those who wear white coats or **GREEN PYJAMAS**, and that professional administrators have turned some British hospitals into friendlier and more cheerful places – also into shopping malls and market-places. White coats, incidentally, are not inevitable among clinicians: some consultants examine patients while clad in *sub fusc* suits (in more formal days British consultants favoured black jackets and discreetly striped black trousers, and looked like bank-managers or stock-brokers). Old prints and early photographs of operating-theatre scenes often show surgeons doing their work in outdoor clothes, occasionally protected by rubber aprons if the procedure was gory. The habits, fads and fashions in medical dress would be a subject for a different study; but it may be observed that in British hospitals the junior doctors make a point of *not* turning down the collars of their white coats, as if to imply that they are perpetually rushed off their feet and have no time for niceties of dress. (When I observed that many architects wore bow-ties, and probably did so to avoid smudging the plans on their drawing-boards, a doctor replied, 'Oh, but so do gynaecologists'). Eighteenth-century and earlier physicians carried round-knobbed walking-sticks, which became symbols of their calling, and doctors were often caricatured holding these to the side of their noses. The round tops of the canes were in fact pomanders filled with scented herbs, whose purpose was to ward off infectious vapours and mask foul smells (see also **AROMATHERAPY**): for the same reason English judges carried (and still carry, on ceremonial occasions) small scented posies. (A selection of impressive job titles enjoyed by the grey-suited is listed under **CHIEF/PRINCIPAL NURSING OFFICER** and **HOSPITAL ADMINISTRATOR**). See also under **STETHOSCOPE**.

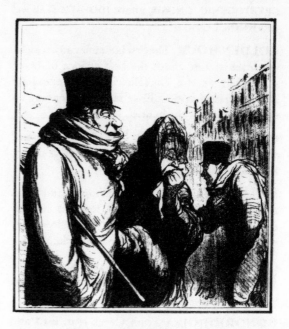

Paris *grippé*

Parisians in the grip of *La grippe*. Lithograph by Daumier

(LA) GRIPPE The French name for **INFLUENZA**. Up to the Second World War the word was commonly used by English-speaking people who considered themselves too grand to be suffering from the common **FLU**. It comes from the French *gripper*, to seize, or grab, and was well described in 1776 by a traveller. 'An epidemic cold seems to have spread itself from London to Barcelona. In passing through this [French] kingdom it has obtained the name of *grippe* – a term significant enough from the nature of its attack upon the throat'. It was also, at different times, called 'The Spanish Flu' (not to be confused with the **SPANISH FLY**), for like the **(FRENCH) POX** the influenza was traditionally thought to be an **ADVENTITIOUS** disease which could be blamed on other nations. Today its provenance is traced scientifically rather than xenophobically, and many different strains have been isolated in different countries, so that their progress can be followed across the world: 'Asian flu' really *is* Asian. See under **PRUNELLA** for a 'Hungarian Camp Fever', and of course the **(FRENCH) POX**.

(THE) GROCKLE TRADE Grockle is a disparaging Devonshire/Cornish slang-word for a holidaymaker; and the majority of local people think of grockles as those whose cars clog up the roads and who drop litter, less as tourists who patronise local shops. But grockles who fall ill while on holiday, especially in southwest England, and sign on as temporary patients, are welcomed by family doctors for the fee they generate.

GROG-BLOSSOM A form of **RHINOPHYMA** – a **ROSACEA** of the nose, which is usually elderly and male, but the condition not necessarily caused by an excess of grog.

GROWING-PAINS A form of **ARTHRALGIA**, or rheumatism-like pains experienced by children or adolescents. The term is also occasionally used for the emotional or psychological problems encountered by the young. The hyphen between the two words is essential, although several respected and authoritative books, like *The Merck Manual* and *Mosby's Pocket Dictionary*, regrettably omit it: growing-pains are associated with growing, whereas growing pains are increasing pains.

GULF SYNDROME Veterans who in 1991 took part in the action against Iraq in the Arabian Gulf complained years later of a variety of symptoms that fitted no known disease. Possible causes put forward included a hitherto undetected use of nerve gas by Iraqi forces, fumes from the oil-wells these set alight, and that elusive but powerful bacterium transmitted by a handshake with a lawyer.

GUNE- The Greek 'woman' prefix: see **GYNE-**.

GURGULATIONS An old word for rumblings in the belly, e.g. the **WOMBLES**. The 16th-century Dr Andrew Boorde, in his *Dyetary*, wrote that 'cows' and ewes' milke are 'not good for them the which haue gurgulacyons in the bely...'. See also **BOR-BORYGM(US)**.

GUSTUS Latin for taste – hence medicine that tastes disgusting. The Greek equivalent is **GEUSIS**.

GUTTAE Latin for drops or drips, as prescribed by pharmacists: singular *gutta*, from which the gout is named. It would be convenient to derive dropsy from it, too, but it is a contraction of the word hydropsy.

GUTTUR(O)- The 'throat' prefix: Latin *guttur*, the throat.

GUY'S HOSPITAL One of the younger London hospitals, founded as recently as 1721 by the bookseller and successful South Sea Bubble speculator Thomas Guy (c.1645–1724) at a cost of £238,295. In 1818 the surgeon James Blundel carried out the first blood transfusion there, using a syringe. Later he invented special apparatus to perform the procedure, which led the way to modern transfusion.

GYN(A)ECOLOGY The word can be dismantled into its components thus: Greek *gune*, above +*oikion*, house, making the Greek/Latin *gynaeceum*, or women's apartments. With the *-ology* 'knowledge' suffix it means the branch of medicine dealing with women. The equivalent male prefix is **ANDR(O)-** although this seems not to be as popular for words about men's troubles (see also androgynous and **HERMAPHRODITE**).

GYN(A)ECOMASTIA Literally, 'womens'-breasts-condition': an abnormal enlargement of the breasts in men, often temporary and usually benign, and sometimes associated with disorders of the **TESTES** or **PITUITARY**. Some say it may also be acquired after years of ingesting recycled drinking-water from which the hormones of the female contraceptive-pill have not been filtered; and/or from eating the meat of animals which farmers have illicitly fed with female hormones to stimulate the growth of the animals and their own profits. See also **BEER BELLY**.

GYNE-/GUNE- The Greek 'woman' prefix, which helped to form numerous words, e.g. **GYN(A)ECOLOGY**. Purists prefer to transliterate it into English characters as *gune-*, while medical English always uses *gyn(a)e-*.

H*h*

HAC NOCTE Pharmacists' code for 'tonight'. See also **NOCTE** – and **HOR. DEC**. for medicines to be taken at bed-time.

H(A)EM(O)-, H(A)EMA-, -(A)EMIA The blood-related prefixes and suffixes, from Greek *haima(t)-*, blood, see below: e.g. anaemia, lack of blood; leukaemia, (an excess of) white blood (-cells); septicaemia, bad blood, etc. American simplified spelling prefers 'hem(o)' etc. – thus risking confusion with words made from *hemera*, Greek for 'day'. See also **LEUK-** and **SANGUIS**.

H(A)EMOPHILIA This combination of two Greek words literally means 'love of blood', as shown by Dracula, for example. In real life it refers to a condition affecting mostly males who suffer from a tendency to bleed, either spontaneously or from the slightest injuries. See **-PHILIA**.

H(A)EMOPTYSIS The coughing-up or spitting of blood. For the spitting connection see under **PITUITA**.

H(A)EMORRHAGE Literally, a raging of blood: see **RHAGIA**.

H(A)EMORRHAGING Most people are familiar with the word from newspaper reports and know what it means, just as they know from advertisements what **H(A)EMORRHOIDS** are; and that **HYPERVENTILATING** means 'breathing hard' because sports commentators have taken to using it. Women often say 'I was haemorrhaging' when referring to their **MENSES** and mean 'a very heavy period'. Why not say 'bleeding'? Perhaps it is because misunderstandings could arise. If, say, a Liverpool woman went to her GP and said 'Doctor, I'm bleeding', he might pose the counter-question, 'Where are you bleeding from?' – and she would then reply, 'From Knotty Ash, doctor'.

H(A)EMORRHOIDS For once the **-OID** suffix ('something resembling the shape or nature of...') is misleading and does not mean 'in the shape of'. Most authorities say that the word comes from the Latin *haemorrhoïs*, a kind of poisonous serpent whose bite was thought to produce unstaunchable bleeding. 'Emerois is a ma[n]ner [of] adder...' declared an author in 1398, 'and hath that name, for he suckyth the blood out of hym that he smyteth'. See also **PILES**.

HAIMA/HAEMA Greek for blood – hence all the prefixes, above.

HALITUS Latin for breath or vapour. With the **-OSIS** (or 'condition') suffix it becomes *bad* breath but only by association: literally translated it merely means 'breath condition'. Halitosis is, however, more than merely the result of too much beer or garlic, etc. having been consumed, or poor dental hygiene, and the word should be used only when there is a medical cause for bad breath. See also **MALARIA** – originally 'bad air'.

HALLUX Modern Latin for the big toe, corrupted from *allex*. But see also **POLLEX** and **DIGITUS**.

HANGMAN'S FRACTURE A fanciful name for the dislocation of the 1st and 2nd cervical vertebrae. But I have it on impeccable authority that when hangmen execute their victims they break different ones – *and* the spinal cord. For occupational conditions, real or imagined, see under **BREWER'S DROOP** and its cross-references to others – e.g. below.

HARE LIP An old but insensitive term for what is better called a **CLEFT LIP**.

HATTER'S SHAKES An occupational disease akin to **ST. VITUS'S DANCE** (and see also **CHOREIA**) caused by mercury poisoning and formerly mistaken for a form of madness. Mercurous nitrate was widely used in the making of felt hats and slowly poisoned the workers who were exposed to it (hence the Mad Hatter in Lewis Carroll's *Alice in Wonderland* (1865). Some Japanese people suffer from its equivalent, Minamata Disease, a degenerative neurological disorder caused by poisoning with a mercury compound found in seafood obtained from waters contaminated with mercury-containing industrial waste. After Minamata, a town of western Kyushu, Japan.

HD High Dependency wards, for hospital patients requiring a greater degree of attention than others. See also **IT**.

HEAD-MOULD-SHOT An old English term for a condition which now doubtless has a more accurate, scientific name. It was described in 1719 as occurring '...when the Sutures of the Skull, generally the Coronal, ride; that is, have their Edges shoot over one another'.

HEARTSINKS GPs' name for patients whose appearance in the surgery is greeted by – one hopes inward – dismay. Sometimes abbreviated to HSPs. See also **DOORHANDLES**.

HEBE- The Greek prefix denoting youth or puberty, mostly used in botanical terms but also hebephrenia, a form of mental disturbance that occurs at or around puberty. And see **EPHEBIATRICS**.

HEIMLICH MANOEUVRE Named after the American surgeon Henry J. Heimlich (born 1920): an emergency technique every diner should learn and which is used to eject an object, such as food, from the trachea of a choking person. The technique employs firm upward thrusts just below the rib cage to force air from the lungs, and with it, it is hoped, the obstructing morsel.

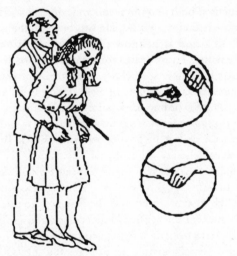

1. Stand behind victim and wrap arms around waist.
2. Grasp your hands as shown, with thumb of fist against victim's abdomen, above the navel and just below the sternum.
3. Press your fists into victim's abdomen with quick, abrupt jerks.

Microsoft Multimedia Reference Library with permision

HELP FOR POLICE TO FIND THE MISSING PERSONS Mnemonic for the bones of the lower limb: Hip, Femur, Patella, Tibia, Fibula, Tarsals, Metatarsals, Phalanges.

HEMICORPORECTOMY A Greek–Latin hybrid (like 'television'): *hemi*, half; *corpus*, body; *ectomy*, cut off. A rare operation indeed – after which only one half of the body remains viable. See also **BASKET CASE**.

HEPA(T)- The prefix for the liver, for which organ the Greek word is *hepar*, adopted into Roman Latin as *hepaticus*.

HERMAPHRODITOS The son of **HERMES** and Aphrodite, who must have been one of the earliest to carry an acronymic name (like Bill and Shirley calling their offspring Birley). Hermaphroditos bathed in the fountain of the nymph Salmacis, got physically too close to her and thus acquired some of her sexual characteristics, hence hermaphroditism, the condition of a person with both male and female sexual characteritics. When our genes misbehave in some spectacular manner, folk-wisdom always finds a ready excuse, like the old superstition that if a pregnant woman got a fright, mental illness could results in her offspring. Hermaphroditism is not uncommon and may occur in various degrees, especially in babies whose mothers received fertility treatment. Mixed bathing is definitely not a risk. The term hermaphrodite was also allusively used in the British Navy in days of sail ('A sailing vessel that combines the characters of two kinds of craft ... one that is square-rigged like a brig forward, and schooner-rigged aft...'); and Dr Douglas D.C. Howat reports having heard it used in a Lincolnshire farmyard, of a four-wheeled cart, the front part of which could be removed to make a small two-wheeled vehicle, leaving a serviceable two-wheeled cart at the rear (and by this reckoning a bicycle that can be taken apart into two monocycles might be called a 'hermaphrobike').

HERMES Son of Zeus and Maia; better known by his Roman name, Mercury, he was the Greek Messenger of the Gods, God of Communications, and a sort of Tour-Guide of souls to Hades. His son by **APHRODITE** (alias **VENUS**) was the first hermaphrodite – see above. Hermes was one of the most overworked gods in the classical religious system: God of Travellers, of Luck, Music, Eloquence, Commerce, Young Men, Cheats, and Thieves. He was also said to have invented the lyre and flute – presumably in his spare time. Hermes is represented with winged hat and sandals, carrying the Caduceus, the wing-topped staff, wound about by two snakes. The staff was carried by Greek officials and became a Roman symbol for truce and neutrality. But snakes-on-a-stick were a common ancient emblem, and resulted in the naming of a constellation in Sagittarius, Ophiuchus, 'the Serpent-holder' (from

Greek *ophis*, a serpent – his Latin name is Serpentarius), a star-sign unaccountably ignored by astrologers. In earlier cultures, notably the Babylonian, the intertwined snakes symbolised fertility, wisdom – and healing, for which reason it has, since the 16th century, served as the symbol of medicine and is the insignia of just about every medical organisation in the world; the medical branch of the United States Army as well as the Royal Medical Corps of the British Army. Hermes/Mercury also gave his name to the chemical substance **MERCURY** or 'quicksilver', used in clinical thermometers and, formerly, as a cure for **VENEREAL** diseases.

HERNIA So pretty a word it might be the name of a female character in a novel or play (like **AMELIA**, **CANDIDA, PRUNELLA**, etc.) but no, it is the everyday Latin word for a break or rupture. It comes from the Greek word *hernos*, a sprout or shoot (in this case one breaking through the abdominal wall). For some reason the condition, which is caused by muscle weaknesses, often gives rise to levity, although jokes about trusses and 'first careless ruptures' have somewhat abated since hernia repair has become a simple operation, often now performed laparoscopically (see **LAPAR(O)-** and **-SCOPE**), under local anaesthetic and on a one-day hospital visit. (A Scottish surgeon who pioneered such hernia repairs was said to insist that his patients wore the kilt, so that they did not have to remove their trousers). The levity may be part of folk-tradition, for it was believed that hernias were caused by a surfeit of sexual activity: Nestor was said (by Juvenal) to have ruptured himself after too much sport with his numerous girl-friends. See also **ANEURYSM** and **DIVERTICULUM**.

HERPES The name of this inflammatory (sometimes sexually transmitted) disease comes from the Greek word *herpein*, creep; which should please the feminists who believe that all men are creeps. For herpes zoster see under **SHINGLES**.

HETERO- Greek *heteros* means different, making various formations that denote or imply difference, e.g. heteroblastic, heterocephalus, **HETEROGRAFT**, a graft from a different person or species (which, says the distinguished transplant surgeon Robert Sells, has now been largely superseded by xenograft). See also **ALLO-, HOMO/HOMEO** and **XENO-**.

HETEROGRAFT See above.

HIDROSIS A politer word for sweating, for those who find even the polite 'perspiration' too populist or unscientific-sounding. From the Greek *hudor*, sweat. The Latin equivalent is **SUDOR**. According to an old English saying, 'Horses sweat, men perspire – but ladies glow'.

HIPPOCAMPUS Greek *hippos* is a horse. Two words immediately spring to mind: the hippodrome – literally a race-course for horses (see **DROME**) though later applied to circuses; and the hippopotamus: literally a river-horse. *Campos* in Greek is a monster, so the hippocampus would be a horse-like monster (but see also **TERATO-**, the 'monster' prefix). The brain has two hippocampi, so named because they were thought to resemble a sea-horse. The word is not connected with **HIPPOCRATES**, below.

HIPPOCRATES Greek doctor–priest who practised both as a physician and surgeon and lived from c. 460 to c. 375 BC. He was born on the island of Kos and is acknowledged as the Father of Medicine. Hippocrates formulated the oath that bears his name (see below), a fragmentary copy of which exists on papyrus pieces dating from about 300 BC. According to popular belief the oath, in a Christianised form, is administered to every graduate in medicine, but this has not been so (at least in British medical schools) within anyone's living memory; and besides, the oath is in many respects now outdated. At present (1995) a new form is being discussed. It was Hippocrates who took the first steps to turn the treatment of the sick from a superstition into a science. His predecessor, in a sense, was the God the Greeks called Aesculapius and the Romans **ASKLEPIOS**. The *Hippocratic Sleeve* was a triangularly-folded flannel bag used by apothecaries to strain liquids, a kind of filter. See also **ARS LONGA**, **VITA BREVIS** and **ALCOHOL**.

HIPPOCRATIC OATH 'I SWEAR by Apollo the physician and Asklepios and Hygieia and Panacea, invoking all the gods and goddesses to be my witnesses, making them witnesses, that I will fulfil this Oath and this written covenant to the best of my powers and ability. I will look upon him who shall have taught me this art even as on mine own parents; I will share with him my substance, and supply his necessities if he be in need; I will regard my teacher in this art as equal to my parents, to make him a partner in my livelihood, and when he is in need of money, to share mine with him; to consider his offspring as my brethren and will teach them this art, if they desire to learn it, without fee or covenant. I WILL IMPART it by precept, by lecture and by all manner of teaching, not only to my own sons but also to the sons of him who has taught me, and to disciples bound by covenant and oath according to the law of the physicians but to none other. THE REGIMEN I adopt shall be for the benefit of the patients to the best of my power and judgment, not for their injury or for any wrongful purpose. I will not give a deadly drug to any one, though it be asked of me, nor will I suggest such counsel; and likewise I will not give a woman a pessary to procure an abortion. But I will keep my life and my art in purity and holiness. I will not use the knife, not even, verily, on sufferers from stone, but I will give place to such as are craftsmen therein. WHATSOEVER HOUSE I enter, I will enter for the benefit of the sick, refraining from all voluntary wrongdoing and corruption, especially fornication with any woman or man, in bond or free. WHATSOEVER THINGS I see or hear concerning the life of men, in my attendance on the sick or even apart from my attendance, which ought not to be published abroad, I will keep silence on them, counting such things to be holy secrets. NOW IF I FULFIL this oath and confound it not, be it mine to enjoy life and art alike, with honour and good repute among all men for all time to come; but if I transgress and violate my oath may the contrary befall me'. On the other hand, the patient has responsibilities, too, and might take Ecclesiasticus xxxviii,1-3 to heart: 'Honour a physician with the honour due unto him for the uses which ye may have of him: for the Lord hath created him. For of the most High cometh healing, and ye shall receive honour of the king. The skill of the physician shall lift up his head: and in the sight of great men he shall be in admiration'. See also **BEDSIDE MANNER**.

HIPPOLAGNIA An unnatural sexual attraction for horses, going far beyond the love many children and young girls feel for ponies and horses. Sufferers from the condition (who appear always to be men or adolescent boys) are often driven by some strange impulse to mutilate horses, usually in the area of their sex organs. Cases were reported from the Middle Ages (though perhaps the earliest recorded instance occurs in the story of *The Golden Ass* by Apulaeius. Peter Shaffer's play *Equus* provides a horrifying modern example of these strange compulsions. Outbreaks of such attacks are reported in the newspapers with increasing frequency – and each instance sparks off others, in the copycat way of news epidemics. See also **KLEPTO-** and other -lagnias, including **UROLAGNIA** and **PYROMANIA**.

HIRSUTISM From Latin hirsutus, rough, shaggy, bristly. See **HYPERTRICHOSIS**, below.

HIRUDO Also **SANGUISUGA**, the generic names of the blood-sucking **LEECH**, which please see.

HISTOLOGY The science or knowledge of organic tissue – from Greek *histos*, a loom, thence tissue.

HIV Abbreviation of Human Immunodeficiency Virus. It is not, as often heard, the 'HIV virus', which duplicates the last word and would make it the Human Immunodeficiency Virus Virus. See also under **AIDS** – or, as it is often called, 'full-blown' **AIDS**.

HIVES The English word for urticaria, a skin eruption. It is of uncertain origin and has nothing to do with beehives – although **ALVEUS** has.

HOLIDAY HEART SYNDROME The phenomenon of **ARSD** – Alcohol-Related Sudden Death Syndrome – among heavy drinkers who over-indulge (perhaps, abroad, where alcohol may be cheap) or at home at weekends (in spite of its higher cost). See also **SATURDAY NIGHT PALSY**.

HOME DOCTOR Not **MY SON THE DOCTOR** but a medical book for self-instruction and reference. Early editions of Mrs Isabella Beaton's *Household Management* mixed cookery with health hints, so the index read, 'Kidneys, broiled; Kidneys, fried; Kidneys, inflamed; Kidneys, roasted...' etc. A four-volume edition of *Cassel's Book of the Household* of about 1880 goes so far as to include hints as to how 'Operation in the Home' should be performed. This is a slightly abbreviated extract:

> Although sickness of all kinds is a source of anxiety, an illness which necessitates a surgical operation is still worse. As it has to be done, and cannot be avoided, every effort should be made to bring it to a successful issue. The result depends very much on attention to a number of minute details, some of which fall entirely within the province of the surgeon; whilst others should engage the attention of the nurse and friends. If the choice of a sick-room is important, the selection of a house for the performance of a surgical operation is of still greater moment. Much will depend on the condition of the drains. A small operation, such

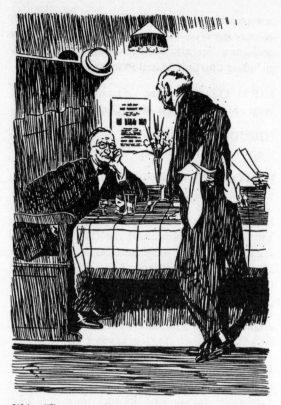

Waiter. "I'VE GOT STEWED KIDNEYS, DEVILLED BONES, FRIED
LIVER, STUFFED CALVES' HEAD -"
Customer. "MY SYMPTOMS EXACTLY."

Punch, May 10, 1933

as the opening of an abscess or removing piles,
would be performed on the bed or sofa; but for
operations of greater magnitude, such as the
amputation of a limb or of the breast, a good,
firm table will be needed. The bed or table must
be placed in a good light, and a thin curtain before
the window will prevent the possibility of an
audience collecting in the street. If there is a
carpet, it will be best to protect it with a
mackintosh sheet. Plenty of clean towels and hot
and cold water will be needed, and really that is
all – except, perhaps, that it is just as well to have
a bottle of good brandy at hand in case of
emergency...

This is followed by a section on anaesthetics – ether,
chloroform and nitrous oxide or **LAUGHING-GAS**, with
the helpful information that 'in most large towns there
are specialists who do nothing but administer
anaesthetics...' See also under **CLOACINA** and **AMELIA**.

HOMEO- Prefix, from Greek *homios*, meaning
similar: This is a simplified spelling of *homeo* (see
below).

HOMEOPATHY An allegedly natural way of
healing by 'treating like with like'. From the Greek
homoeo, likeness. 'Homeopathy' is the now standard,
simplified spelling, though to be etymologically
correct it should be 'homoeopathy', as even the latest,
and increasingly tolerant, edition of the *Oxford English
Dictionary* points out. But so long as we don't further
simplify it to 'homopathy' (which could be as
confusing as the spurious **'HOMOPHOBIA'**) there is
little risk of a misunderstanding. Homeopathy (see
PATH-) is a method, devised at the end of the 18th
century by the German physician Samuel
Hahnemann (1755–1843), of treating diseases by
administering, in very small doses, substances that in
a healthy person would produce symptoms closely
resembling the same disease – hence the *homoeo-*, or
'sameness', connection. I accidentally came across a
'homeopathic' quotation in Lyly's *Euphues* of 1580:
'The roote Rubarbe, which being full of choler,
purgeth choler'. Ambrose Bierce's *A Devil's Dictionary*
defined it, somewhat ambivalently, as 'A theory and
practice of medicine which aims to cure the diseases
of fools. As it does not cure them, and does sometimes

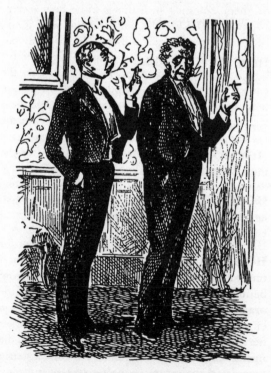

UNCONSCIOUS HOMEOPATHY
"I WAS VACCINATED STRAIGHT FROM THE CALF, YOU KNOW!"
"AH! SIMILIA SIMILIBUS!"

Punch, AUGUST 2, 1884

kill the fools, it is ridiculed by the thoughtless, but commended by the wise'; and Bierce defined a homoeopathist as 'the humorist of the medical profession'. There is evidence that Beethoven turned to it in the hope of alleviating his deafness. See also **ALLOS** for allopathy; and **RHUBARB**.

HOMO- Prefix, from Greek *homos*, the same, hence homolateral, (on) the same side, and numerous other formations indicating sameness, including homosexual.

HOMO is also the Latin word for man – the species, not the gender – and therefore a constant source of confusion with **HOMEO** (above) and the notion that it means *man* as opposed to *woman* – one that has been especially galling to feminists and man-hating women.

HOMOPHOBIA A new and much over-used nonsense-word used as if it meant 'fear of, or discrimination against, homosexuals'. The only proper application of it would be to describe animals that run away when man approaches: they are truly homophobic, because they fear *man* – whether male or female, hetero- or homosexual, is immaterial to them.

HOR. DEC. Pharmacists' abbreviation of Latin *hora decubitus*, 'to be taken at the hour of lying down', i.e. at bedtime. Latin *cubare*, to lie – but see also **ACCOUCHEMENT**. Cubare also turns up under **INCUBATION**.

HORMONE From Greek *hormaein*, to stimulate, to urge. See **PHEROMONE**.

HORRENDOMA Informal hospital slang for an aggressive malignancy – or any unpleasant experience or encounter, e.g. with an obnoxious patient.

HOSPITAL ADMINISTRATOR Once upon a time any statement to the press or television would be made by a senior hospital doctor, but with the dramatic rise during the 1970s in the newsworthiness of medicine and surgery a profligate National Health Service started to engage specialists to 'deal with the media' (presumably the professional medics might have 'said the wrong thing') – one of a group collectively known as **GREY SUITS**. The title now pales beside a growing number of more impressive ones, some of which will be found under **CHIEF NURSING**

OFFICER. I recall seeing a newspaper cartoon showing father and small son leaving a toy shop. The child carries under his arm a box labelled *Little Doctor Set*. The father is saying, 'And who knows, son. One day perhaps even a *Hospital Administrator!*'.

(TO) HOSPITALISE To take or consign a patient to hospital for treatment or rest (and for excessive self-hospitalisation see **MÜNCHHAUSEN SYNDROME**). The *Oxford English Dictionary* lists 'hospitalise' but prefaces the entry with a warning, 'Frequently commented on as an unhappy formation'. However, the word appeared in written English as early as 1902 and has been popularised by newspapers. Following its early acceptance into American English hostile comments have become more muted in British English – or been abandoned as hopeless. The creation of verbs from nouns is an ancient process: wounds are cauterised and bandaged, patients stretchered (especially those injured on sports fields), to be hospitalised, where their records will be accessed and they will be ministered to, nursed, pampered and medicated – though not, one hopes, **DOCTORED**.

HOSPITAL NAMES In 1824 Ludwig van Beethoven, who throughout his life suffered from chronic hypochondria, was told by some of his friends who tried to persuade him to move to England, 'You know, in England they have a hospital for every disease' (and we know this because Beethoven was deaf, so that much of what was said to him was written down and survives in his Conversation Books). The speaker was not far wrong, for the UK pioneered specialist hospitals (and Beethoven was also told, 'In England there is a sect whose members eat nothing but fruit and vegetables!'). British hospital names were usually factual, specifying the diseases they were intended for with brutal frankness. In addition to Lunatic Asylums, which survived well into the 20th century, there were numerous Hospitals for Imbeciles, for the Indigent Poor, for Consumptives, for Cripples, etc. The change from stark names to **PC** euphemisms accelerated from the middle of the 20th century, as the new **WELFARE STATE** led the way in kindness and compassion. In Liverpool the Hospital for the Incurables was renamed, first, The Cancer Hospital, then The Liverpool Radium Institute – and when people understood the purpose of radiation treatment, The Liverpool Clinic. (Then it was closed down, which saved any further changes.) Lunatic

Asylums and Hospitals for the Insane underwent even more drastic renamings. Again in Liverpool, The Venereal Diseases Clinic became the Seamen's Clinic, which was soon changed to Special Clinic or abbreviated to STD Clinic. Psychiatric prisons, for what used to be called Criminal Lunatics, became 'hospitals', their inmates being redefined as 'patients', not prisoners (with the advent of 'market forces' they are probably now 'customers'). Such institutions usually took the names of the locality in which they were situated, much to the chagrin of local inhabitants, who had not only to cope with the fear from escaping patients but having their area turned into a byword for criminal madness (in Northern English slang, *winnucky*, for mad, is derived from Winwick, the site of a mental-hospital; and near London, *Colney Hatch* suffered the same fate). One psychiatric 'hospital' (*recte* prison) near Liverpool has seen three radical name-changes in the space of a dozen years. Old-established names may be compromised by changes in verbal usage, e.g. the National Hospital for Nervous Diseases (in Queen Square, London) which, overtaken by an altered public perception of the word 'nervous', is now the National Hospital for Neurology and Neurosurgery. It certainly gives a better idea of its functions. But venerable names of ancient British hospitals have been abolished or submerged in the bureaucratic verbiage of the **GREY SUITS**, e.g. Guy's Hospital, founded in London in 1721 by the bookseller and philantropist Thomas Guy, now carries the leaden name 'Lewisham and District Health Authority Guys Branch'. Asylums disappeared much earlier, probably with the abolition of the word **LUNATIC** and the change of use of the word **BEDLAM**. See also **RELEASE INTO THE COMMUNITY**.

HOSPITARE 'To entertain' in Latin. *Hospis* could mean either a guest or a host. Thus a hospital became, first, a place for guests, later for travellers, then a place devoted to the education of the young (i.e. a school) and, finally, for treating sick people. The word is also related to *hostes*, a stranger (and thence enemy – for the line between welcoming a stranger and killing him if he behaved badly must have been a finely-drawn one).

HOUSEMAID'S KNEE The informal name for an inflammation of the **BURSA** over the kneecap, caused by kneeling on hard floors. According to the *Oxford English Dictionary* the term was first recorded in 1831, in the *London Medical and Physical Journal*, although it is there referred to in such a way as to suggest that it was already known: 'The bursa slightly thickened, but distended with fluid, uneasy, and painful, the most ordinary state of the housemaid's knee' (surely not every housemaid's knee?). Less is heard of it today: not only are there fewer domestic servants but they are better informed of the risks. 'Carpet-layer's Knee' may be more common, although they are obliged to wear knee-pads. Parson's Knee, suffered by priests, monks and nuns has also been described. Other forms of 'occupational rheumatism', are Golfer's Shoulder, Miner's Elbow and Weaver's Bottom (*Textbook of Pathology* by Adami and McCrae, 1912), though one might think the compression caused by kneeling and the tension produced by swinging a golf-club would produce different effects. See also numerous other occupational diseases cross-referenced or mentioned under **BREWER'S DROOP**. And **SMOKER'S FACE**.

HOUSEMAN The old, traditional name for a young house physician or surgeon resident in a British hospital who, having passed all the qualifying examinations, works under supervision before being fully registered (when he becomes a **SENIOR HOUSE OFFICER**) as an independent medical practitioner (see **INTERN** for the American equivalent). In Britain he will most likely be part of a **FIRM**. Although the word 'houseman' has happily embraced young doctors of both sexes for well over a century, sexual equality and **PC** awareness during the 1980s demanded a change to House *Officer*. Similar neologisms were forced upon the posts of **MATRON** and the **ALMONER**, to name only two.

HOUSE OFFICER See above.

HOW'S YOUR FATHER? It is difficult to believe in these brutally frank times that a generation or two ago, doctors questioning a patient about matters they might have considered embarrassing, e.g. 'How about your sex life?' might have said (at any rate to male patients), 'What about the old How's Your Father?' It comes from the English music-hall, where a lewd punchline could be side-tracked, the comedian breaking off (at a point where everyone knew it anyway) and enquiring about Father.

HRT Hormone Replacement Therapy, normally as given to menopausal women for cosmetic or health reasons; though the same term could be used if men had their waning hormones replaced. In Chinese medicine this is allegedly achieved by the administration of ground rhinoceros horn – RHT?

HSP See **HEARTSINKS**.

HUALOS (HYALOS) Greek for glass, producing the *hyalo-* prefix – as in the hyaloid artery, hyaloplasm, hyaluronidase, etc. For the Latin equivalent see **IN VITRO**.

HUMBY According to *The Deeper Meaning of Liff* by Douglas Adams and John Lloyd (who have enriched the English language with their ingenious namings of conditions everyone knows about but no-one has bothered to describe) this is 'an erection which won't go down when a gentleman has to go to the lavatory in the middle of dallying with a lady'. This mildly distressing condition obviously has a clinical cause, related to the **PROSTATE** (see also **LOVER'S BALLS**), but has it ever been clinically named?

HUMERUS The bone of the upper arm from the shoulder to the elbow. This is another word of confusing origin: the Latin is really *umerus*, but at some point it sprouted an *h*, causing endless confusion with the word for moisture or fluid, as in humid, from *humidus*: and with humour, which in ancient medicine denoted a body fluid and was no laughing-matter.

HUNCHBACK One of the words, like **CRIPPLE**, which are now considered too stark for general use. Doctors would in any case be more specific, and speak of **KYPHOSIS**. They might also mention the **DOWAGER'S HUMP** – though not in front of a dowager.

HYGIEIA In Greek mythology, the Goddess of Health, daughter of **ASKLEPIOS**. Hence *hygiene*, the word for sanitary health, the promotion of healthy habits, cleanliness, etc.

HYMEN It sounds as if there should be a connection between Hymen, the Greek God of Marriage, and the hymen, the virginal membrane, a fold of skin which partially closes the external opening of the vagina and which women were supposed to keep intact until deflowered on their honeymoon. But the Greek word *hymen/humen* originally meant *any* kind of membrane or skin-fold, and Hymen's name was unrelated to it, though he did give his name to the word hymn, which was originally a wedding-song.

As for defloration, I use that old-fashioned word (for what seems now to be an old-fashioned way of losing one's virginity) only to cross-refer the reader to another forgotten word, **FLOWERS**.

HYOID BONE A small U-shaped bone in the neck, from *hyoïdes*, meaning shaped like the letter upsilon. In the Middle Ages it was considered the source of the voice and a hyoid bone that is alleged to have belonged to St. Boniface (b. Crediton, Devon, c. 675, d. Friesland 754 or 755), a saint famous for his eloquent vocal prowess when preaching, is preserved in the Romanesque Saxon church at Brixworth. See **-OID**, the 'in-the-shape-of' suffix.

HYPER/HUPER Greek for over, above, high, something higher than normal. As in hyperthermia, too much heat, too hot (but see below). The Latin equivalent is **SUPER-** or **SUPRA-**.

HYPERTENSION High blood-pressure.

HYPERTRICHOSIS An excess growth of hair, often all over the body (*hyper* or *huper*, above + *tricho-*, the 'hairy' prefix. Also hirsutism and, more dramatically, the werewolf syndrome.

HYPERVENTILATING After a brave train-driver on the London Underground had narrowly averted a collision he said to an interviewer, 'I was hyperventilating like mad'. To the layman, who has copied the expression from sports commentators, this is a posh way of saying 'I was breathing hard'.

HYPNOS/HUPNOS Greek for sleep. See also **SOPOR** and **SOMNUS-** and the deepest sort, **COMA**. The Greek-based equivalent of the Latin **SOMNAMBULIST**, a sleep-walker, is hypnobate. In general the *hypno-* prefix is applied more to matters relating to:

HYPNOSIS An artificially induced sleep, from **HYPO/HUPO**, Greek for below, under, less or lower than normal **HYPER**, above. The difference between hypertension and hypotension is therefore crucial – and is yet another example of how important it is to know the origin or words. The same goes for **HYPOTHERMIA**, a condition afflicting the **GERIATRIC** – who might be even more uncomfortable if they suffered from hyperthermia. See **-IATR(O)-**. Hypodermic means beneath the skin (See **DERM-**).

HYPOCHONDRIA The most common disease known to man – and probably the only one for which no-one has yet succeeded in obtaining legal compensation. Hypochondriacs are convinced they have a dreadful disease, and probably several. Their condition is made worse by an addiction to health-columns in newspapers and magazines and even medical books (though not this one, I hope). Hypochondria literally means 'under the breast-bone' or **STERNUM**. The ancients thought that this was the place where human emotions are generated – and that it was made of gristle, for which the Greek word is **CHONDROS**. See also **COUNSELLING**, **RSI**, **DAY TRIPPERS** and **WHIPLASH**, etc.

HYPOTHERMIA From *hypo*, below, and *therme*, heat. The meaning is self-explanatory, but the word is often used ignorantly in the press (even confused with *hyper*thermia) or employed emotively by politicians when referring to the old, poor or hungry. What may be required is a **CALEFACIENT**.

HYSTER-/HUSTER- From the Greek *hustera*, womb, its removal, hysterectomy (sometimes explained as 'taking away the nursery but leaving the playpen'). Hysteria was originally thought to be a sickness brought on by a malfunction of the reproductive organs, or the 'female' condition in general, and is also misused to describe anything thought to be extremely funny, as in 'You should have heard his lecture. It was *hysterical!*' (See also **DELIRIUM** for alleged happiness); also **-TOM-** and **-ECT-**.

HYSTERICAL FUGUE See **FUGUE**.

I*i*

IANTHINE From Greek *ianthos*, violet-coloured.

IATR(O)- From Greek *iatros*, a physician. Hence the many *-atry* and *-atric* endings, such as paediatrics, podiatrics, psychiatry, etc. The *Oxford English Dictionary* cites an 1843 use of the word iatrarchy, meaning the order or hierarchy of physicians. But **GERIATRIC** should strictly be applied only to people who are both old and *sick*, that is, in need of a doctor. The proper adjective for the old and *healthy* is gerontic. An iatrogenic disease is one said to have been caused by a doctor, by his treatment or prescriptions. See also **EPHEBIATRICS**.

ICP Abbreviation of intracranial pressure.

ICTERUS Jaundice. From Greek *icteros*, a yellowish-green bird, by looking at which persons were supposed to be cured of jaundice. Whether the bird's name came before that of the sickness is not certain.

ICTUS A blow or thrust, hence also the name for a stroke: originally also the heartbeat. From Latin *ictere*, to strike or smite.

ICTUS SOLIS Literally, in Latin, a blow or stroke from the sun – in other words, sun-stroke. Not to be confused with **RICTUS**.

IDIO- The 'self' prefix. See also **AUTO-** and below.

IDIOPATHIC From Greek *idios*, itself + pathos, disease, suffering. An idiopathic disease is one without a known cause.

IDIO(T) Unlike **MORON**, which gained an official definition of mental impairment, the original idiots were reticent and private persons of ancient times who kept themselves to themselves: *idios* means self, own, private. Perhaps it was thought they were foolish not to take part in public affairs but it was not until the 14th century that idiots were considered fools (in English spelt 'idgets', leading to the charming, mild and almost affectionate, term of abuse 'a nidget' – and among Irish people 'eejit' is still used). In medicine the old meaning prevails, as in idiopathic, describing a disease arising by itself in a particular part of the body; and idiosyncratic, of a condition due to an individual's disposition or susceptibility, etc. See also **CRETIN**; **LERESIS**, for foolish talk.

ILEUM Latin for the groin or flank; one of the three portions of the small intestine, prefix *ileo-*.

ILEUS Obstruction of the ileum.

IM- Latin negative prefix, like **IN-**.

IMMUNISATION From Latin *immunis*, free. A process which induces or augments resistance to infectious or contagious disease, e.g. by **INOCULATION** or other methods. It goes back as far as the 18th century and the **COWPOX**, and its annals contain many stories of dedicated and intuitive discovery. The father of modern immunisation is probably Sir Almroth Wright (1861–1947), who founded the Inoculation Department at St. Mary's Hospital, Paddington, London. Mr Michael Reilly writes: 'He was best known for his work on immunisation against typhoid and paratyphoid (TAB inoculations). I trained at St. Mary's in the 1930s – his Inoculation Department is now called the Wright–Fleming Institute of Microbiology – and was privileged to hear Wright's farewell address – a masterly and erudite exposition of what makes a true scientist tick. It was from him that I first heard the term "saltus empiricus", which describes the empirical, imaginative leap that reveals the answer to one's problem, but after which one has to go back and work hard to prove that the answer is correct. Alexander Fleming was his pupil and successor – a nice little man, who taught us bacteriology. He was President of our Swimming Club, having been a swimmer and water-polo player, which I was, too. He was a good but uninspiring teacher. We all learned how to differentiate various types of staphylococci on an agar plate by the use of *Penicillium notatum*, but none of us – and I honestly believe that includes Fleming – realised that his discovery would prove to be a "breakthrough" in the treatment of diseases caused by bacteria'. (Another reminiscence: the present compiler's late and former father-in-law, Dr Rowdon Marrion Fry, was one of Fleming's younger colleagues under Wright in the Bacteriology Department at St. Mary's between 1924 and 1931, that is, during the penicillin period).

IMPETIGO Various pustular skin-conditions, from Latin *impetere*, to assail, attack.

IMPOTENCE Another of those polite, euphemistic abbreviations that have ruined a good and formerly more widely useful word. It comes from Latin *potentia*, power, preceded by the *im-* 'not' prefix and really means *any* loss of power. But today it is used to refer to an adult male's inability to achieve penile erection. The proper term is sexual impotence (alternatively impotency), which may be caused by psychological, anatomical or neuromuscular factors; by exposure to certain chemicals (see **BREWER'S** and **DERBYSHIRE DROOP**), or by the consumption of too much alcoholic drink, which, as Shakespeare said in *Macbeth* ('The Scotch Play'?), '... provokes the desire but it takes away the performance'; or by old age, i.e. **GERONTIC** impotence. Here Shakespeare gets it right again, in *Henry IV Part II*: 'Strange that desire should so many years outlive performance'.

IN- The Latin negative prefix, of which **IM-**, above, is a later modification evolving naturally because it is quicker and easier to say, for example 'immaculate' than 'inmaculate'.

INCUBATION The period between the first symptoms of a (usually infectious or contagious) disease and its full development: Latin *in* + *cubare*, to lie upon, to brood (in the sense of hatching out eggs). Hence also incubus, a nightmare thought to manifest itself in a male spirit or devil that 'lay upon' the sleeper (always female, except presumably in very unusual circumstances) and had sexual intercourse with her: in other words in the man-on-top position. The female equivalent is succubus (from *sub*, beneath + *cubare*, to lie: Latin *succuba*, a whore). There appears to be no 'succubation period', except death itself: to succumb is derived from *sub* + *cumbere*, to sink under pressure or be overwhelmed by it. There is, however, **SUCCUSSION**, which please see, but which is unrelated. See also **PRODROMAL**.

INCUBUS See above. Also **DECUBITUS** and **SUC-CUBUS**.

INCUS Latin for an anvil, and also the name for a component of the middle ear. The **MALLEUS**, or hammer, strikes it.

INFARCT(ION) A localised area of **NECROSIS** resulting from tissue **ANOXIA**. There are various kinds of infarction but the one we laymen hear most about concerns **CORONARY** disease. The word comes from the Latin *infarctus*, a stuffing-up or stuffing-in, an obstruction or interpolation, from *farcire*, to stuff or cram. All the delectable dishes in French cookery described as *farcis* (see also under **CEREBR-**) come from the same word, as does 'forced' – more prop-

erly 'farced' – meat. Even the theatrical farce is related – literally 'stopping the show' (when Beethoven died his last words were reported to be *La commoedia finita est*) but the *Oxford English Dictionary* offers the conjectural information that from the 13th century onwards extemporaneous interludes of buffoonery were interpolated in – or stuffed into – liturgical works in order to amuse worshippers. See also the equally unamusing **EMBOLISM** and **THROMBOS(IS)**.

INFECTIOUS/CONTAGIOUS Often used to mean the same thing but *infection*, strictly, is the transmission of a disease by airborne droplets and/or bacteria, while in *contagion* it is passed on by touch, from the Latin *con* + *tangere*, touch: *contagio*, contact. See also **(THE) PEST** and **INCUBATION** and its potentially entertaining ramifications.

INFESTATION Although Latin *infestare* means to assail, harass or persistently molest, infestation is now understood to refer to an attack by a living organism, and usually one that is bigger than a germ, virus or bacterium, for example a worm or mite.

INFIBULATION The closing-off of part of an opening, usually to prevent sexual intercourse or to make it painful. The assault is practised in primitive, male-dominated cultures (*cultures?*), nearly always on young girls and women, whose **NYMPHAE** are sewn together, leaving just enough of an opening to allow them to menstruate. This is to ensure that they keep their virginity for their future husband, and to increase his pleasure when he first rapes her on their wedding-night (report cases of such operations being illicitly performed in Western countries at the request of immigrants or visitors are not infrequent). Infibulation has also been practised on males to perform the function of a **CHASTITY-BELT** – note that the Latin word fibula means a buckle or clasp – as it prevents both masturbation and full sex. A quotation of 1650 speaks of the 'art of Infibulation, or buttoning up of the Prepuce with a Brasse or Silver button'; and a 1779 reference, taken from the *Monthly Review*, describes '... an operation performed on young boys and singers by the Romans, who used it as a muzzle to human [sexual] incontinence'. See **CIR-CUMCISION** and – for another example of musicians suffering for their art, the **CASTRATION** of singers.

INFLUENZA In 1743 the *London Magazine* reported '...news from Rome of a contagious Distemper raging there called the *Influenza*'. The Italian word is much

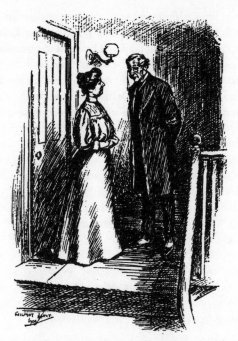

Patient's Wife. "WELL, DOCTOR. I SAY IT'S INFLUENZA.
WHAT'S YOUR HUMBLE OPINION?"

Punch, March 10, 1909

the same as the English 'influence' but means, in addition, a visitation or outbreak; and was short for *influenza di febbre* (an outbreak of fever). In this sense the Italians have used it since the beginning of the 1500s. The French call it **(LA) GRIPPE**. Like the **FRENCH POX** (always a good vehicle for international insults) the flu has usually been blamed on foreigners. But only recently has this been done for good scientific reasons, as international facilities have become available for the local testing of different strains of viruses according to the places in which they occur. Easterners therefore no longer need to feel insulted when Westerners speak of 'Asian flu'.

INGUINAL From Latin *inguen*, groin.

INJURIES/WOUNDS Modern carelessness with language, especially among journalists, has obscured a useful distinction. A soldier who trips over a stone on the parade-ground and sprains his ankle is *injured*. So is a tank-commander who falls off his vehicle while on exercise. But should they be so much as grazed by a bullet in war or insurrection (whether from enemy or 'friendly' fire) they are *wounded*. See also **TRAUMA**.

INOCULATION Literally means 'inserting an eye' (see **OCULUS**) and derived from horticulture, where

it has since at least 1589 meant the placing of a bud or eye (remember potatoes also have 'eyes') of one plant under the bark of another. When, in the early 1700s, the intentional subcutaneous introduction of the smallpox virus was developed, the gardening term was pressed into service.

INSTANT POSTUM A quasi-medicinal 'food drink', or cereal beverage, developed for his own use by the American Charles William Post while convalescing from an illness in 1894, though the Instant element (indicating ready solubility) was added a little later. Room suggests that the *-um* ending may have been intended to suggest a **NOSTRUM**.

INSULIN The 'insular' element in the word comes from the Islets of Langerhans, first described by the German anatomist Paul Langerhans (1847–88) – and ultimately from the Latin *insula*, an island. See also **BANTING** and **DIABETES**.

INTENTION TREMOR A fine, rhythmic, purposeless tremor associated with voluntary movement. See **BASIN**.

INTER Latin for between.

INTERN The comparatively recent American equivalent of what the English (and formerly Americans, too) used to call a houseman – applied to either sex – but officially described as a Junior House Officer: a recent medical graduate working under supervision in a hospital (and often residing there) as part of his training, prior to gaining hospital promotion or becoming a general practitioner. Some of the young doctors performing the arduous duties of a live-in, on-call, intern or houseman may note the semantic closeness of 'intern' to 'internment'.

INTESTINUS Latin for the intestine, for which the Greek is *enteron* – both producing much-used derivations.

IN THE CLUB When an uneducated Englishwoman tells her GP she is 'in the club' she means she is pregnant. The club in question is the 'pudding club' – a popular old euphemism which goes back well into the 19th century but is still used even when no euphemism is intended or expected. Other 19th-century expressions are 'bow-windowed' (c. 1840), 'in the family way' (since 1890), 'in trouble', 'in an interesting condition' and, in places like Liverpool and Glasgow, where many Irish immigrants settled, 'the Irish toothache'.

INTRA- Latin for within. Not to be confused with:–

INTRO- Latin for into.

IN VITRO When applied to fertilisation, one which is achieved 'by test-tube' – see the words for glass, Latin **VITRUM** and Greek **HUALOS (HYALOS)**.

IRIS This part of the eye is so called, rather fancifully, after the Greek goddess Iris, who appeared as a rainbow. It is the iris which determines a person's eye colour – blue, brown, grey, etc.

IRRUMATION See under **FELLARE**.

ISCHIA Latin, from Greek, for the hip-joints or hips. Another Latin name is *coxa*.

ISCHIACUS Latin for 'one who has gout in the hip'.

ISCHION Greek for the hip: see above, and **SCIATICA**.

ISLETIN What **BANTING** at first called **INSULIN**.

ISLETS OF LANGERHANS See the preceding entry and its cross-references.

ISO- The Greek prefix denoting equality. In isodactylism all fingers on one hand are the same length. Lord Smith (violinist as well as surgeon) says that the famous British violinist Albert Sammons owed some of his remarkable technical facility to the fact that he was isodactylic – and having an extremely long little finger is especially helpful in violin-playing. Isograft, an Anglo-Greek word mixture meaning a graft between genetically identical, or isogenic, individuals. For other kinds of graft see also **ALLO-** and **XENO-**. The Latin equivalent of *iso-* is **EQUI-**. For more about fingers in music and other applications see **DIGITUS**.

ISOTONIC Although this has a proper meaning in physiology (meaning, *inter alia*, that all muscles under discussion are equally stretched) the word has been appropriated by the soft-drinks industry and nonsensically applied to 'Isotonic Drinks', which, it is claimed, replenish energy expended by sportsmen and women. The use of proprietary soft-drinks to speed convalescence may deserve closer socio-medico-historical study. For example, in British hospitals the traditional drink brought to patients by friends and relatives has for most of the 20th century been one called Lucozade: no table beside a sickbed is thought to be complete without it. Lucozade, which indeed performs a useful function, has an impeccable medical pedigree. It was invented in about 1930 by a Newcastle upon Tyne chemist, W. W. Hunter, whose daughter was suffering from jaundice and had been advised to take as much glucose and fluid as possible. To make the drink more palatable he developed one containing glucose dissolved in carbonated water, with the addition of citrus flavours. Later he sold the formula and its name to the **BEECHAM** Pharmaceutical Company of St. Helens. Lucozade is even enshrined in English folk-humour. Wounded Soldier in a field hospital: 'I hear we've got a case of syphilis coming in'. Second Soldier: 'Good. It'll make a change from Lucozade'. See also **TONIC**.

ISSUE A rather old-fashioned word for anything that flows out or emerges, e.g. blood, pus, etc., from Latin *exire*, to go out; also for offspring. 'Issues' have unfortunately become an over-used and fashionable word in politics and sociology – gender issues, race issues, etc., *ad nauseam,* and pronounced 'ishoos'. Only a generation or two ago a female worried about 'women's issues' would have been sent to her gynaecologist.

IT Intensive Therapy. See also **HD**.

-ITIS Suffix usually denoting an affection, affliction or inflammation, e.g. cystitis, enteritis, fasciitis, gastritis, etc. But not **PRURITUS**, which is often erroneously written 'pruritis'.

ITU Intensive Therapy Unit.

IUXTA See **JUXTA**.

IV Abbreviation of intravenous.

'I WALKED INTO A DOOR' Every urban GP knows what this usually means when a patient has a black eye. If said by a man it means, 'I was in a brawl', if by a woman, 'My husband/boyfriend beat me'.

J*j*

JAB Slang for an injection, or to inject, probably coined in the first place by the press for its headline-useful brevity but now in almost universal use, though it might occasionally frighten a nervous patient, or child, fearful of a **LITTLE PRICK**.

JEEP-DRIVER'S BOTTOM One of the occupational conditions (for others see **BREWER'S DROOP**) but for this one see under **PILONIDAL SINUS**.

JEJUNUM In full, *jejunum intestinum*, from Latin *jejunus*, empty, fasting, starving: the second part of the small intestine: for the first, see **DUODENUM** – probably because after death (i.e. during **POST-MORTEM**) the upper small bowel is always found to be empty as **PERISTALSIS** continues after the heart stops. In English intellectual jargon *jejune* is a favourite word, used to describe something (usually a work of art) the speaker considers dull, insipid or unsatisfying.

JEWISH PENICILLIN Clear chicken soup, usually made with barley. Jewish mothers traditionally prepare this for invalids, as this **BROTH** is believed to have strong curative powers. There is an old Russian saying, 'If a poor Jewish farmer cooks a chicken, one of them is ill'. See also under **IMMUNISATION** and **PENICILLIN** itself.

JOGGER'S NIPPLE A preventable, easily cured, self-inflicted discomfort first described in the United States, where jogging, like every other health fad, has become a national craze. Further explanation is hardly necessary but if you need to know, Jogger's Nipple is caused by the chafing of insufficiently-supported, bouncing breasts against the fabric of a garment – usually nothing more than a T-shirt. It is aggravated by cold weather, which tends to bring out the **MAMMILLAE** – to their owner's discomfort and some bystanders' delight. What jogging does to pectoral muscles is nobody's business (except their owners'): in heavily-addicted and well-endowed women it is probably responsible for more drooping breasts than childbirth. See also **CELLIST'S NIPPLE**, an occupational complaint rather than a recreational one.

JOHNS HOPKINS American financier and philanthropist who in 1867 gave his name – and $7m – to the hospital and university he founded in Baltimore, MD. It was inaugurated in 1876 and became a noted centre for postgraduate research, especially its Medical School, which was established in 1893. Johns Hopkins (1795–1873) really was called Johns, though he is frequently 'corrected' to 'John'.

J. P. FROG Acronymic code used by American medical persons of some terminally ill **GERIATRIC** patients. It means 'Just Plain F..... Run Out of Gas'. See also **DNR**, **(THE) OLD MAN'S FRIEND** and other euphemisms/abbreviations.

JUGULUM Latin for the collar-bone, from *jugum*, a yoke or collar, for horses or oxen; it therefore means, literally, 'a little yoke'. The five jugular blood-vessels are those near the jugulum. None is indispensable to life unless allowed to bleed uncontrolled, and there is no *one* jugular to 'go for', as the popular saying would have it. However, the opportunities which that part of the body affords to murderers, either by throttling or throat-cutting, produced the words *jugulatio*, murder (by either method), and *jugulo*, I slay – the neck being the most vulnerable part of an adversary, easier to find than his heart. All five jugulars can be safely removed, writes Mr Michael Reilly, who adds, 'I suppose that the assonance between 'jugular' and the 'glug-glug' of impending dissolution impresses the journalists'.

JUNIOR HOUSE OFFICER A newly qualified doctor, provisionally registered for a year after he has taken his final examinations. See also **HOUSEMAN** and **INTERN**.

JUXTA Latin for next-to, adjoining, neighbouring.

K*k*

KAOLIN From the Chinese *kao*, high + *ling*, hill. Also known as China clay, it is used in the manufacture of porcelain and the treatment of **DIARRHOEA**, for which it is a superb remedy, either on its own dissolved in water or in conjunction with some other medicinal substance (e.g. morphine) on prescription: every family medicine cupboard should have some, especially for the nursery.

KARYOKINESIS Not an apparatus you can sing along to but (from Greek *karyon*, nut + *kinesis*, motion) something to do with the division of cell nuclei, for which see a proper medical reference book.

KAUSTIKOS Capable of burning by fire or acid corrosion and the origin of *caustic* prefixes/suffixes. *Holocaust* means 'burn all – everything and everyone'.

KAUTERION A branding-iron, with which the Greeks would mark slaves and animals – hence cautery and cauterize.

KELOID As in a keloid scar: from the Greek *chele*, claw. Cheloid, the older way of spelling it, seems therefore more appropriate. Not related to a keel-like manifestation, for which see **CARINA**.

KERATIN Fibrous proteins that form the chemical basis of horny epidermal tissue, i.e. a corn. It accounts for the second element of 'rhinocerous' – and see **RHIS/RHINOS** for the first.

KERAT(O)- Prefix relating, *inter alia*, to the cornea (a word derived from the same root) – the transparent circular part in the front of the eyeball. From the Greek word for horn, a substance it resembles. The prefix is also used in relation to other horny bits, e.g. on the skin, perhaps the hands (of the 'sons of toil'?). Keratectomy means cutting the cornea – but see under **PRK**.

KERBSIDE CONSULTATION The accosting of a medical man of one's acquaintance, usually the family physician, in the hope of an informal consultation. It happens also at parties and other social gatherings, and not only to doctors – though dentists seem strangely immune to the practice.

God and the doctor we alike adore
But only when in danger, not before
The danger o'er, both are alike requited:
God is forgotten, and the doctor slighted.
 John Owen (?1560–1622) *Epigrams.*

KEYHOLE SURGERY The popular name for a minimally invasive method of surgery described under **LAPAR(O)**.

KINE- *Kinema* is Greek for movement, and led to our cinema, which was often spelt with a *k* in the early picture-palaces. Many words are made with *kine*-prefixes, e.g. kinesthesia, the sense of movement kinanesthesia, lack of awareness of it.

KING EDWARD VII'S HOSPITAL FOR OFFICERS This grandly named institution was founded by two upper-class English nursing-sisters (and sisters in real life) Agnes and Fanny Keyser, at the suggestion of the Prince of Wales, 'whose friendship they enjoyed' – and the Prince enjoyed many female friendships both before and after he became Edward VII. In 1899 the Misses Keyser, keen to 'do their bit' for the Boer War effort, took wounded officers into their house at 17 Grosvenor Crescent, London, to nurse them back to health. As so often happened in British charitable health-care, the institution remained long after the original need had passed, and the King Edward VII is now a large private hospital situated in the West End of London, with a roll of distinguished consultants. It ministers to anyone who can pay its fees or is suitably insured, though officers of the armed forces (serving or retired) and Ministers of the Crown still enjoy special rates. For another manifestation of British upper-class nursing see under **FANNY**; also **HOSPITAL NAMES** and its cross-references.

KITING In the *Oxford English Dictionary* this is given as a slang term used by thieves and their pursuers for the passing of forged cheques. Now it also means, among drug addicts and English NHS scroungers, altering a medical prescription so as to obtain illegally a greater quantity of a drug than was prescribed by the physician.

KJ A test of a patient's reflexes, in the form of a Kneejerk. Also a sardonic description of a person's expected and predictable (nowadays probably also **PC**) reaction. See **KNEEJERK**, below.

KLEPTOLAGNIA Sexual excitement generated by theft (in the thief, not the beholder, still less the

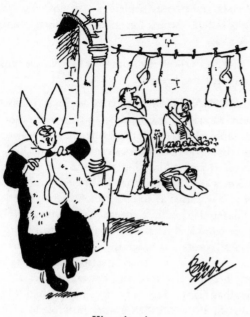

Kleptolagnia

victim), from Greek *kleptein*, to steal and *lagneia*, lust – perhaps a more extreme form of kleptomania, the abnormal, neurotic, recurring urge to steal articles, not for their value or for financial gain but for the thrill: a condition sometimes observed in **MENOPAUSAL** women.

KLEPTOMANIA See above: literally, 'mad about stealing', but apparently without any sex interest.

KNEEJERK The word has almost lost its original meaning related to the familiar test of reflexes and is now used by most people to describe any automatic and predictable reaction. See **GENU-**, under **PAVLOV'S DOG** and **TUNNEL VISION**, and previous page.

KNIFE AND FORK BRIGADE Medical **REP**s' name for **GP**s who make a habit of enjoying as many free meals as possible at the expense of pharmaceutical companies.

KNIFE AND GUN CLUB In inner-city hospitals, the accident and emergency department.

KRUSCHEN SALTS One of many aperient salts formerly popular in the United Kingdom: 'Enough to cover a Sixpence' being the recommended dose. A long-running and successful advertising campaign, with its slogan 'That Kruschen Feeling', captured the British public's imagination and became something of a catch-phrase; and to describe some drastic and rapid action people would say, 'It went like a dose of Kruschen's' (or '...like a dose of Eno's' or simply '...like a dose of salts'). Other patent medicines were/are **ANDREWS LIVER SALTS, ENO'S**, and Dr William Kitchiner's once celebrated **GENTLE PERAMBULATORS** and **PERISTALTIC PERSUADERS**.

KURU 'Trembling Disease' which affects only members of the Fore tribe in New Guinea who ritually eat/ate the brains of their dead, usually of women. Another form of trembling disease is observed among members of the public who give impromptu 'vox pop' interviews on television: they usually punctuate or amplify their statements with rapid, tremulous shakes of the head, a particularly distracting sight in women who wear dangling earrings. For other selectively-racist diseases see **FAVISM, SICKLE-CELL AN(A)EMIA, TAY–SACHS DISEASE** and **THALASS-(ANA)EMIA.**

KYPHOSIS From Greek *kyphos*, crooked, humpbacked: excessive outward curvature of the spine. See also **DOWAGER'S HUMP** – and its accidentally aristocratic-sounding opposite, **LORDOSIS**. Also **SCOLIOSIS**.

L*l*

LABIA Latin for the lips, singular labium, often used as an abbreviated form of *labia pudendi* – 'the lips of shame' – see **PUDENDA**; also **NYMPHAE**.

LACHESIS The name of one of the Three Cruel Fates, who arbitrarily controlled the birth, life and death of man (man in the **HOMO** sense); also the name of a genus of American rattlesnake whose tails are/ were used in **HOMEOPATHY**. The other two Fates were *Clotho* and *Atropos* – for whom see under **ATROPINE**.

LACT- The Latin milk prefix. See **(GA)LACT-**.

LADY ALMONER See **ALMONER**.

LAEVUS Latin, on the left side. See also **SINISTER**.

LAGNEIA Greek for lust – producing the useful suffix -*lagnia* for describing some of the more unusual forms of sexual desire, several of which will be found under their own or related headings, e.g. **HIPPOLAGNIA**, **KLEPTOLAGNIA** and **UROLAGNIA**. The Romans' word for lust was **LIBIDO** but this now seems to have acquired gentler, more **NORMAL**, connotations. See also **MANIA**.

LALA Greek for speech: another word rooted in onomatopoeia, because it mimics the movement of the tongue; 'mama' is the sound of the infant seeking the **MAMMAE**. For 'talking dirty' see under **COPRO-LALIA** and **GILLES DE LA TOURETTE**.

LANDICA The classical Romans' name for the **CLITORIS**.

LAPAR(O)- From Greek *lapara* the flank, itself from *laparos* soft, slack – in effect the soft underbelly. Combined in the usual way with **-(O)TOMY** and **-(O)SCOPY** to denote cutting and looking, respectively. Although the word now suggests a certain specialised modern operation which is performed with the help of fine, illuminating fibre-optic tubes and miniature cameras, the term goes back to the middle of the 19th century and *Laparoskopie* was first coined by a Munich surgeon, H. C. Jakobaeus, in 1910.

LAPSUS A fall or slip, hence prolapse, the falling-forward/slipping-down of any part of the body from its normal position, or a collapse, literally, falling-together. In theology prolapsion was 'a falling or slipping-away into error'. See also the Greek equivalent,

PTOMA and **PTOSIS**, which gave us not only symptoms but also words for death – the final collapse. See **SYM-**.

LARYNG(O)- Prefix from Greek *larynx*, the throat; modern Latin *laryngeus*.

LAUGHING-GAS Nitrous oxide of gazote, discovered in 1799 by the English scientist and inventor Sir Humphry Davy (1778–1829) when he was only 20 or 21. He carried out various experiments on himself, on one occasion 'drinking' 16 quarts of it for nearly 7 minutes and reporting that 'it absolutely intoxicated' him. It was used as an an(a)esthetic which when administered in less than anaesthetising amounts (Davy once completely lost consciousness and had to be revived) produced happiness and giggles – but was soon being abused, causing serious damage to takers' health. The English poet and writer Robert Southey (1774–1843) must have almost had a fit of **GIGGLE-INCONTINENCE** when he wrote to a friend 'Oh Tom! Such a gas has Davy discovered, the gaseous oxide. Oh Tom! I've had some. It made me laugh and tingle in every toe and fingertip: a new pleasure for which the language has no name. Oh Tom! I'm going for more this evening. It makes me so strong and so happy. So gloriously happy.' An addict in the making. Laughing-Gas in its early days became the subject for comic songs. See also **ETHER**.

LAXATIVE An aperient, from the Latin *laxus*, loose, *laxare*, to loosen, when said of the bowels. See also **CATHARTIC** and **CASCARA** as well as other cross-references: **ENO'S** and **KRUSCHEN SALTS,** and **PERISTALTIC PERSUADERS**, etc.

LAZAR Nothing to do with the laser (which is sometimes erroneously written 'lazer') but an archaic word meaning a pitiable and diseased person, e.g. a **LEPER** or sore-ridden beggar. For Shakespeare's use of it, see under **TETTER**. The word is derived from Lazarus, who was raised from the dead, Luke XVI, 20. One of the old English terms for a hospital was Lazarus House (*Lazarett* in current German) and as most of their diseases were contagious, lazars were obliged to carry a Lazarus Clapper to give warning of their approach.

LAZY FRENCH TARTS LIE NAKED IN ANTICIPATION Mnemonic for the order of the nerves that pass through the superior orbital tissue of the skull: Lacrimal, Frontal, Trochlear, Lateral, Nasociliary, Internal, Abducent.

LE See under **LUPUS**.

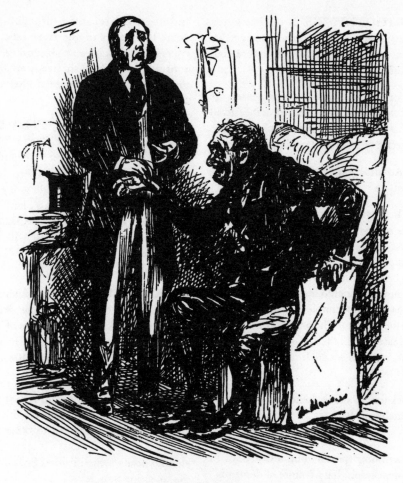

OH, HORROR!

Surgeon. "Your Pulse is still very high, my Friend!
Did you get those Leeches all right I sent the Day before Yesterday?"
Patient. "Yes, Sir, I got 'em right enough. But mightn't I have 'em biled next time, Sir?"

Punch, July 14, 1877

LEECH Usually taken to be a disrespectful nickname for a physician, a transferred term arising mistakenly from the fact that the aquatic blood-sucking worm hirudo or **SANGUISUGA** formerly played an important part in the healing arts. In fact, the transfer is in the opposite direction. Numerous references exist from AD 900 onwards to the leech meaning a physician or healer, in Old Norse and Teutonic languages: modern Swedish has *läka*, to heal, Old Irish *liaig*; and many other related words are listed in the *Oxford English Dictionary*. See also **BLOOD–LETTING** and **CUPPING**.

> *A skilful leech is better far*
> *Than half a hundred men of war.*
> Samuel Butler (1612–1618), English poet.

LEGIONELLA A hybrid, almost **HERMAPHRODITE**, word for a bacterium of the *Legionella* genus. The word combines the last bit of salmon*ella* with the first two syllables of *Legion*nnaire and refers to Legionnaires' Disease, so named after an outbreak of a severe form of bacterial pneumonia in July 1976 among veterans attending a legionnaires' convention in Philadelphia.

LEISHMANIA Nothing to do with madness or **MANIA** but a kind of parasite causing the disease *leishmaniasis*, once common in the tropics and subtropics. It was discovered by a Dr Leishman, who was a Scottish professor and Brigadier in the British Army during the First World War and is therefore pronounced 'Leeshman', not in the German manner sometimes heard.

LEMON-ON-TOOTHPICKS A reference to a certain body-shape of which the term is (exaggeratedly) descriptive, not unlike a **DOWAGER'S HUMP** but caused by cortisone treatment.

LENS Latin for a lentil, whose shape suggested the name for one of the facets of the eye as well as the curved piece of glass that refracts rays of light. In old medicine a lentil was a freckle or other spot on the skin.

LENTIGO An affliction of the skin, from **LENS**, above, via lentil.

LEPROSY The origin of the name of the skin disease leprosy is uncertain, possibly from medieval Latin, but it first occurs in Coverdale's translation of the Bible, (Leviticus XIII, 3). See also **LUPUS**, of which the word may be a corruption. Like **MONGOLS** the word 'leper' is now considered insensitive because of its connotations of untouchable outcasts: 'patients with leprosy' is the **PC** term. The proper medical term is Hanson's disease; or, in the *Oxford English Dictionary, elephantiasis graecorum* – which may offend both elephants and Greeks.

LEPSIS Greek for an attack, hence also a seizure, e.g. epilepsy, catalepsy, etc.

LERESIS The *Concise Oxford Medical Dictionary* says this means 'rambling speech, immature both in syntax and pronunciation. It is a feature of dementia'. Perhaps not only in dementia. Foolish talk is a feature of much of the present impromptu output of radio and television, where it is called, without a hint of irony, 'unstructured speech'. The word comes from the Greek *leros*, silly talk, *lereo*, I speak foolishy. And is it a coincidence or an example of the gruesome humour of officialdom that Europe's most notorious psychiatric camp, the Greek State Therapeutic and General Hospital, is situated on the island of Leros? The 1989 edition of the big *Oxford English Dictionary* does not list the word.

LESION From Latin *laedere*, to hurt: damage or injury, or 'any morbid change in the exercise of functions or the texture of organs'.

LETHAL From Latin *lethum*, death, has a subtly different shade of meaning from 'deadly' and is usually applied to drugs or poisons, e.g. 'a lethal **COCKTAIL**'.

LETHARGY From Latin *lethargia*, itself from Greek and originally meaning forgetfulness: those who drank the waters of the river *Lethe* in Hades ('the Waters of Oblivion') were able to forget the past. Later it meant a dull, sluggish, sleepy apathy or laziness – curable perhaps with a dose of **ENO'S** or **KRUSCHEN SALTS**?

'LET ME THROUGH, I'M A DOCTOR' A quotation from the same collection of apocrypha as 'Come up and see me sometime' and 'Play it again, Sam'. In truth, doctors tend to keep their heads down unless there is a serious accident or emergency): the medical person travelling on a plane or train may be a senior **CONSULTANT** in a **SPECIALTY** far removed from any **A&E** work he last dealt with decades earlier. Today the cry is more likely to be 'Let me through, I'm a counsellor'. Or a lawyer.

LEUK(O)-LEUC(O)- The whiteness prefix, from Greek *leukos*, white. For example, leukocytes, white blood cells; leukaemia, an excess of these, etc., and leukorrhoea, a white discharge ('the whites' or, from the Latin word for white, **CANDIDA**).

LEVATOR From Latin *levare*, to raise: the 'lifting' muscle which raises and constricts the **RECTUM** and therefore maintains continence. With various syllabic additions it is also applied to other muscles of the body, e.g. that which raises the upper lip and/or wrinkles the nose – which Robert Sells says is also called the 'sneering muscle'.

LFT Abbrevition of Liver Function Test – see **TMA**.

LIBIDO The straightforward Latin word for sexual desire, or lust, from *libet*, 'it pleases, it's wonderful, it's lovely!' (well, isn't it?) – but see also the Greek equivalent, **LAGNIA**, which is usually associated with less 'normal' manifestations of desire. Alleged 'loss of libido' is one of the most frequently sued-for conditions, as it is also the feignable and least provable. The loss usually afflicts people after they have suffered alleged **TRAUMA** and is a source of useful income for those looking for an untestable condition for which to claim – see also **AMBULANCE-CHASERS**. For this reason rather than the spread of do-it-yourself sex instruction manuals the word *libido* has entered the public imagination. For another and less commonly used word meaning lust see **CONCUPISCENCE**.

LIENAL Relating to the spleen, for which the Latin is *lien*, Greek **SPLEN**.

LIG- The 'binding' or 'fastening' element, hence words like ligament, ligand, ligases, ligation and ligature, etc. From Latin *ligare*, to bind.

LIP(O)- The 'fatty' prefix, from Greek *lipos*, fat. For example, *lipoma*, a fatty tumour; and the Anglo-Greek hybrid, *liposuction*, for the cosmetic removal of human blubber. See also **-OMA, PINGUESCENCE.**

LIQ. Pharmacists' abbreviation for liquor, a solution.

LIQUAMEN A fluid in which a medicinal substance is suspended to be drunk as medicine. The word has now almost fallen into disuse but recalls the Romans' *liquamen*, which was a sauce made from the raw entrails of fish and used in place of salt. The fish were collected in a vessel and left for weeks to ferment and rot: the resulting liquid would be strained and used as a condiment to give flavour and saltiness to their diet. The ancient South East Asian equivalent (now widely obtainable in the West) is *blachan* or *trasi* – made from prawns or shrimps, salted, dried, pounded and rotted. The modern descendant of these, and liquamen, would be anchovy sauce, or canned anchovies ground and liquefied in their own oil, perhaps with a dash of dark soya sauce.

LISTERELLA Another possibility for a pretty girl's name like **LISTERIA**, below, **MYRINGA**, and numerous others. The name – an alternative for **LISTERIA** – was coined in 1927 by J. H. Pirie, who wrote, 'I propose the specific name *hepatolytica*, and the generic name *Listerella*, dedicating it in honour of Lord Lister, one of the most distinguished of those connected with bacteriology whose name has not been commemorated in bacteriological nomenclature'.

LISTERIA A bacterium (formerly called **LISTERELLA** – above) also named after the eminent English surgeon Joseph (later Lord) Lister (1827–1912), who demonstrated that carbolic acid was an effective antiseptic agent, decreasing post-operative deaths from infection. It was called Listerian Antiseptic Surgery and the carbolic disinfectant, whose odour was once so noticeable in hospitals, Listerine. Lister was, however, influenced by the work Louis Pasteur carried out four years earlier. Lord Smith says that Lister's Day Books in the Royal College of Surgeons show that he observed the bactericidal effect of mould before, and unknown to, Sir Alexander Fleming (see **PENICILLIN** and cross-references).

LITH(O)- The prefix denoting a stone, Greek *lithos*

– Latin **CALCULUS**. In certain connotations used as a suffix, *-lith*.

LITHOTOMY Purists say that this should really be *lithectomy*, as the stone is cut out – see **-TOM-**, not into. The 17th-century French composer Marin Marais (1656–1728) composed a *Lithotomy Sonata* – full title *Le Tableau de l'Opération de la Taille* – describing the procedure for the cutting of the stone and including a kind of running-commentary text descriptive of the surgeon's actions as well as the patient's demeanour. In 1658 the English diarist Samuel Pepys (1633–1703) underwent a similar operation – and thereafter annually celebrated its successful outcome with a party, which he called his 'Stone Feast'.

LITHOTRIPSY From Greek **LITH(O)-**, stone + *triptikos*, to rub or wear away. Modern lithotripter (also lithotriptor) machines work by the application of non-invasive, extra-corporeal shock-waves that break up stones; but the word goes back to the late 1830s, when a lithotriptor would be introduced into the body to rub away or crush stones. The procedure itself is even earlier, and the *Oxford English Dictionary* quotes a manual of 1846: 'In the year 1827, when lithotripsy was yet in its infancy'.

LITTLE PRICK Facetious euphemism for an injection and, an old medical joke. As early as the 18th century there was a three-part catch (i.e. part-song) about it, composed in 1770 for the 23rd anniversary of the Catch Club by Dr Francis Hutcheson (1721–80), an Irish doctor–composer:

> *Mother: Oh Doctor, Oh Doctor, I'm terrify'd out of my wits!*
> *Poor Nancy my Daughter is fall'n into Fits.*
> *But you come, Dear Doctor, just in the Nick, etc.*

to which the Doctor sings in reply:

> *The first Step in cases like this to be sure,*
> *is breathing a Vein: I'll engage for a cure*
> *If you'll let me but give her a Prick... etc. etc.*

LIVERPOOL SLIPPER A form of bedpan pioneered in 1836 by doctors and nurses at the Liverpool (Royal) Northern Hospital (founded in 1833, closed in the late 1980s) and made of the finest porcelain by the Thomas Minton pottery company of Stoke-on-Trent. From the 1830s onwards until the advent of the disposable bedpan, receptacles of this kind were described as of the 'Liverpool shape', though differently shaped bedpans had previously been made by Wedgwood. A surviving Liverpool Slipper in my possession (another is preserved in the Liverpool Museum's collection) is inscribed 'The Bed Slipper of Liverpool Northern Hospital 1836' and under its glaze gives printed instructions for use: 'The slipper must not be inserted under the side of the body as the common bedpan but be passed under in front. A flannel cap for the toe part [of the Slipper] held on by strings round the heel will afford access with comfort to the patient'. Most of the remaining instructions are worn away but they end with the words '...comfort will be afforded to the Patient'. Among other Liverpool medical 'firsts' are several important innovations in social medicine, hastened perhaps by Liverpool's unenviable reputation as the most unhealthy city in Victorian England, largely through uncontrolled mass-immigration of destitute Irish famine victims, who in the space of 10 years doubled the city's population. In 1846 Liverpool appointed the first municipal Medical Officer of Health, Dr W.H. Duncan, who worked in the South Dispensary (a perfectly-proportioned early Georgian building destroyed in the 1980s by municipal **MORONS**). Liverpool opened the first Municipal Wash-house and Public Baths in 1842. To this pioneering work in public health must be added important early discoveries in tropical medicine and orthopaedic surgery. See also **MANCHESTER** and **GLASGOW**.

LMF Abbreviation used in time of war for what to-day's litigious civilians (and, increasingly, members of the armed forces) call **POST-TRAUMATIC STRESS DIS-ORDER/SYNDROME**, which please see. LMF stands for Lack of Moral Fibre and may appear thus in the patient-files of some of the more candid family physicians, especially those who served in the forces.

LOBOTOMY Although this appears to be an example, like **LUMPECTOMY**, of the mixing of English with Greek or Latin, the English 'lobe' does in fact come from Greek, via Latin *lobus*, so this description of a form of brain surgery is etymologically sound.

LOCUM Short for *locum tenens*, which is Latin for 'one who acts for another', and also gave us the lieutenant, which (like so many warlike terms) comes from French: *lieu*, place + *tenant*, holding – one who holds the place of another.

-(O)LOGY One of the commonest and most useful suffixes, from Greek *logos*, word but embracing also knowledge.

LORDOSIS This has nothing to do with the British titled aristocracy or Lords of the Realm. It is named from the Greek *lordos*, meaning bent backwards; and is, curiously enough, a kind of mirror-image condition of **KYPHOSIS** (i.e. anterior curvature of the spine, producing convexity in front) which British doctors in a certain manifestation call **DOWAGER'S HUMP**.

LOT. Pharmacists' abbreviation for Latin *lotio*, lotion. See **LIQUAMEN**, above, and **LOTIUM**, below.

LOTIUM Latin for urine, especially when stale. The Romans understood the cleansing power of the ammonia it generates and used it for washing clothes – hence the ingenious layout of Roman urinals, which were designed for recycling this plentiful material. Men would stand on the *outside* and urinate *in* – through conduits or channels that conveyed the liquid into the building. This doubled as a laundry, where togas would be soaked in lotium (and, one hopes, afterwards well rinsed in plain water, especially those worn by **CANDIDATES** for office) – perhaps the first 'cottage' industry – and it puts a different – and older – complexion on the familiar saying about the principle of giving corporate jobs to potential enemies or critics: 'Better to have him *inside* pissing *out* than outside pissing in'. Effective, chemical-based soap as we know it had yet to be invented in Roman times (though they had a cleansing substance called *sapo*) and barbers (i.e. barber-**SURGEONS**) as late as the Middle Ages still applied lotium to the hair as a kind of shampoo: old English plays are full of lotium jokes against barbers and surgeons. Lotium was also known as **LYE** (i.e. urine used for its detergent alkaline qualities: alkali = lye), or else 'chamber-lye' (urine from chamber-pots): 'We leak in the chimney; and our chamber-lye breeds fleas like a loach' (Shakespeare: *Henry IV Part I*); an earlier authority quoted in the *Oxford English Dictionary* defines the three substances as one: 'Locium, lye or pysse'. And another passing-note: the delightful 17th-century English diarist Samuel Pepys was given to 'pissing into the chimney', as the fire neutralised unpleasant odours. Shakespeare echoed the practice of urine-conveyance by conduit in *Henry VI Part II* (though with particular reference to one in the City of London which was used only as a urinal, not a Roman-style laundry): 'I charge and command, that of the Cities cost the pissing conduit run nothing but Clarret Wine'.

LOVER'S BALLS An often **EXQUISITE** testicular pain, perhaps associated with a temporary inability to pass urine and also known as 'Petting Pain'. It is experienced by boys and men during or after a 'heavy petting' session involving prolonged erection but no ejaculation (constricting clothing may also play a part): in other words, foreplay which is not succeeded by play – an overture without the opera, a prelude but no fugue. The condition probably gave us the vulgar expressions 'balls-aching' and 'ball-breaking', for anything considered painfully tedious. There appears to be no classical name for it, so perhaps the ancients, who wore fewer clothes, did not suffer from it, although 17th- and 18th-century English love poetry is full of delicate pleas from swains asking nymphs to 'ease my pain and give me relief' (an appeal to **ONAN** would also do the trick). It might, however, be classed as a form of orchitis (see **ORCHIS**). According to Dr Stephen Lock the condition is now rare, as 'we live in an era of instant consent'. The manifestation on the neck of one or both participants of a **SPAMMIE** may be a feature.

LUB-DUP Sometimes written 'lubb-dupp': the normal heart-sounds as heard through a stethoscope, coinciding with the closure and opening, respectively, of heart valves.

LUBRICITY From Latin *lubricus*, smooth, slimy and slippery (hence lubrication). More often used figuratively and opprobriously than medically – e.g. when referring to an allegedly lubricious person's elusive shiftiness – but Andrew Boorde's *Breviarie of Health* (1547) has 'lubricite of humours in the matryx' and Dr Johnson (1755) wrote of 'lubricity of the bowels'.

LUES See **LYSIS**. Luetic is the same as syphilitic, which see under **SYPHILIS**.

LUMBAGO This, with other *lumb-* words, comes from Latin *lumbus*, a loin. The Romans suffered from something they named *lumbago* but which Julius Paulus in AD 200 defined as '*vitium et debilitas lumborum*' – 'a twisted and weakened loin'. See also **SCIATICA**.

LUMPECTOMY Polyglot formation from the English word *lump* + the Greek **-ECTOMY**: the removal of a lump. According to the *Oxford English Dictionary* it was coined in Canada in 1972, but Mr Robert Sells writes, 'I suspect earlier than this, by Mr (later Sir) Geoffrey Keynes, bibliophile and biographer, and (almost incidentally) consultant surgeon at Barts, the first man to perform a simple lumpectomy instead of radical mastectomy'.

LUNATIC The discredited word for someone suffering from impaired mental health and probably confined to a Lunatic Asylum. The word originated in the days when the moon and its phases, especially full-moon, were thought to induce temporary or permanent madness. For other brutal, catch-all hospital descriptions see under **HOSPITAL NAMES** and **STD**.

LUPUS Latin for 'wolf'. From the middle ages it was the colloquial word for various skin diseases, some possibly **LEPROSY**: 'Lupus is a malignant vlcer quickly consuming the neather parts and it is verie hungrie like vnto a woolfe'. (Barrough, 1590), quoted by the *Oxford English Dictionary*. The name now indicates a tubercular infection of the skin and comes with added qualifications, e.g. lupus erythematosus (LE) verrucosis and vulgaris – for which see a proper medical treatise.

LURGY 'A fictitious, highly infectious disease invented (?) and made a byword by the Radio Goons', says the *Oxford English Dictionary*, but draws attention to a possibly related word for idleness, 'feverlurgy' or 'feverlargie', defined in 1808 as 'Two stomachs to eat, and none to work'. Now often heard when speakers describe any suspected infection (usually their own) for which they have no explanation ('I must have picked up a lurgy...'). See also **ALLERGY**.

LYE The limpid fluid which runs from a blister, or the 'water' which collects in the body when a person has the **DROPSY**. For another meaning see **LOTIUM**.

LYMPHA The Greek equivalent of the Latin *limpidus*, or clear water, sometimes water in general, or a stream – hence both lymph and the poets' limpid brooks, etc.

LYSIS/LUSIS Greek *lysein*, to loosen, to break down, hence analysis – often called, literally and correctly, a breakdown (see the **ANA-** prefix). The Latin equivalent is **LUES** – a plague, one that causes the breaking-down of tissue with consequent disfigurement. *Lues venerea* is an old name for syphilis.

LYSOL A creosote-based, water-soluble disinfectant patented in 1891 (but now in the public domain), its name a combination of **LYSIS/LUSIS** above, and the -ol suffix denoting oil.

LYSOZYME From Greek *lysein* (above) + *zyme*, ferment. An enzyme having antiseptic actions that destroy some organisms foreign to the body. Normally present in saliva, tears, sweat and breast milk.

M*m*

M'NAGHTEN RULES In psychiatric medicine, a rule about criminal insanity determining whether an accused person is responsible for his actions. Named after Daniel McNaghten, who was tried for murder in 1843 and acquitted on a plea of insanity. Pedants often insist that his name should be written McNaghten but the substitution of a single apostrophe for the c in 'Mc' is merely a 19th-century typographical quirk: McNaghten is intended.

MACRO- The large-size prefix: Greek *makros* means long, big or large.

MACROBIOTICS Now usually applied to food that claims to be 'whole', unadulterated and 'organically' grown, but this definition is an invention of the health-food industry. Macrobiotic literally means 'long life' (makros, *long* + *bios*, life), with the implication of prolonging it – whether by good doctoring or a healthy lifestyle. Ludwig van Beethoven was interested in the subject (who is not?) and in 1820 owned a book called *Die Makrobiotik* by Dr Christoph Wilhelm Hufeland (1762–1836), then in its 3rd edition, published in Berlin in 1820), which recommended among other measure the consumption of 'three or four whole white peppercorns to aid the digestion'. Beethoven lived to be 56 years and three months, having drunk too much, eaten unwisely, been constantly angry with the world and a regular visitor to whorehouses. General life-expectancy among males in Biedermeier Vienna was about 45 years, so he did not do badly, though not as well as Hufeland himself. But Beethoven was a moderate pipe-smoker, hated passive smoking and avoided smoke-filled taverns whenever he could. See also **BIO-/(BIOT)** and **MICRO-**.

MACULE A spot, or blemish, pimple or zit, for which the Latin is *macula*. In spite of the *-a* ending the word is singular (as is **VERTEBRA**) so the plural is *maculae*. However, all suggestion of pedantry would be avoided if we were to use the old English colloquial form mackle (plural mackles), which the *Oxford English Dictionary* describes as 'obsolete'. With the **IM-** negating prefix we get immaculate, spotless, as in virgins and the allegedly **PARTHENOGENIC** conception. See also **MOLE**.

MAD COW DISEASE The popular, certainly easier to spell, name of bovine spongiform ecephalopathy.

MADNESS One of the oldest English names for mental illness, now not only superseded by more specific terms but also devalued by popular American usage in which 'I am mad' means 'I am angry'.

MAGIC BULLETS Journalists' cliché useful for describing scientific medical treatment, usually radiotherapy making use of isotopes and 'bombardment' with particles. But the expression was first used in 1910 by the German Nobel Prizewinner Dr Paul Ehrlich (1854–1915) the discoverer of a diphtheria antitoxin and of **SALVARSAN**, which was helpful against **SYPHILIS**. Magic Bullets also appear, tangentially, under the heading **WEBER'S TEST**.

MALARIA This insect-borne disease was at first thought to be caused by 'bad air': *mal* + *aria*. Not to be confused with 'bad singing' (a different kind of air!) or halitosis ('bad breath'), for which see under **HALITUS**. And see also **MILARIA**. See also **QUININE**, an ancient Peruvian remedy for it.

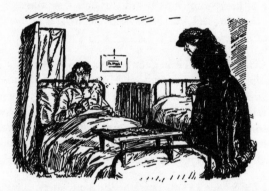

VISITOR. "BUT THOSE ATTACKS OF MALARIA DON'T LAST LONG DO THEY?"
TOMMY. "MINE ISN'T ORDINARY MALARIA. THE DOCTOR CALLS IT 'MALINGERING MALARIA' "

Punch, January 29, 1919

MALINGERER From French *malingre*, sickly, ailing (and an earlier English definition of *malingre* was 'ugly, scabby, loathsome'); but unlike the **HYPOCHON-DRIAC**, who *believes* he is ill, the malingerer knows he is not. He merely pretends to be unwell (sometimes hoping to persuade his doctor that a condition of which he has in fact been cured is still afflicting him) perhaps to escape duty or work: a likely case of **PLOMBOSCILLOSIS**. The British Welfare State and the ever-increasing ingenuity of claimants for industrial and other injuries who threaten to overwhelm the **NHS** have brought about a veritable epidemic of malingering. **GPs'** notes about some *malade imaginaire* may contain a coded abbreviation recording their only recommended treatment: **TTFO**. See also **BED-HOPPERS** and **MÜNCHHAUSEN SYNDROME** – and Abram-men under **BEDLAM**.

MALLEUS A hammer, and the name of a bony component in the ear. See also **INCUS**.

MALUM Latin for bad, evil, misfortune, calamity, injury, etc. – hence malformations, etc. But it also means 'apple' – which has led to countless Latin puns and, doubtless, early medical jests. Benjamin Britten immortalised it in music, in Miles's song to the Governess in *The Turn of the Screw*, after Henry James.

MAMMA(E) Latin for the breast(s); *mammillae*, literally 'little breasts', for which see a separate entry under **NIPPLE(S)**, also **AREOLA**. 'Mamma' doubtless preceded the invention of language, as it is formed from the instinctive sucking motions of the lips as they seek milk from the mammillae. ('Dada' and 'papa' come slightly later in their development – see also **PAPILLA(E)**). Mammoplasty is plastic surgery to the breast, mammography an X-ray or other photographic investigation. See also **JOGGER'S NIPPLE**, above, and **MAST(O)-**, below.

MAMMILLAE Literally a small breast but see the entry above. See also the analogous papilla(e).

MANCHESTER OPERATION Or the Manchester Repair, of a prolapse of the womb (see also **LAPSUS**) developed in Manchester. Another northern-English contribution to medicine is a bedpan called the **LIVERPOOL SLIPPER**, and there is the **GLASGOW COMA SCALE**.

MANCINISM From Italian *mancino*, left-handed, the state of being so. See also **LAEVUS** and **SINISTER**.

MANDIBLE The large bone constituting the lower jaw is named after the Latin *mandere*, to chew.

MANE Pharmacists' direction: 'in the morning'.

MANIA Greek for madness. See also **LAGNIA**.

MANU- The hand prefix, from Latin *manus*, the hand – see **CHEIR-** for the Greek equivalent – and **SURGEON**.

MAPLE SYRUP URINE DISEASE An anomaly in amino acid metabolism which gives the urine an odour like maple syrup. Under **MENU CONDITIONS** will be found other unappetising namings. It is also called the Menkes Syndrome.

MARKETING MANAGER According to a news item printed in the *Daily Telegraph* on July 29, 1992, such a post is held by a **GREY SUIT** at St. Anthony's Hospital, Cheam, in the South of England. Its existence is perhaps not as inappropriate as may at first appear, as the entrance-halls of most large hospitals now resemble shopping malls; but at St. Anthony's the hapless marketing manager proposed making the 'environment' more user-friendly for heart patients by piping rock 'music' to them, and was reported as saying that 'it is very pleasant and serves to relax patients'. His colleagues in Psychiatry might have told him that loud and repetitive drum rhythms raise the heartbeat rate and increase the flow of **ADRENALINE** (something leaders of armies have known since the dawn of time, and organisers of rave parties know today). Rock music is the last thing (and might well *be* the last thing) to inflict on heart patients, especially that of a group which the Marketing Manager favoured, appropriately called 'The Stranglers': see the origin of the word **ANGINA**.

MARSUPIALISATION An operative technique for curing a **CYST** by creating a pouch-like opening. From Greek *marsupion*, a purse (the English sense, a small container for money, not a handbag, as has become the American meaning).

MASTECTOMY See the entry below, as well as the **TOM-** 'cutting' prefix. Also, for an early reference to it, under **DUODENUM**.

MAST(O)- The breast prefix. Greek for breast is *mastos*, in Latin *mamma* – see above. Hence, with the **-OID** 'in-the-shape-of' suffix:–

MASTOID Literally, in the form of the female breast: 'a nipple-shaped, conical prominence of the temporal bone', the bony protuberance behind the ear.

MASTURBATION 'The primary sexual activity of mankind and some of the higher animals. In the nineteenth century it was a disease; in the twentieth, it's a cure', said the American psychiatrist Thomas Szasz (in his book *The Second Sin*, 'Sex', 1973) – or else, in the words of the entertainer Woody Allen, 'Don't knock it, it's sex with someone you love'; and indeed, like no other human activity, it has progressed from the sinful to the therapeutically recreational. The word is a corruption of mastrupation, itself a contraction of manustupration, which you will find mentioned as 'self-abuse' in the entry on **ABUSE** and under **STUPRATION** as 'hand-rape' (note the **MANU-** manual prefix); and also referred to under **ONAN**. The 17th-century English antiquary and gossip John Aubrey (1626–97) relates an incident involving the philosopher Thomas Hobbes and his pupil, the young Duke of Buckingham: 'Mr Hobbes told me, that G(eorge) Duke of Buckingham had at Paris when about twenty yeares old, desired Him to reade Geometrie to him: his Grace had great naturall parts, and quicknesse of witt; Mr Hobbes read; and his Grace did not apprehend, which Mr Hobbes wondered at: at last, Mr Hobbes observed that his Grace was at mastrupation, his hand in his Codpiece. This is a very improper age...'

MATERIA MEDICA In Latin literally, 'medical matters', and often used as a generic title in books and articles about medicine. It comes from the writings *De Materia Medica* by the Greek botanist Pedanios Dioscorides, compiled in about AD 55, which lists the properties of some 600 medicinal plants and animal products with alleged dietetic or medicinal value. Dioscorides served as a surgeon in Nero's army.

MATRON Until the late middle of the 20th century, and for some years beyond, this was the senior nurse in a British hospital, but the post was renamed in the interest of sexual equality **CHIEF** or **PRINCIPAL NURSING OFFICER**. The Latin *matrona* means a mother or married woman, literally 'big mother'.

MATULA Classical and medical Latin for a chamber-pot, *matula vas urinae*. See also **CHAMBER-POT PRACTICE**.

MAXILLA Latin for the jaw, used in various forms and prefix adaptations. The Greek is *gnatho*, which please see for a curious theory: **GNATHOS**.

ME (Pronounced as separate letters, M.E., not 'me'): **MYALGIC ENCEPHALITIS**.

MEATUS Latin, from *meare*, to flow or pass: a natural channel or tubular passage, an opening. The prefix is *meato-*.

MEDIC In Britain generally a medical student or **INTERN**, whereas in America this can also mean a member of a military medical corps, a physician or surgeon.

MEDICARE The United States equivalent of the British NHS, or at any rate part of it. The Medicare Act was signed by President Johnson on July 30th 1964 at Independence, Mo., and was the first government-operated health-insurance scheme for Americans aged 65 or over.

MEDICASTER An old English word for an incompetent physician, a pretender to medical skill, a **QUACK, CHARLATAN** or **STERCORARIAN**. A feminine form, medicastra, also exists. The word occasionally occurs in English literature from 1602 but unfortunately fell into disuse in the 19th century. Anyone embarking on a polemic against his colleagues might find it worth reviving. The *-aster* ending seems always to have indicated incompetence, or at any rate belittlement, most commonly in the 17th and 18th centuries, when many a poet was ridiculed by critics as 'a mere poetaster'– though, of course, they might themselves have been criticasters. Alas, the same process cannot be applied to weather forecasters, tempting though it may be, for it is a different formation.

MEDIO-. MEDI- The Latin prefixes indicating 'middle'. See **MESO-, MES-, MESIO-** for the Greek.

MEDULLA Latin for pith or marrow, probably from *medius*, middle, and therefore used in different applications to distinguish the inner region of any organ, etc. when different from the outer.

MEGA(LO)- From the Greek word for big, great. Hence megalomania, a form of madness involving delusions of grandeur.

MELA(N)(O)- The 'blackness' prefix. Melancholia, or a 'black' depression, comes from the conjunction of Greek *melas*, black + *chole*, bile – for the bile was thought to be the seat of man's mood-changes: more specifically, and according to the ancient theory of humours, an excess of black bile was characteristic of a melancholic temperament. Melanoma (*mela* + the *-oma* 'tumour' suffix) refers to the often dark-coloured aspect of skin-cancers. See also **CHOL(E)-**.

MELOS Greek for a limb. Not to be confused with *melas*, in the previous entry.

MEMBRANA Latin for the skin that covers the body; also for thin sheets of tissue, or membranes, that cover some parts of it.

MENARCHE Combined from the Greek *men*, month/moon and *archaios*, from the beginning: the onset of menstruation (see **MENSES**). The word *looks* as though it should be pronounced in the French manner but it was in fact coined by a German doctor, E. H. Kisch, in 1900, as a professional euphemism. He would have pronounced it 'men-arkay', which is still appropriate (not 'main-arsh'). The 'men' prefix has nothing to do with the male of the species (as even the *Bias-free Word Finder* accepts), but some feminists, who prefer to call themselves 'wimmin' or 'womyn' to avoid the 'men' syllable, also dislike the first syllable of *men*struation.

MENDELISM The concept of heredity as applied in the laws of the pioneering Austrian geneticist, Gregor Johann Mendel, 1822–84). A popular definition is enshrined in a limerick about a young fellow named Starkie, 'who had an affair with a 'darkie'. The result of his sins were quadruplets, not twins: one black and one white and two khaki'.

MENINX Greek/Latin for a membrane. Prefix *mening-*, producing meningitis when it is inflamed.

MENISCUS The medical Latin name for curved fibrous cartilege in the knee and other joints is derived from Greek *meniskos*, a crescent, which is the diminutive of *men*, moon.

MENOPAUSE From Greek *men*, moon, hence *mene*, month + *pausis* (Latin *pausa*, also from the Greek, *pauein* to stop, cease). The English word 'pause', for a temporary cessation, is therefore a modified derivation. See also **CLIMACTERIC**.

MENS, MENTIS Latin for the mind, hence mental. But see also the other 'mental', under **MENTUM** below.

MENOPAUSE/MENSES/MENSTRUATION From the Greek and Latin words for the moon and the month (see above). As stated, there is no connection whatever with *men*, and suggested alternatives are based on ignorance. As with the **(FRENCH) POX**, nations use menstruation as an opportunity for flinging abuse at each other. According to *Vocabula Amatoria*, a French woman unavailable to her lover would say to him, 'Not tonight, my dear, the English have landed' *(Il n'a a pas moyen ce soir, mon cheri: les Anglais ont débarqué)* and the *Vocabula* helpfully explains that this is 'in allusion to the colour of the uniform of English soldiers'. When the English redcoats went into khaki the

expression would have fallen into disuse – or else drastically changed its meaning. The French also provided the English euphemism 'flowers', from *flueurs*, itself from Latin *fluere*, to flow. Others include 'the curse' (i.e. that which God brought down on Eve), the 'monthlies', the 'monthly courses', 'feeling poorly' or, most commonly, 'having a period'. In Liverpool slang the saying is, 'I've got the painters in' or, 'I got visitors'; or, when periods have been missed, 'I haven't had no visitors for eight weeks, doctor'. In response to which those unfamiliar with the local argot may send them for counselling to alleviate their loneliness. (Another Liverpudlianism will be found under **H(A)EMMORRHAGING**). A report from an Edinburgh hospital says that Scottish women say, 'I haven't seen anything for three months, doctor' – possibly risking referral to the ophthalmologist; and I am told that women students at Oxford University would say they were 'laying an egg'.

MENTUM Latin for the chin, producing the word mental in its less usual meaning, of and pertaining to the chin. Thus 'mental deficiency' could mean a sub-average intelligence function – or chinlessness.

MENU CONDITIONS See under **BEER BELLY, CHERRY ANGIOMA, COFFEE GROUNDS, CORNED BEEF RASH, CRANBERRY JELLY STOOLS, MAPLE SYRUP URINE, PIGEON CHEST, PIGEON TOES, PORT-WINE STAIN, PRUNE BELLY SYNDROME, RICE WATER STOOLS, SPAMMIE, STRAWBERRY GALLBLADDER, STRAWBERRY N(A)EVUS, STRAWBERRY NOSE** and, if you can bear to, **SMEGMA**. See also **PATELLA**, for a relation of the delectable Spanish rice dish paella. All the foregoing perhaps washed down with **CAFÉ AU LAIT SPOTS**. But 'mulibrey', as in **MULIBREY NANISM**, is not a misprint for 'mulberry'.

MERCURY The son of Zeus, and the Greek Messenger of the Gods, and therefore God of Communications, Commerce – and Thievery. He was also known as **HERMES**. His son by **APHRODITE** was the first **HERMAPHRODITE**. See also **HATTER'S SHAKES** and **VENUS** for the substance named after him.

MERDA The old Latin word for excrement. It was used by medieval English doctors: '...for this sekenese take merde of a dove...' (1486) and, in an epigram of 1587 they recommend a drastic way of ridding oneself of the smell of garlic, which was – by some still is – taken medicinally: 'If after thou of Garlike strong/

The sauour wilt expell/ A Mard is sure the onely meane/ To put away the smell'. This might almost be an example of **AROMATHERAPY** before its time, or else a kind of **BEZOAR**. The French have not forgotten *merda*, for they use *merde* both as description and an exclamation – and the English might well revive it: 'merd' would make a change from the starker 'turd' and cause less offence than 'shit'. But see also **STERCUS, CLOACA** and **CLOACINA**.

MESMERISM A form of hypnosis pioneered in the 18th century by the Austrian physician Franz Anton Mesmer (1734–1815), who produced states of genuine insensibility to pain, rigidity of the body, etc. He also thought he could cure the sick by holding magnets over them to 'draw' sickness from their bodies. Mozart makes fun of this in the opera *Cosi fan tutte*, in which the spinning of magnets is accompanied and illustrated by frenzied trills on the woodwind. Magnetism and its allegedly curative or preventive properties never left the public's consciousness and returned scientifically with the introduction of **MRI**, or Magnetic-Resonance Imaging, and people still and some claim to feel better for wearing copper bracelets. For another survivor see **GALVANISM**.

MESO-, MES-, MESIO- The Greek prefix indicating the middle, producing numerous anatomical and medicinal terms – remember that Mesopotamia is '(the land) *between* two rivers, the Euphrates and Tigris'. The equivalent Latin prefix is *medio-*.

META- This widely used Greek prefix expresses the notions of sharing, having action in common, pursuit, quest or change: not unlike the Latin *trans-*.

METACARPUS From Greek *meta*, above + *karpos*, wrist. The middle portion of the hand, five slender bones numbered from the thumb side, I to V.

METAPHRASIS Again from *meta*, above + *phrasis*, speech: originally a linguistic term but applicable to the **SPOONERISM**.

METATARSUS From Greek *meta* + *tarsos*, plate: the group of five long bones of the foot lying between the **TARSUS** and the toes. **METATARSUS VARUS** is more popularly known, and better explained, as **PIGEON TOES**, while metatarsus valgus is the opposite condition.

METATARSUS VALGUS A congenital deformity of the foot in which the forepart rotates outwards – the opposite of

METATARSUS VARUS See **PIGEON TOES**.

METRA Greek for the uterus, related to *mater*, mother. Hence endometrium.

METRON Greek for a measure. From this are derived various formations, including emmetropic, ametropic and hypermetropic – normal, defective and excessive size (respectively) of the eye.

MIASMA The Greek word for pollution, infectious, noxious or putrid exhalations. Early Victorians thought miasmata caused **CHOLERA**. Purists say that the only correct plural is *miasmata* but 'miasmas' is commonly accepted.

MICRO- From the Greek *mikros*, small – a prefix with many hundreds of applications both ancient and modern. The *mini-* prefix, on the other hand, dates from only about 1930, when the piano manufacturers Eavestaff & Co. produced their famous Minipiano: the miniskirt and mini car did not arrive until the early 1960s, to turn the prefix into a craze. See also **TABLOID** and **MACRO-**.

MICROBE Any micro-organism, whether **BACTERIUM** or **VIRUS**. The word literally means 'small living thing', from *mikros* (above) + *bios*, life.

MICROMELIA From *mikros*, small + *melos*, limb: insufficiently developed hands/arms or legs/feet. See also **AMELIA** and **PHOCOMELIA**.

MICTITION Latin *mictionem*, also *minctionem*, from *mingere*, the action of urinating. Hence also minge, a now rare dysphemism for the female pudenda. See also the **UR-** prefix. Not to be confused with:–

MICTURITION The *desire* to pass urine, or a morbid frequency in the voiding of it. For the plain, uncomplicated action see above.

MIGRAINE The word for the old enemy which so many people carry in their head comes from the Greek-based *hemikrania*, literally 'half of the head', because symptoms often include a headache on one side of the **CRANIUM** (see also **SODA**). Older English forms include (the) megrim(s) – which was the main headword in the original edition of the *Oxford English*

Dictionary. It also lists magryme, maigram, megroome, migrimme, mygrine, migraime, migramme, mygrane ... altogether some 30 variants. Probably more than the Eskimo have for snow.

MILARIA Prickly heat, and the name of the small skin eruptions that look like millet-seeds, for which the Latin is *milium*. It should really be written miliaria, which would avoid a possible confusion with malaria. Another version appeared in an article by a well-known English music critic, who declared that 'Mozart died of military fever' – a kind of foreign legionnaire's disease, presumably.

MILIARY FEVER One of the miliary conditions (see above), which include miliary carcinosis and miliary tuberculosis.

MILKMAN SYNDROME 'Ostomalacia due to decreased tubular reabsorption of phosphate often on an hereditary basis (autosomal recessive)', explain Drs Firkin and Whitworth in the *Dictionary of Medical Eponyms* (Parthenon Publishers, 1987). It is named after the American radiologist Dr L.A. Milkman (1895–1951) and has nothing to do with that treasured and long-established British institution, the early-morning domestic milk-delivery; which is sad, as the milkman is as much part of British amatory folklore as the travelling salesman in rural America.

MILLER'S THUMB An occupational condition harking back to pre-industrial flour production (for others see under **BREWER'S DROOP** and cross-references). It was suffered by millers as a result of their feeling the flour for unground grains. Miller's thumb is also the name of a small freshwater fish.

MINAMATA DISEASE See under **HATTER'S SHAKES**.

MINER'S ELBOW One of the professional or activity-based conditions recounted under **BREWER'S DROOP**.

MIST. Pharmacists' abbreviation for *mistura*, mixture.

MITTE Pharmacists' word for a 'dose to be taken, supplied: more literally 'sent' (e.g. 'Send this **BOTTLE** round to the gentleman's house'); or perhaps just a doctors' code to mystify the patient if their handwriting does not.

MITTELSCHMERZ German for 'pain in the middle' – not the middle of the body but midway between two menstrual periods (see **MENSES**), when the ovum (see **OV-**) is being released from the ovary. The phenomenon was discovered by a doctor in Germany, hence its German name, but 'ovulation pain' is just as good if not better. See also **PMT**.

MNEME The Greek for memory, hence mnesia and, with the **A**-for-absence prefix, amnesia, loss or absence of memory; also mnemonics, a kind of *aide-mémoire* with the help of rhymes, jingles or acronyms.

MNEMONIC Adapted into English in the 18th century from the Greek *mnemonikon*, a device to aid memory. Such aids are much used by medics, who have much to learn and remember, and some will be found in the appropriate places in this book.

MOHEL See under **CIRCUMCISION**.

MOLAR The grinding tooth, from Latin *mola*, a millstone. The incisor is the cutting tooth.

MOLE A discoloured spot on the skin, or **MACULE**, possibly a pigmented prominence, originally also used for a distinguishing sign, from the Germanic word *maal* (*cf* German *Merkmal*, distinguishing sign). 'My father had a moale upon his brow', said Shakespeare in *Twelfth Night*.

MONGOL(ISM) Thus described by the English physician J. L. H. Down in 1866. It was not until almost a century later (1961) that the condition was named **DOWN'S SYNDROME** after him.

MONOZYGOTIC Abbreviated MZ, of twins or larger numbers of multiple-birth children derived from a single ovum, and therefore identical twins (triplets, etc.) – literally 'single-yoked' (not 'yolked'!): see **ZYGOTE** for the origin of the second element. Unalike twins are called dizygotic, or **DZ** for short.

MONS VENERIS The romantic, classical name for the rounded fatty eminence that covers a woman's **PUBIC** bone, an area so often and so lovingly depicted by sculptors (on classical statues always inaccurately bald and unfunctionally cleftless). The straight translation is mount (surely better 'mound'?) of Venus, and it is named after the Romans' Goddess of Love (Aphrodite to the Greeks). Shakespeare calls this pubic area pillicock hill (*King Lear*, III, iv, 76). In men it is more prosaically the *mons pubis*.

MONTEZUMA'S REVENGE Travellers' **DIARRH(O)E(I)A**, which Mexicans and other South Americans in fact call **TURISTA**. It is the same as **DELHI BELLY, BOMBAY CRUD, GIPPY TUMMY** and the **TURKEY TROTS**. Montezuma's alleged revenge is a stomach-upset specifically contracted in Mexico, which repays Europeans in this manner for the slaughter in 1520 of the Aztec ruler and his people by the Spanish conquerors. But see also under **PRAYER'S KNEE**.

MOON-CALF An abortive, shapeless fleshy mass in the womb; a false conception. The word appears to be a direct translation from the German *Mondkalb* (Luther), meaning either a mole or what the *Collins German Dictionary* translates as a *Dummkopf*. In 1658 an English writer reported that 'A certain woman brought forth in stead of a child, four creatures like to frogs... this was a kind of Moon-calf'. The quotation comes from the *Oxford English Dictionary*, where I stumbled upon the 'mooncalf' by accident. I have failed to find it in a modern medical dictionary, so the expression is probably obsolete. But *Mosby's Pocket Dictionary* includes:–

MOON FACE A condition characterised by a round, puffy face, occurring in people treated with corticosteroids; and Firkin and Whitworth's *Medical Eponyms* has:–

MOON MOLARS Cusps of first molars looking like mulberries, a result of congenital syphilis, named after H. Moon (1845–92), a dental surgeon at **GUY'S HOSPITAL**.

MORBID Of the nature of, or indicative of, or else productive of, disease. From Latin *morbus*, disease, *morbosus*, sickly, ailing; related to *mors*, death.

MORBID ANATOMY The anatomy of diseased organs or structures, as opposed to general anatomy. Hence the somewhat unhappy appellation, Morbid Anatomist, who is not necessarily a sickly one.

MORON Now a term of contempt and abuse aimed at a supposedly stupid person (from Greek *moros*, dull or stupid); but in 1910 the American Association for the Study of the Feeble-minded adopted it as the official description of 'an adult person having a mental age of between eight and twelve', who was therefore 'one of the highest class of the feeble-minded'. See also **IDIO(T)**.

MORPH- The 'change' word element, and one of the most useful Greek building-blocks which is often combined with others: *endo-, ecto-, meta-, -osis*, etc.

MORPHINE The pain-relieving substance is named after Morpheus, Greek God of Dreams (not sleep, as often erroneously said); related also to *morph*, the root meaning shape or form.

MORS, MORTIS Latin for death, hence post-mortem, mortality, etc.

MOTOR Agent-noun from the Latin *movere*, to move – something which imparts motion (another formation from the same), i.e. makes a muscle move. It predates the electric motor and motor-car by at least two millennia. A glance at early patent specifications reveals how well-educated the ingenious 19th-century engineers were, who so carefully and allusively named many of their discoveries.

MR (MRS) BROWN A fictitious patient sometimes called for in an out-patients' department when a doctor requires a tea-break.

MRI Magnetic Resonance Imaging. For an early use of magnetism see **MESMERISM**.

MSW Medical Social Worker, formerly called **ALMONER**.

MUCOUS MEMBRANE DISEASE (SYNDROME) A recently described recruit to the group of medico-legal complaints which **PRESENTS** like a mild cold: a stuffy or runny nose and/or a sore throat. The **SICK BUILDING SYNDROME** may or may not be the cause of it.

MUCUS Latin for slime or glue – from which comes also the old-fashioned word for an adhesive – mucilage, via Latin *mucilago*. But the Greek for a nose is *mukter*, and to blow it, *mussesthai*, so we could here have another chicken-and-egg situation on our hands.

MULIBREY NANISM A rare genetic disorder whose symptoms include dwarfism, as well as other signs found in *mu*scle, *li*ver, *br*ain, and *ey*es – the name being an acronym (which is at the same time a mnemonic) formed from the letters italicised above.

MUMPS The popular name for infectious *parotitis*, an acute viral disease, comes from the Dutch *mompen*, to mope or sulk. Parotid means 'situated near or beside the ear', in this case referring to a pair of glands: *par(a)*, beside, *ot(o)-*, the ear prefix/suffix.

MÜNCHHAUSEN SYNDROME One of the few name-based conditions not eponymously named after its discoverer. Those 'suffering' from this syndrome (inevitably often called 'Munchies') make malingering their full-time pursuit. They try to get themselves admitted to hospital by pretending to one or several illnesses: they claim to have taken overdoses, swallowed foreign objects, or have 'excruciating' pain in various parts of the body; and are often recognised as soon as they take off their shirt, by the multiplicity of operation scars they display. Some are 'genuine' psychotic/hysterical **HYPOCHONDRIACS** or **NOSOPHILES**, others merely love the comfort, warmth and attention they get in hospitals, especially (if male) from female nurses. They are also known as **BED HOPPERS** and may acquire a remarkable knowledge of symptoms, which they learn from family medical books, and develop acting skills for simulating them. A Münchhausen subject well known in Liverpool and black-listed in all hospitals, met a sad but appropriate end. He witnessed a road accident in the city and, seeing casualties lying on the ground, decided to lie down in the road also, expecting to be taken to hospital with them. At that moment the rescue services arrived, and one vehicle unfortunately ran over him. The correct spelling of the word is Münchhausen, with an umlaut *ü* and two adjacent *h*s. It is not, however, 'Münchhausen's Syndrome' as

Count von M. did not discover the condition, much as he might have liked to boast of having done so. It is named after a German nobleman much given to bragging and exaggeration about his own exploits and accomplishments – social, military and sporting. His adventures include the cutting-in-two of a horse (if there were a medical name for this it would be *hipposchismatism*), which was afterwards sewn together again and lived; and a story about a stag shot with a cherry-stone which seeded itself inside the animal's head and caused a cherry-tree to grow from it (perhaps related to the cherry-stone stories associated with appendicitis). The Münchhausen stories were the work of a German, Rudolf Erich Raspe (1720–97), who fled to England after some civil misdemeanour. They were therefore published first in the English language (*Münchhausen: Narrative of his Marvellous Travels*, 1785) in order to earn some money, and only later translated into German. The syndrome was named by Dr Richard Asher in *The Lancet* (10 February 1959): 'Here is described a common syndrome which most doctors have seen, but about which little has been written. Like the famous Baron von Munchausen [Asher misspelt the name], the persons affected have always travelled widely; and their stories, like those attributed to him, are both dramatic and untruthful. Accordingly the syndrome is respectfully dedicated to the baron, and named after him'. Had this distinguished medical man been a braggart himself he could have revealed that he nearly became the father-in-law of one of the Beatles (if that is a matter for boasting). And a couple of musical footnotes: Münchhausen was a real name borne by a real German family, one of whose members married J.S. Bach's nephew, J.C.F. Bach and another, Baron Adolphe von Münchhausen, chamberlain to Frederick II of Prussia, composed and published music between about 1790 and c. 1800. If he was *the* Baron he probably had the works written for him so that he could boast about them...composition-by-proxy? See also **MALINGERER**, **PLOMBOSCILLOSIS** and **SUPRATENTORIUM** and, no doubt, many instances of the **REPETITIVE STRAIN INJURY**.

MÜNCHHAUSEN SYNDROME-BY-PROXY
The first case so described involved a man who had '...deliberately smothered children to the verge of death in the hope of winning sympathy by his skill in reviving them'; since. When numerous other incidents have been fitted up with the 'proxy' description, some

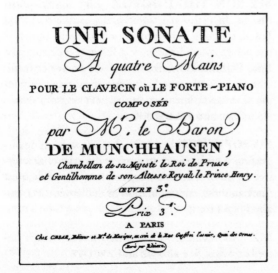

Did he really write it, or was he just boasting?

rather fanciful, especially in press reports. Once a condition is given a name, and that name is exposed in the media, sufferers from it multiply.

MUS- The muscle prefix. In Greek and Latin *mus* is the word for both a muscle and a mouse – *musculus*, 'little mouse' – perhaps because the rippling of muscles looks a little like a subcutaneous mouse running about. The Greek-based prefix is *my(o-)*, hence myocardium, a heart muscle; myalgia, muscle pain; myasthenia, muscle weakness; etc. In medieval English 'mouse' was still used to mean a muscle.

MUSICLE When I was compiling this book **PAVLOV'S DOG**, conspiring with what remained of my previous profession, decided that every attempt at my typing the word 'muscle' should result in the non-word 'musicle', to be subsequently corrected. I feel therefore that it should get a once-and-for-all entry in its own right.

MUTTON DRESSED AS LAMB This colloquial description of a – usually ridiculous and unsuccessful – attempt at recapturing lost youth by wearing inappropriate clothes may indicate a clinical condition: **CISVESTISM**.

MYALGIC ENCEPHALITIS A newly-coined name, popularly abbreviated ME and much described in the health columns of magazines and newspapers. Each time they devote space to it, more and more sufferers crowd the waiting-rooms. There was after the First World War an illness called *encephalitis lethargica*, which reached epidemic proportion in English-speaking countries and was popularly known as the Sleepy Sickness (not to be confused with the African Sleeping Sickness, or trypanosomiasis). This was marked by headaches and drowsiness and in extreme cases resulted in coma and death. Great wars give rise to mysterious demographic manifestations (such as the proportion of male to female children born) but if ME is part of a reaction to the almost superhuman efforts expended by the West during the Second World War it has waited a long time before manifesting itself. Some doctors flatly deny its existence and declare it is nothing more than the condition they describe as **TATT** ('I'm tired all the time, doctor!'), and part of the **STRESS** that afflicts many who are exposed to the hurlyburly of modern life. Others say it may be a

mild form of viral encephalitis. Others, again, keep an open mind and acknowledge that there are some conditions which as yet cannot be recognised by any existing pathological process.

MYC-, MYCET- Prefixes denoting *antibiotics*, from Greek *muces, muket-*, mushroom or fungus. Such word elements often help to make the names of proprietary drugs, e.g. Erythromycin – see **ERYTHRO-**. Also **PENICILLIN** and **PENIS**.

MY(O)- The muscle prefix – see also **MUS-**, above.

MYOPIA Greek for 'screwing up the eyes' – an action which helps them to focus better, from Greek *muein*, to close + *ops*, the eye (see also the **MUS-/MYS-** muscle prefixes, above). This is how it became the word for shortsightedness: really 'screwed-up-eyes-sightedness'.

MYOTONIA The inability to relax a voluntary muscle for a period following its use, and which when it affects the face may lend it a certain mask-like aspect. This evidently affects some television actors who go in for the Long Meaningful Look cliché. More information about the *-tonia* ending will be found under **TONIC**.

MYRINGA Modern Latin for the ear-drum, old Latin *tympanum*: perhaps one of the 'pretty girls' names' group of conditions, like **AMELIA, CANDIDA, CARINA, HERNIA, LISTERELLA, PRUNELLA**, etc.

MY SON THE DOCTOR Like many quips-turned-cliché this one, traditionally ascribed to proud Jewish mothers, is soundly based on social history – the persecution of the Jews in Europe, especially the East. Portable skills, like that of the doctor or musician (or indeed comedian), were important for people who never knew when the next pogrom would occur. See also **FELDSHER**.

MYSOPHOBIA From Greek *mysos*, something disgusting + *phobia*, fear: an anxiety disorder characterised by an over-reaction to, and fear of, the slightest uncleanliness, contamination or defilement. Personally I'm all for it.

MZ Abbreviation of **MONOZYGOTIC**, which describes twins. See also **DZ** and **ZYGOTE**.

N*n*

NAD Abbreviation of 'No Abnormality Detected' and/or 'Nicotinamide adenine dinucleotide' – but has also been used, in respect to a patient's examination or other procedure, to mean 'Not Actually Done'.

N(A)EVUS A pigmented, congenital skin blemish.

N(A)EVUS FLAMMEUS A birthmark varying in colour from a pale red to a deep, reddish purple, also called a **PORT-WINE STAIN** (not to be confused with a **SPAMMIE**) though in polite English society the expression 'port-*wine*' is considered a solecism, like '*horse*-riding'. But 'port stain' would have been too vague a term.

NARES Latin for the nostrils and/or nasal passages. See also **SEPTUM**.

NASUS Latin for the nose, hence several words with the prefix *naso*-. See also **AROMATHERAPY, MUCUS, RHIS**, and **OSME/OLERE**, to smell.

-NATE The 'birth' suffix. Latin *natus*, born.

NATES Latin for the rump or buttocks, *puge/pyge* in Greek – as in callipygian, 'having beautiful buttocks' (like the famous statue, the Callipygian Venus). The English 'buttock' adjective is, confusingly, natal, which is apparently unconnected to the natal word that relates to the birth process, let alone to a province in South Africa.

NAUSEA A feeling of sickness in the stomach, combined with a loathing of food and an inclination to vomit. The Greek word *nausia* or *nautia*, from *naus*, ship, literally means seasickness. *Nausea* is the Latin form but origin and meaning are the same in both. See also **WOMBLES** and cross-references.

NECRO- The Greek 'death' prefix, from *nekros*, dead, or a dead body. The examination of a corpse should really be described as a necropsy (a biopsy when of a living body) rather than an **AUTOPSY**, which has a different literal meaning (see also the **-OPS-** and **BIO-** suffixes/prefixes) and is considered by purists to be an erroneous formation. Necrophilia is a morbid preoccupation for dead bodies, sometimes even to have sexual feelings for them. See also **MORS, PTOMA** and **THANATOS**.

NECROPSY Purists maintain that this, together with **THANATOPSY**, is a better and more accurate word for the inspection of a **CADAVER** than **AUTOPSY**.

NECROSIS Mortification, or the death or dying of (or dying-off of), usually, tissue. The English derivatives are necrosing/necrotising.

NECROTISING FASCIITIS This (see also **FASCIA**) enjoyed a sudden burst of publicity in the Spring of 1994 after what was described as a 'cluster' of cases, and sensationalised in the press as a progressive 'flesh-eating' disease – as if to suggest that armies of flesh-eating streptococci were relentlessly making their way along the motorways. The streptococcal gangrenous outbreak was, of course, nothing new. In a letter to *The Times* (28 May 1994) the Consultant Radiologist Mr A.C. Lamont recalled his student notes on plastic surgery of 1971: 'If infection is not rigorously excluded during and after skin grafting, when the dressing is removed you will find no graft and a lot of fat little streptococci', and:–

> He prayeth best
> Who loveth best
> All creatures great and small.
> The streptococcus is the test,
> I love him least of all.

NEMATODE A thread-like worm, from Greek *nema*, thread + the **-ODE** 'in-the-form-of' suffix, Greek *odos, eidos* (see also **-OID**). See also **VERMIFORM**.

NEO- The Greek prefix of newness, from *neos*, new, with the Latin *natus*, birth. Hence neonatal, pertaining to the new-born, and:–

NEONATE A fancy – and surely unnecessary – word for a new-born baby: see both elements, **NEO-** and **NATE**.

NEPHR- Prefix denoting the kidney, for which the Greek is *nephros*. The equivalent Latin word is *renes*, and both contribute a share of derivations concerning nephritic or renal matters (and see **ADRENALIN**). The mineral nephrite, or jade, was considered effective against diseases of the kidneys: perhaps another chicken-and-egg problem?

NERVUS Latin for nerve – and see below.

NEURASTHENIA A formerly common but vague diagnosis, meaning literally 'lack of strength, or weakness, of the nerves' (*sthenos*, Greek for strength; *asthenes*, weak). It gradually went out of fashion and by 1965 an authority (quoted in the *Oxford English Dictionary*) wrote: 'Neurasthenia is observed with such frequency in housewives who are bored and feel neglected by their husbands that it has often been called "housewives' neurosis". The condition is, of course, constantly being joined by other and newer complaints equally vague or disputable: the newspapers (and soon afterwards the waiting-rooms) are full of them. See also **SAD** and **TATT**.

NEUR(O)- The 'nerve' prefix – see below.

NEURON Greek for a sinew, nerve or tendon – hence numerous words like neurosis, neuralgia, etc., but also aponeurosis, which has to do with fibrous connective tissue. Perhaps two different words are needed – one for a tangible sinew or visible nerve, e.g. the little worm-like thing the dentist extracts from a tooth, and another for 'the nerves' as a state of mind. As early as AD 260 the doctor Erasistratus of Ceos, who also understood the action of the heart, distinguished between motor and sensory nerves, a discovery he made by dissecting living criminals – for more about which see under **DUODENUM**. The Latin equivalent, *nervus*, accounts for another crop of derivations. Aneurin is the name of vitamin B_1 (see the **A(N)-** prefix): did that vehement and outspoken Welsh politician Aneurin Bevan know that whatever his forename means in his own language*, to the Greeks it would have meant 'lacking in muscle'?

*In fact the Welsh name Aneurin comes from the Latin Honorius and was adopted by a Welsh bard in about AD 600.

NHS The British National Health Service, which forms the largest part of the Welfare State, was the world's first practical national scheme offering universal free health and social insurance to its citizens as well as to visitors. It was based on the principle that those in possession of health and wealth would through modest contributions pay for the sick, the poor and their own retirement pension. Its architect was the social reformer and economist William Henry Beveridge (born in 1879), first Baron Beveridge, although much of it is believed to have been the work of his even more idealistic Personal Assistant, the Labour peer Lord Longford (born in 1905). The Beveridge/Longford scheme set out to ensure that the state would look after its citizens from the cradle to the grave, without their having to pay a single penny towards treatment, not even for a couple of aspirins to cure a headache or adhesive tape to cover a small graze. 'It's on the NHS'

became a catchphrase. But even before Beveridge's death in 1963 the impracticality of the scheme was becoming evident, and charges had to be introduced. As the years went by and the post-war employment boom first faded and then turned into recession, the number of claimants rose with the increase in unemployment, and therefore the number of people requiring benefits began to overtake that of those able to pay contributions – which spells death for any insurance scheme. Population growth was swelled by immigrants, mostly poor and unskilled, which further upset the balance between contributors and claimants. Meanwhile medical and surgical advances brought newer, better and more expensive forms of diagnosis and treatment, and kept more patients alive longer (it has been said that the second half of the 20th century saw more advances in diagnostic and surgical techniques than the previous 500 years). In spite of all these self-evident truths, politicians (who promise anything to get themselves elected) encouraged the population to expect more and more benefits and services, from free contraception to generous death benefits – protection not so much from the cradle to the grave as from the erection to the resurrection. By the late 1970s Beveridge's futuristic dreams had turned into a fiscal and administrative nightmare, and by the end of the 1980s the **NHS** was approaching collapse. See also **CARING, COUNSELLING, GREY SUITS** and cross-references.

NICOTINE Named after the 16th-century French diplomat Jacques Nicot, Ambassador to Lisbon, who introduced the tobacco plant into France from America in 1560. The earliest known reference to tobacco is dated 1492 and credited to two Spaniards, Luis de Torres and Rodrigo de Jerez, who reported to Columbus that they saw natives who 'drank smoke'. Rodrigo evidently caught the habit, for he was imprisoned for the 'devilish habit' by the Inquisition in 1518. It was thought at first that tobacco possessed beneficial medicinal properties: 'It cleeres the sight ...the oile or juyce dropped into the eares is good against deafnesse ... layd upon the face taketh away ... spots thereof', says John Gerard in his *Herball* (1636); claiming even that 'many notable medicines are made hereof against the old and inveterat cough, against asthmaticall or pectorall griefs... against griefe in the brest and lungs: against catarrhs and rheums, and such as have gotten cold and hoarsenesse...' but adds by way of warning, 'Some use to drink it (as it is termed) for wantonnesse, or rather custome, and cannot forbeare it, no not in the midst of their dinner; which kinde of taking it is unwholesome and very dangerous...'.

It was not until the mid-20th century that its devastating effects on health were fully understood.

NICTARE Latin, to wink. Hence the nictating eyelid, often observed in some television performers, in whom it is an affectation, not a nervous **TIC**.

NIDUS Latin for a nest, but also used figuratively – as in English – for a dwelling or home, as well as a receptacle. In medicine, a place in which bacteria have settled because of its suitable conditions for their growth; also the nucleus round which a gallstone forms. See also **PILONIDAL** and **PSEUDOFOLLICULITIS**.

NIGHTINGALE WARD Hospital wards designed after the recommendations of Florence Nightingale (1820–1910) – 'austere open dormitories', as Dr G.L. Cohen called them in his report *What's Wrong with Hospitals?* (1964). In one of her letters (to John Stuart Mill) and dated September 12th 1860, Florence Nightingale made a curiously narrow-minded statement about women in the medical profession, un-perceptive even for her time: 'Instead of wishing to see more doctors made by women joining what there are [i.e. what doctors there are in the profession], I wish to see as few doctors, either male or female, as possible. For, mark you, the women have made no improvement – they have only tried to be 'men' and they have only succeeded in being third-rate men' (from *Forever Yours, Florence Nightingale*, Selected Letters, published in 1989).

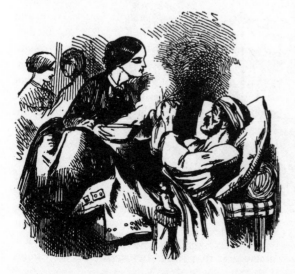

Punch, October, 1854

NIGHTINGALE WRAP A cheap kind of bed-jacket – originally 'a flannel wrap designed to cover the shoulders and arms of a patient while confined to bed'.

NIPPLE(S) The *Oxford English Dictionary* describes these, the **MAMMILLAE**, as 'the small prominences, composed of vascular erectile tissue, in which the ducts of the mammary glands terminate externally in nearly all mammals of both sexes; esp. that of a woman's breast', adding (perhaps with relief) that 'there is no clear connection with Old English *nypel*, used by Aelfric of an elephant's trunk'. There is, however, a charming and interesting connection

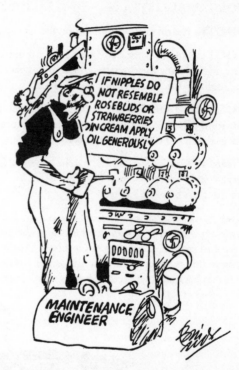

with 'nibble': Haydocke, translating Lomazzi in 1598, says, 'The heades or extuberances whence the milke is sucked out, are called Nibbles'. Variant spellings include neble, neapil and neaple. Their attraction for infants is best described by anthropologists, and their fascination for men of all ages by poets, who liken them to rosebuds, fruits, flowers and other pretty things. This description is by the English poet–priest Robert Herrick (1591–1674):

> *Have ye beheld (with much delight)*
> *A red rose peeping through a white?*
> *Or else a cherry (double grac'd)*
> *Within a lily, centre-plac'd?*

Or ever mark'd the pretty beam
A strawberry shows, half drown'd in cream?
Or seen rich rubies blushing through
A pure smooth pearl, and orient, too?

So like to this, nay all the rest,
Is each neat niplet of her breast.

It should be added that although German men share these sentiments their poets may lack the appropriate language to express them, for in German a nipple is called *Brustwarze*, literally 'breast wart' (see **VERRUCA**).

NMR Nuclear Magnetic Resonance scan.

NOCTAMBULIST A sleepwalker. See **AMB-**.

NOCTE Pharmacists' abbreviation for 'at night'.

NOCTURIA A compound word for the need to pass urine during the night, from *nox*, night (*noctis*, of the night) + **UR-** (from Greek *ouron*) urine.

NOLI ME TANGERE Latin for 'touch me not' (St John XX, 17). Medieval name for an ulcerative disease akin to **LUPUS** or **LEPROSY**.

-NOMY The 'laws-of' suffix, e.g. in *taxonomy*, from Greek *taxis*, order + *nomos*, custom, law. Not to be confused with *onoma*, name.

NORMAL Of a saline solution: one containing the same concentration of sodium chloride as the blood. Apart from that, medical people often hesitate to declare things either normal or abnormal. Some say that they have spent a lifetime looking for a 'normal'

man, and when they find him he will probably prove to be quite abnormal. Latin (and Italian) *norma* means square (both noun and adjective – and how apt for many a soprano in the title role in Bellini's opera *Norma*). In Latin *normalis* is applied to something that is made in accordance with the measurement of a carpenter's or mason's square.

NO-SHOW(S) A patient who misses an appointment without bothering to cancel it. From airline slang? See also **DNA**.

NOSO- A useful prefix, from the Greek *nosos*, disease. Its under-use is probably due to the erroneous association it is likely to suggest with the nose.

NOSOCOMIAL INFECTION That found in, and possibly generated by, a hospital environment or conditions in one. See also **IATROGENIC**.

NOSOLOGY The branch of medical science that deals with the classification of diseases.

NOSOPHILE A person who is morbidly attracted to sickness or disease, or to hospitals, perhaps one suffering from (*suffering?* – no, probably *enjoying*) the **MÜNCHHAUSEN SYNDROME**.

NOSOPHOBIA Fear of sickness, particularly of hospitals.

NOSTALGIA Just as **NAUSEA** was originally and specifically *sea*sickness, so was nostalgia *home*sickness: from Greek *nostos*, return home + *algia*, pain. When homesickness is so severe as to become a physical illness it is called nostomania. See also **ANAMNESIS**.

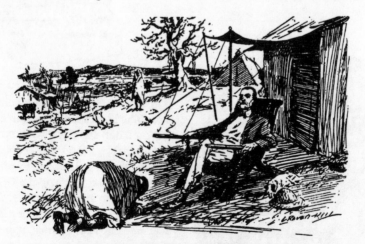

ENGLISH AS SHE IS COMPREHENDED.
Babu. "SIR. I BEG THAT YOU WILL TRANSFER ME FROM THIS PLACE. I AM HOME-SICK."
Deputy Commissioner. "BUT AM I NOT CORRECT IN SUPPOSING THAT THIS *IS* YOUR HOME?"
Babu (with conviction). "YES, SIR, IT IS - AND I AM SICK OF IT."

Punch, May 29, 1907

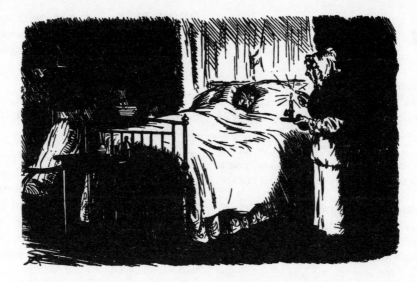

OUR NURSES

Experienced Night Nurse (sternly). "Come, come, Sir! You must stop
that horrid Noise. If you keep Wheezing and Snoring like that
all Night, how am I to get to Sleep!!"

Punch, 25 November, 1871

NOSTRUM A medicine or medical application prepared by the person recommending it, especially a **QUACK** remedy or **PATENT** medicine, *nostrum* being the neuter singular of *noster*, our. Many pharmacists are still able to offer a **BOTTLE** or mixture of their own devising.

NOXA Damage. Latin *nocere*, to hurt. Hence noxious, hurtful or harmful; and its opposite innocuous, not hurtful, harmless; and indeed in*noc*ent – an everyday English word with a Latin past – see the **IN-** prefix; also the ancient medical precept, *Primum non nocere*.

NUCHA The nape of the neck; but in obsolete terminology it denoted the spinal cord, from the Arabic *nucha*, adopted into medieval Latin.

NURSE The word, now meaning a sickroom or hospital attendant, is derived from the same source as 'nourishment', hence the 'wet' nurse employed to suckle infants (in French *nourice*). In the sense of attending to the sick the word is probably not much older than Shakespeare, who wrote in *A Comedy of Errors* (1590): 'I will attend my husband, be his nurse, Diet in his sicknesse, for it is my Office', meaning a bringer and preparer of food.

NUSTAGMOS Greek for nodding; but as one can nod sideways as well as up-and-down the word gave us nystagmus, a rapid, involuntary, lateral movement of the eye – in derived formations the letters *y* and *u* are often alternatives for each other.

NYC/NOC The two 'night' prefixes, the first from the Greek for night, as in nyctalopia, night-blindness (see below), the second from the Latin, *nox/noctis*.

NYCTALOPIA From Greek *nyx*, night + **OP(T)** 'sight' element. Poor night vision, incorrectly called 'night-blindness'. But in the etymological dictionaries a nyctalope, paradoxically, is 'one who has the power of seeing by night'.

NYCTOPHOBIA The above + the 'fear' suffix: an irrational or obsessive fear of the dark.

NYD Not Yet Diagnosed (perhaps a case of **GOK**); or Not Yet Done.

NYMPHAE From Greek *numphe, nympha*, a bride, which is the social meaning. Anatomically, they are the inner lips or **LABIA** of the **VULVA**.

O*o*

OAC Notes-abbreviation for a 'horrible hacking cough', but said with the aspirated *h* omitted, as is the habit of many patients from the South East of England. When a man with a broad cockney (i.e. London) accent told his doctor he had 'An orrible acking cough', the physician advised him to 'take a couple of aspirates'. For the Latin name see **TUSSIS**.

OB- The Latin directional prefix, which can indicate towards, in-front-of, closing-off, blocking, 'away' (in the sense below), etc. Obstruction is derived from *ob + struere*, to pile or build up; obstetrics comes from 'standing before' (or between the legs of) a woman giving birth: *obstetricus* and *obstetrix* mean, respectively, a male and female birth-helper.

OB (Pronounced as separate letters, i.e. O.B.: abbreviation of Open Bowels.

OBESITY Latin *obesus*: one who has been 'eating away' – merrily, or perhaps sadly; from *ob-* (see above) and *edere*, to eat. This is a word which changed its allegiance: the first sense of the Latin *obesus* was 'wasted away, lean and meagre', in other words, eaten away. See also **BANTING, BULIMIA, CELLULITE** and **OREXIS**, for different words related to appetite or slimming; and **PYKNIC** for a resulting fatness. See also **PINGUESCENCE**.

OBSTETRICS See above, under **OB-**.

OCULUS Latin for eye, anatomical, botanical or horticultural (e.g. a bud, as on a potato). Hence **INOCULATE**, to insert a graft from one plant into another, or a germ or virus into the body to produce immunity from disease. The Greek eye word is **OPHTHALMOS**. See also **OPTOMETRIST**.

OD Abbreviation for 'Took an (intentional or accidental) overdose' (and at the bank it stands for an overdraft). Also pharmacist's abbreviation of *omne die*, every day.

ODA Operating Department Assistant.

-ODE Like **-OID** this is a 'likeness' suffix, from Greek *aeides* (or *oidos*) in-the-shape-of, e.g. **NEMATODE**.

ODORARE Latin: to perfume, to imbue with fragrance. A deodorant takes smells away – good and bad ones – see **REEKER**. See also **AROMATHERAPY**.

ODUNE From Greek *odune*, pain – see **ANODYNE**.

OEDEMA Greek-based word for a swelling or tumour. Americans prefer to spell it edema. See also **DROPSY**.

(O)ESOPHAGUS The gullet. Of uncertain Greek origin but *phagein*, to eat, has something to do with it (see also the **-PHAG(E)-** prefix/suffix). Americans simplify the spelling by omitting the intial *o*; and Ambrose Bierce, the American author of *The Devil's Dictionary*, defined the (o)esophagus as 'That portion of the alimentary canal that lies between pleasure and business'.

(O)ESTR- The prefix relating to the female sex hormone (o)estrogen or to oestrus, the condition of being sexually on heat (usually reserved for animals, in which this is more easily discernible). From *oistros*, the Greek word for a gadfly: to be stung by one was thought to send people, especially females, into a frenzy.

-OID Greek suffix for 'in the shape of', from *aeides* (or *oidos*) in the shape of, e.g. humanoid, android (see **ANDR-**), ovoid, in the shape of an egg, asteroid, in the shape of a star, etc. Related to the **-ODE** suffix. See also **TABLOID**.

OLD CHARLIE FOSTER HATES WOMEN HAVING DOWDY CLOTHES A slightly unconvincing mnemonic for the functions of the blood: Oxygen (transport), Carbon dioxide (transport), Food, Heat, Waste, Hormones, Disease, Clotting.

(THE) OLD MAN'S FRIEND Doctors' name for pneumonia, which often eases the terminally old into death. See also **J. P. FROG**.

OLERE Latin *oleo*, I (emit a) smell. It is tempting to draw a parallel with *oleum*, oil, for the ancients' habit of cleansing themselves and each other by anointment with olive oil must have produced some rancidly sticky moments, especially as they had little or no chemically-effective soap. See **REEKER**.

OLFACTORY Of or pertaining to the sense of smell (Latin *olere*, above), so an olfactor is, literally, he who, or that which, smells; a smelling-agent. See also **OSME, AROMATHERAPY**.

OLIGOS Greek for 'few', making a useful prefix, e.g. oligospermia, etc. – and oligarchy, rule by a few people.

-OMA The Greek-based swelling, mass or tumour suffix. See also **ATHERE, CARCINOMA, LIPOMA** and **ONCOLOGY**. Also the 'blackness' prefix **MELAN(O)-**.

OMOS Greek for the shoulder. Hence omalgia, pain or rheumatism in the shoulder.

OMPHALOS Greek for the navel (Latin *umbilicus*). Omphale was the Queen of Lydia, a very masculine lady to whom Hercules was for three years bound as a slave. He fell in love with her in spite of her mannishness (or because of it – psychosexual troubles were not invented last week) and led a submissive life, wearing female garments and spinning wool for her. She, however, wore a lion's skin (normally worn only by men) and followed masculine pursuits – surely the first recorded instance of couple trans-sexualism, cross-dressing, and role-reversal, and an example of the avoidance of sexual stereotyping. According to some accounts Hercules had several children by Omphale, so at some points in their relationship they must have abandoned their comical role-playing. If Omphale as a baby suffered from an omphalocele (a protruding navel) it might account for her given name (see the chicken-and-egg situation regarding **CLAUDICATION**) though not for her subsequent behaviour, which was eccentric, to say the least. *Omphalos* also means a centre, boss, or hub, e.g. the central, rounded bit on a shield (and she was nothing if not self-centred). The *omphalos* in the Temple of Apollo at Delphi was thought to be the centre, or navel, of the earth. Hence also *omphalism*, excessive centralisation of administration, usually of government. Some said the British National Health Service suffered from it until power was devolved to those institutions which opted for it. It is a well-known but as yet unexplained fact that any small quantity of fluff found in the recesses of the navel is invariably composed of blue woolly fibres.

ONAN A biblical character who in the first book of the Old Testament 'spilled his seed upon the ground' and so gave his name to *onanism*, 'the crime of self-pollution' (*Chambers's Cyclopaedia*). But it was all a big misunderstanding, officer, and I can explain everything. Onan was no masturbator, and *Genesis*, Verse 9, Chapter 38, makes this quite clear. God had slain Onan's brother Er ('who was wicked in the sight of the Lord' – no reason given), so Onan was asked to take his sister-in-law 'and perform the duty of an husband's brother unto her' (Verse 8). This he was evidently willing to do, but did not wish to make her pregnant: 'And Onan knew that the seed should not be his; and it came to pass, when he went in unto his brother's wife, that he spilled it on the ground [*sic*: not the bed?], lest he should give seed to his brother'. It was a clear case of coitus interruptus, not masturbation. In modern terms this would have been the equivalent of smoking but not inhaling. Nevertheless, 'the thing which he did was evil in the sight of the Lord: and He slew him also' (Verse 10). So much for early attempts at birth control. And in any case, after centuries of fierce condemnation, with threats ranging from blindness to death, even straightforward, recreational masturbation has been declared not only harmless but positively therapeutic. It is also an inescapable requirement of Artificial Insemination by Donor, so that Onan should be rehabilitated forthwith and be declared patron saint of **AID**. On top of all that, and in spite of the severe misgivings expressed 2000-odd years ago, it is now perfectly legal to marry one's deceased brother's wife. See also **GENESIS**, for a reference to all the 'begetting' that goes on in the First Book of the Old Testament.

ONCOLOGY The study of tumours, from Greek *onkos*, a mass or swelling. Various formations include oncofetal, oncogene, oncogenesis, oncologist, oncovirus, etc. – all combined with recognisable suffixes which please see. See also **CARCINOMA**.

OOOTTAFAVGVAH Letters spelling out the names of the nerves of the **CRANIUM** (for an account of which please see a real medical dictionary): they are almost impossible to remember unless turned into a mnemonic of the kind used by medical students and nurses. This one – somewhat male-orientated – stands for 'O,O,O, To Touch And Feel A Virgin Girl's Vagina And Hymen!'

OPEN-SPHINCTER 'POOH' TYPE A type of **FLATULENCE**, which please see for the connection.

OP(H)-/-OPS-/OPT- The 'eye' prefixes/suffixes, occurring in various forms. See also below.

OPHTHALMOS The Greek word for eye (Latin **OCULUS**), hence the *opth-* prefix denoting eyesight and seeing, from Greek *opsis*, sight. Autopsy literally means 'seeing for oneself' (which, some say, should correctly be called **NECROPSY**); synopsis, 'seeing everything together' (i.e. what is called an 'overview' in the USA, from the German *Übersicht*); and myopia, short-sightedness, is literally 'a screwing-up' of the eye-muscles, which gives the shortsighted a small improvement in vision. See also **OPTOMETRIST**, below.

OPTOMETRIST The optometer, an instrument for measuring or testing vision, its acuteness, perception, range, etc., was invented and so named in the 18th century but for some reason the person trained in the use of it has always been called, in British English, an Ophthalmic Optician, more often just Optician. Now, however, the (surely more accurate, simpler and therefore preferrable) American word optometrist is gaining ground, so perhaps we could reserve optician for the person who makes, or assembles and fits, the lenses and frames of the spectacles. See also **SNELLEN CHART**.

ORCHIDECTOMY The removal of the **TESTES**, see below.

ORCHIS Greek for testicle; genitive *orchidis*, orchidectomy their removal: (see also **-ECTOMY**). The *orchi-*, *orchido-* and *orchio-* prefixes, as well as the adjective orchic, all refer to the testes. The horticultural orchids are so named because of the supposed similarity in shape of their roots to testicles. Thus a gardener 'deadheading' his or her orchids is in a way performing an orchidectomy. English gardeners and country people call the wild orchid 'ballock-grass', also 'hare's ballocks' and 'sweet ballocks'. There is, however, no connection between *orchis* and 'orchestra', in its vulgar use, as in 'I kicked him in the orchestras', which is English rhyming slang, used in the traditional abbreviated way with the rhyming word omitted: 'orchestra stalls'. Triorchidism means having three testicles – but again there is no musical connection between this and the Treorchy Male Voice Choir, which is not a group of singing supermen (the very opposite of castrati?) but is named after a place in Wales with a fine musical tradition. It all gives a new slant to the title of James Hadley Chase's novel, *No Orchids for Miss Blandish*. See also **DIDYMUS** and **CRYPTORCHIDISM** – and **LOVER'S BALLS**.

OREXIS Greek for appetite. Hence *anorexia* – lack, loss or absence of it. The adjective (and noun) for sufferers from this condition should really be *anorec-tic*, not 'anorexic' – and for more about this see under **DYSPEPSIA** and **OBESITY**.

ORGANON Greek for an *organ*, but the word literally means 'that with which one works' – which is why it can mean a bodily organ as well as a musical instrument. The Latin equivalent is *viscus*, which has also produced numerous derivatives, none of them musical.

ORGASM Latin *orgasmus*, from the Greek word for a swelling, but because the word has gained such strong sexual connotations doctors tend to use other words or suffixes for non-sexual swellings, e.g. words constructed from *kele/cele*. We now also have the time-saving verb 'to orgasm', coined by expensive doctors for whom time is money. When one of them said of a patient, 'She orgasmed in a non-coital situation' his British colleague asked, 'Do you mean she came unscrewed?' In 19th-century English having an orgasm was called 'to spend' (both for men and women) and in the 17th and 18th centuries it was euphemised as 'a little death' – hence the disconcerting and sometimes misunderstood 18th-century euphemism 'to die' – for which see under **PRAE-COX**. According to Ernest Hemingway (1899–1961) the force of an orgasm can be measured on some kind of personal Richter scale – after a much-quoted passage in Chapter 13 of *For whom the Bell Tolls*, in which an orgasm allegedly made the earth move.

ORTHO- The Greek prefix denoting straightness, correctness, normality. Orthodontics means 'straight teeth', but orthop(a)edics (from *orthos* + *pais*, child) has been widened to mean the removal of all deformities, the straightening or repair of limbs, and especially bones, of adults as well as children. But orthopnoea is not 'correct breathing' but a condition which a short-of-breath patient is best able to alleviate by being propped up on pillows. Orthoptics involves the correction of vision defects without surgery, e.g. by means of exercises; orthotopic is, literally, a term for 'in the right place', as opposed to ectopic, outside the right place (see **TOPICAL**). And indeed orthography, too, is important in medicine, meaning correct writing or spelling.

ORTHOPOD Nickname for an orthopaedic surgeon, current among the members of that specialty. In 1982 it was accepted into the *Oxford English Dictionary*, where, on the same page, I encountered the giant word below:–

ORTHOROENTGENOGRAPHY which, when divided into its components, ortho-, Roentgen, and -(o)graphy (see **-GRAPH**) is found to mean 'A technique for producing radiographs showing the exact sizes of organs or bones by using a narrow beam of X-rays perpendicular to the plate or film'. The German surgeon Wilhelm Konrad Roentgen (1845–1923) was the discoverer, in 1895, of X-rays, which have always been known in German-speaking countries as *Roentgenstrahlen* – Roentgen rays. He received the first Nobel Prize for physics in 1901. Another German surgeon, Georg Clemens Perthes, made the first observations that X-rays can inhibit carcinomas and other cancerous growths.

ORTHOTICS A comparatively new term, usually coupled with **PROSTHETICS**: a technician who makes splints and artificial limbs, etc.

OS Latin for mouth, genitive oris, hence all the *orificial* pursuits described under **PROLETARIAN**. For the Greek see **STOMA**.

OS Latin for bone, genitive *ossis*. The Greek is *osteon*, hence the presence of a *t* in many derivations, e.g. *osteo-*.

(O)SCOPY The 'looking' suffix. See **-SCOPE**.

O-SIGN In **GERONTICS**, an old patient whose mouth hangs open – often a sign of impending death, when it might become a **Q-SIGN**.

-OSIS Suffix which usually indicates a diseased condition of whatever precedes it (just as -itis often indicates inflammation). Thus **HALITOSIS** is not in itself foul breath, as often supposed, but an indication of the possible disease. See also **-ITIS**.

OSME Greek for a smell. Anosmia means the inability to smell (i.e. the inability to perceive an odour, not to create one). The Latin equivalent is *olere*, hence olfactory. See also **AROMATHERAPY**.

OSMOS Greek for a (physical) impulse, hence osmosis. From *otheo*, I push, I shove.

OSTEON Greek for bone – *os, ossis* in Latin.

OSTEOPOROSIS The above + *porosis*, here indicating a bone weakness. See also **DOWAGER'S HUMP**.

-OSTOMY, -STOMY The hole-making suffix. See also **STOMA**.

OT(O)- The ear prefix, from Greek *ous, otos*, ear. Hence otology, otoscopy, otalgia and numerous other 'ear' formations.

OT Occupational Therapy.

-OTOMY The 'cutting' suffix.

OTT Over-the-top, i.e. exaggerated – perhaps in a **MÜNCHHAUSEN** 'sufferer'.

OV(O)-(I)- The egg prefix, from Latin *ovum*, egg. Hence ov**OID**, oval, ovulation, oviparous, etc.

OXUS/OXYS Greek for sharp or acute, hence the paroxysm (also, in combination with **MOROS**, which means dull, foolish, the oxymoron, i.e. the mutually contradictory concept 'sharp-dull'). In Latin sharpness is **ACUTUS**. It is therefore tautologous to speak of an 'acute paroxysm'.

P*p*

PABULUM The Latin word for food, or fodder, formerly much used for describing nourishing substances, especially those produced commercially. There is or was a children's patent breakfast-food called *Pablum* [sic].

PACEMAKER See **ARTIFICIAL PACEMAKER**.

PACHY- The Greek 'thick' prefix, hence pachydermia, a thickening of the skin; pachyhaemia (American pachemia), thickening of the blood; pachymeningitis, etc. See the various added elements where cross-referenced.

P(A)ED- The 'boy' or 'child' prefix, hence various formations like paediatrician, literally 'a doctor of children', often called a pediatrist in America, where the *a* is considered dispensable, at the risk of confusion with the 'foot' prefix, *ped-*. The *a* has, however, long been dropped from pedagogy, the teaching of children. See also **PODIATRIST, PUER** and **PROLES**.

P(A)EDIATRICS The branch of medical science dealing with the study of children and their illnesses. See also **EPHEBIATRICS, GERIATRICS** and **GERONTICS**.

P(A)EDOPHILE A self-description of p(a)ederasts and child-molesters which is intended to lend their activities an air of benevolence and gain them respectability; and which, unfortunately, has been adopted by some journalists. It is derived from the two Greek elements for children/boys and love, respectively, (see **P(A)ED** and **-PHILIA**). Dracula missed out there: he might have called himself a **H(A)EMOPHILE**.

PAFO Coded case-note description of injured patients attending a casualty department. It stands for 'Pissed and Fell Over'. Usually **TRIPPERS** are involved.

PALATUM The Latin word for the roof of the mouth, or palate. In transferred use it also stands for a vault (see under **CLAUSTRUM, FAUCES, FOCUS, FORNIX, PHRAGMA, PORTA, THALAMOS**, and **TRABECULUM** for other architectural terms). Many

writers of today seem to be unsure about the difference between a palate, a palette or a pallet – and do not know whether they lick it, mix paint on it or sleep on it. A pallet is a kind of rude mattress, from Latin *palea*, chaff, via the French *paille*, straw, with which such a *palliasse* (from French *paillasse*) would have been stuffed. The palette used by painters for mixing their colours comes from the Italian *paletta*, a flat spoon or trowel.

PALPATE From Latin *palpare*, to touch, stroke gently or caress, hence to examine by touch: a perfectly ordinary English word which is now used mostly by doctors – some say unnecessarily, as there are several English words less likely to confuse the patient, although he would probably not have heard of the direct derivative, to palp: to touch, feel, handle gently. Another Latin-based term that might be replaced by a simpler, vernacular word is **AUSCULTATION**. See under **DIGITUS** for the doctors' 'palpating finger'.

PALPITATE From Latin *palpitare*, to pulsate, throb, tremble or beat rapidly and strongly – hence palpitations, a pounding or racing of the heart.

PALSY Adapted from the Greek **PARALYSIS**, this word was used in various English forms from the Middle Ages onwards (derived via the Old French *paralesie*). A manuscript of about 1300 has 'A man was criplid in parlesie'. In modern usage, palsy and paralysis appear not to have the same connotations, however, and both usually depend on qualifying additions specifying the kind.

PAN- Greek prefix denoting all. A pandemic (with the addition of *demos*, the people) is like an **EPI**demic only worse in being even more widespread, thought to affect all people of a country or the world, whereas an epidemic may be limited to a country, city or district.

PANACEA A heal-all remedy. See **REMEDY/CURE** and **CURE/REMEDY**.

PANCREAS The name of the digestive gland comes from the Greek *pan*, all + *kreas*, flesh; or so all the dictionaries tell us. It is actually fish-shaped, and the all-flesh connection is puzzling, as surely all our soft giblets – human as well as animal – are 'all flesh'. Could there be a connection with Latin *panis*, bread, in view of the fact that the pancreas of lambs, calves, etc., when used in cooking, are called sweetbread(s) – although the pancreas is, of course, neither sweet nor bread? Further etymological investigation seems called for. The pancreas also contains small groups of cells called **ISLETS OF LANGERHANS**, which secrete two hormones, **INSULIN** and glucagon, regulating blood-sugar levels: another connection with sweetness. See **DIABETES**.

PANHYSTERECTOMY 'Having it all taken away', as women say.

PAPERS See under **PUBLISH OR PERISH**.

PAPILLA(E) Diminutive of Latin *papula*, a pimple or swelling, and therefore any small fleshy protuberance or eruption. Also, more rarely, a **NIPPLE**: see also **MAMMILLA**(e): the consequent relation between papillae and mammillae and papa and mama is no doubt both coincidental and fanciful, but worth mentioning.

PAR- The 'birth' element – from Latin *parere*, to bring forth.

PAR(A) An all-purpose prefix that can mean beside, disordered, abnormal, below, above or beyond, i.e. anything but normal, (further confused by words like parachute, from *parare*, Latin to ward off or parry + French *chute*, fall). It should be pointed out that a paramedic is not a disordered doctor but a lay person, perhaps a **FELDSHER**, who works *beside* the doctor.

-PARA The 'number-of-births' suffix (pronounced with a long *a*) from nullipara for a woman who has given birth to no children to a nonipara with a tally of nine live births, and the open-ended multipara, which can be applied to any number greater than two pregnancies followed by the birth of an infant capable of survival.

PARALYSIS Greek *paralyein*, to disable, with the **PARA-** prefix (above), adapted (via Old French) into the English word **PALSY**. See also **PARESIS**.

PARAMEDIC An American-inspired word designed to enable nurses, ambulance-driving first-aiders, chiropodists (podiatrists), masseurs, chiropractors and other highly skilled medical workers to enjoy a name commensurate with their responsible work.

PARANOIA The Greek *paranoos*, distracted mind, is constructed from *para-* + *nous*, mind. In other word, out of the mind, or perhaps, interpreting the prefix in another way, beside oneself.

PARASITE From Latin *parasitus*, 'one who sits beside another' and therefore eats with him, hence a person who lives at another's expense 'and repays him with flattery, etc.', says the *Oxford English Dictionary*. See **ANOPHELES** and **LEISHMANIA** for two common parasites who may eat with us and repay us with sickness or even death; and the **MÜNCHHAUSEN SYNDROME** for a common National Health parasite.

PAREGORIC A soothing medicine, drug or cream – from the Greek word for consoling or soothing. See also **PLACEBO**. A *Paregoric Elixir* was widely sold by chemists from the 18th century to the early years of the 20th. It was a camphorated tincture of opium, flavoured with a little aniseed, and highly addictive.

PARESIS Greek for slackening. Often used interchangeably with **PARALYSIS**, though strictly it indicates a lesser degree of weakness.

PAREUNOS Greek for 'lying together in bed' – with a sexual intent. When this causes pain it can bring about **DYSPAREUNIA**.

PARONYCHIA From Greek **PARA** + *onyx*, the nail. A suppurative infection of the fold of skin at the margin of a nail, more popularly – and more anciently – called a **WHITLOW**.

PAROTID From **PAR(A)-**, beside, + **OT(O)-**, the ear (Greek *ous, otos*) i.e. 'beside the ear'. The parotid gland is the largest of the three salivary glands.

PAROXYSM Greek/Latin *paroxysmos/paroxysmus*, a goad, exasperation or irritation – originally a general term, not relating merely to bodily pain.

PARTHENOGENESIS From the Greek *parthenos*, virgin + the **GEN-**, the origin or generating prefix: reproduction (and subsequent birth) without any concourse of opposite sexes or union of opposite elements. In religion it refers to an immaculate (and therefore miraculous (see **MACULA** for taints and spots) and pure conception, untainted by sex, possibly with the help of the Holy Spirit. However, **IN VITRO** fertilisation does not count as immaculate.

PARTNER The **PC** family physician does not refer to a patient's spouse as his or her husband or wife. Many patients, even those who are lawfully married to each other, will prefer to call them 'My partner...' A homosexual live-in friend, however, remains a partner, at any rate until English-speaking countries follow the example of Holland and legalise one-sex marriage – when partner will become politically incorrect and we shall be obliged to call them wives/husbands. Like the barely-pronounceable courtesy prefix 'Ms' (invented in 1952 by the National Office Management Association of Philadelphia and soon enthusiastically adopted by some feminists) 'partner' belongs to the 'mind-your-own-business' group of words indicating that a person's status, marital or otherwise, is his/her ('their' or 'hos') own business. See also under **POLY-**, as well as a legal–technical note under **BUGGERY**.

PARTURITION The action of bringing forth young, from Latin *partus*, birth; *parere*, to bear, beget, *parturire*, to be in labour. Hence numerous derivatives like post-partum, after the birth; primipara, of a woman who has her first birth, multipara, one who has had many.

PATELLA Latin for a pan, hence the name of the small, moveable bone also called the knee-pan. The Spanish *paella*, a favourite dish of rice, seafood, etc., cooked in a frying-pan, therefore has the same ancestry. See also **MENU CONDITIONS**.

PATENT MEDICINE A proprietary medicine or drug sold under a patent, as opposed to a **GENERIC** preparation. Discoveries by scientists working for pharmaceutical companies can be protected by patent and remain the companies' property for a certain time. The many and various legal implications are beyond the scope of this book but in earlier times the profusion of alleged remedies, elixirs and 'cures' often lent the term 'Patent Medicine' a derogatory flavour.

PATHOLOGY The study (and science) of disease, from Greek *pathos*, suffering (see below) + *logos*, science – the *-logy* suffix being one of the commonest in medicine and other disciplines.

PATHOS The ordinary Greek word for suffering, undergoing, experiencing. *Path(o)-* thus became the prefix of pain, sickness and suffering, resulting in numerous composite words. The strict meaning of pathology is therefore merely the 'science of suffering'; but of course meanings change over the years. See also **PATIENT**.

PATIENT A sufferer, from Latin *patientia*, the quality of enduring, from *pati*, suffer – perhaps also related to the Greek *pathos* (above). It was first adopted by the medieval French, and in 1393 appropriated into English by William Langland for any sort of patient sufferer; then, in 1484, by William Caxton specifically for a sick person: 'Whan the pacyent or seke man sawe her...' If the **GREY SUITS** had their way, British patients would probably be renamed 'clients' or (like British railway passengers) 'customers'. Long waiting-lists and waiting-times sometimes endured by patients intensify the connection with the quality of possessing patience.

PATIENT-DUMPING In the United States, the premature discharge of Medicare or poor patients for economic reasons. For a process in the opposite direction, see **GRANNY-DUMPING**.

PATIENT MANAGER One of the many **GREY SUITS** who help to run the NHS. A person with that title appeared on a television news programme to read a report about a small epidemic. Other splendid new job-names are listed under **CHIEF/PRINCIPAL NURSING OFFICER**.

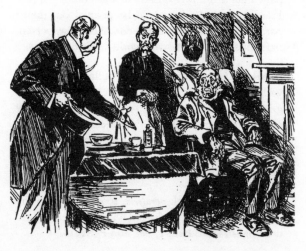

Irate Doctor (finding bottle of quack medicine). "WHY DIDN'T YOU TELL ME YOU WERE TAKING THIS WRETCHED STUFF?"
Patient. "WELL. IT WAS MY MISSIS, SIR. SHE SAYS, I'LL DOSE YOU WITH THIS. AND DOCTOR HE'LL TRY HIS STUFF, AND WE'LL SEE WHICH'LL CURE YOU FIRST."

Punch, October 20, 1909

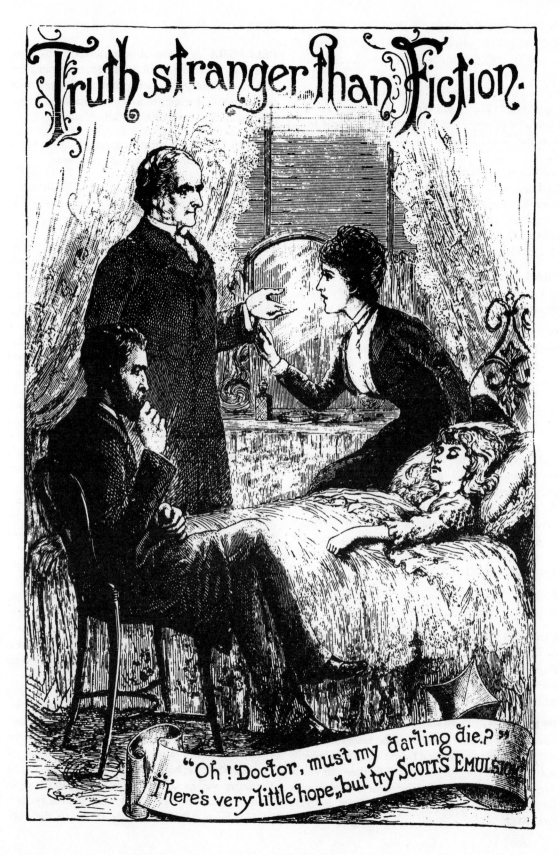

PAVLOV'S DOG What would the press do without him and his master when searching for a way of describing a **KNEEJERK** reaction (even though journalists have composed variations on the theme: '...like Pavlova's dog' and once, through a mishearing by a copytaker, '...like a padlocked dog')? Ivan Petrovich Pavlov (1849–1936) was a Russian physiologist who won the Nobel Prize in 1904 for his work on the nature of digestion. When experimenting on the nervous stimulation of gastric secretions he discovered the conditioned reflex, a physiological reaction to environmental stimuli, which influenced the development of **BEHAVIO(U)RISM**. See also **KJ** and **MUSICLE**. There was, of course, not one Pavlov's Dog but many.

PBAB American doctors' secret code abbreviation of Pine Box At Bedside, meaning that a patient is about to die. See also **CTD** and **J.P. FROG.**

PC Short for politically correct. This kind of alleged rectitude demands that words must be non-discriminatory, non-sexist, non-racist, non-ageist, non-ableist and non-this-that-and-the-otherist. It is an absurd term, as it is neither political nor always correct; but is included here because (thanks to a small but vocal section of the population) the quest for political correctness now pervades our daily life and work. Most big organisations employ **GREY SUITS** whose sole job is the stamping-out of politically-incorrect terms, and who insist on 'equality' (whatever *that* means). Those obliged to use the term may, however, indicate their scepticism by isolating it in quotation-marks, although this, too, may be considered politically incorrect. See **CRIPPLE, DEAF-AND-DUMB, PARTNER**, etc.

PECT- The breast or chest prefix, from Latin *pectus*, the breast *(pectoris,* of the breast*).* But:–

PECTEN Latin for a comb or rake; and for the set of bones in the hand between the wrist and the fingers. Pecten also denotes the pubic region – the pectinal bone being the pubic bone – or the pubic hair, for reasons I am unable to understand.

PED-/POD- The foot prefixes. The two forms have arisen because Greek is *pous, podos* and Latin *pes, pedis* – further confused by the 'children's' prefix **P(A)ED-**, as in p(a)ediatrics – and further still when American spelling simplification turns the last-named into 'pediatrics'. See both **CHIROPODIST** and **PODIATRIST.**

PELL- The skin prefix, from Latin *pella*, skin.

PELLAGRA A disease often attributed to the consumption of diseased maize, and endemic among the peasantry of maize-producing countries or regions of such countries. Perhaps related to the Italian *pelle agra*, rough skin. See also **-AGRA**, the 'attack' suffix.

PELVIS Latin for a basin – pudding or wash – and transferred to describe part of the skeleton.

-PEND- The 'hanging or dangling' suffix, from the Latin *pendere*, to hang. Hence the *appendix*, which is appended to the side of the **CAECUM**.

PENICILLIN The name for, originally, the antibiotic agent obtained from mould-like cultures (see **MYC-**) whose spores resemble brushes or tails (see **PENIS**, below). It was discovered in 1928 by the Scottish-born bacteriologist Sir Alexander Fleming (1881–1955) – 'by accident', as he always pointed out – and first produced in practical form in 1940 by Sir Ernst Chain (1906–79), just in time to save thousands of war casualties from fatal infections, and many millions of people thereafter. Fleming wrote, 'All of us, in our ordinary pursuits, can do research, and valuable research, by continual and critical observation. If something unusual happens, we should think about it, and try to find out what it means... There can be little doubt that the future of humanity depends on the freedom of the researcher to pursue his own line of thought. It is not an unreasonable ambition in a research-worker that he should become famous, but the man who undertakes research with the ultimate aim of wealth or power is in the wrong place... (Quoted in *Alexander Fleming* by Beverley Birch, Exley Publications, London, 1990). For more about Fleming see under **IMMUNISATION**. The hospital room at St. Mary's, Praed Street, London, where Fleming made his discovery, is now the Alexander Fleming Laboratory Museum and is open to the public. For a less scientific, traditional cure-all, see **JEWISH PENICILLIN**.

PENIS Latin for a tail, and in classical times used either facetiously or downright vulgarly. Only much later did it become the polite, medical word for the male sex-organ. *Peniculus* is a little tail, *penicillum* an even smaller one, hence our pencil (also a brush – in the same way as a fox's tail is his 'brush') and, of course, penicillin. The Greek word for the penis is *phallos*. From Chaucer's time down to the 18th century one of the vulgar terms was the – surely somewhat over-optimistic – **YARD**. Numerous other popular terms need not concern us here.

PEPSIS Greek for digestion, from *peptos*, cooked, *peptein*, to digest. Both *peps-* and *pept-*, when prefixed to other word-elements, describe stomach-related conditions, like dyspepsia. Pepsin is the enzyme produced by the **PANCREAS** and causes peptic ulceration of the **DUODENUM**. See also **OREXIS**.

PERAMBULATORS See **GENTLE PERAMBULATORS**.

PERI- The Greek prefix meaning round and about: pericardium, the membranes around the heart; pericranial, about the skull; **PERINATAL** (below); peridontal, around the teeth; periosteum a membrane about the bone, etc. There is, incidentally, a good old English name for the pericardium: it used to be called the 'hull', like the shell of a pea-pod.

PERINATAL Literally, around the (time) of birth.

PERINEORRAPHY A **SUTURE** of the perineum. The *-rhaphy* suffix comes from the Greek word for sewing, *rhaphe*, a seam.

PERINEUM The region between the anus and the scrotum in men and the vulva in women; or, as Blancard's *Dictionary of Physiology* of 1693 put it, 'the Ligamentous Seam betwixt the Cod and the Fundament'.

PERISTALSIS From the Greek *peristellein*, to wrap around, *peristaltikos*, a sending round; which could equally well have been used if Hermes had been despatched and sent round for a take-away of **AMBROSIA**. In medicine it is applied to the digestion, the sending-along by successive waves of involuntary contractions or **VERMICULAR** movements the contents of the bowel, etc. See also below.

PERISTALTIC PERSUADERS An **APERIENT** invented and advertised by Dr William Kitchiner, a delightful early-19th-century quack, cook, dietician, know-all and author of *The Cook's Oracle*. Peristaltic is the English derivation of **PERISTALSIS** (coined not by Kitchiner but **GALEN**) and described above. See also **CASCARA, KRUSCHEN SALTS, GENTLE PERAMBULATORS** and other bowel-opening **PATENT** medicines cross-referenced.

PESSOS Latin word for an oval-shaped stone, from Greek *pesson*, hence the pessary. Pessomancy was a form of divination by reading the chance throw of pebbles, a variation on superstitions like fortune-telling, astrology or the 'reading' of tea-leaves. See also **PR**.

(THE) PEST Latin *pestis*, plague, pestilence, or any **INFECTIOUS** or **CONTAGIOUS** disease. Although it is such an expressive, labially explosive word it is almost completely passed over in favour of **PLAGUE** – apart from expressions like pest-control, which are more concerned with vermin than epidemics.

-PEXY The surgical repairing or fixing suffix, from Greek *pexis*, fastening: cystopexy, enteropexy, nephrosplenopexy, etc. There was a fashionable operation in the late 19th and early 20th centuries vogue among the rich for 'dropped' organs – kidneys, stomachs and colons – from which, says Dr Stephen Lock, Sir Arbuthnot Lane (1856–1943) made a fortune (though his baronetcy was given to him for his other, many and various, achievements in surgery). His students used to mutter, 'It's a weary lane that leaves the colon...' See also **-RHAPHY**, the sewing suffix.

-PHAG(E)- The eating prefix/suffix, from the Greek *phagein*, to eat, e.g. dysphagia an eating-disorder (two words with a vital hyphen between them), etc. A sarcophagus, or stone coffin, was thought to consume the flesh it contained, whereas, of course, the dead matter merely decomposed. The Latin equivalent is *vorare*, to swallow, with implications of *vora*ciousness and greed.

PHAGOCYTE From *phagein* (above) + *kytos*, a cell: literally, therefore, a cell-eater: the white blood cells which swallow and digest bacteria and dead cells.

PHALANGES From Latin *phalanx*, a line of soldiers, hence the lines of 14 tapering bones composing the fingers of each hand and the toes of each foot.

PHALLOS The Greek word for the **PENIS** above.

PHANTOM PATIENT See under **FAF** and **(IT'S) FOR A FRIEND**.

PHARMACY/PHARMACEUTICALS From Greek *pharmakon*, a drug, medicine or poison. In ancient Rome a *pharmakeus* was a poisoner, *pharmacopola* a quack, or vendor of medicines.

PHARYNX From the Greek *pharunx* for the throat or gullet. The related *pharanx* means a chasm or big hole.

PHASIS Greek for speech, hence, with the A-for-absence prefix, aphasia, loss of it, or inability to speak.

PHEROMONE Not 'feramone' or 'feromone' as often written. A substance secreted by animals and humans which influences the behaviour – especially that governing sexual attraction – of other animals or humans, usually of the same species, though experiments have shown that a vacant seat, e.g. in an uncrowded waiting-room in which it (the seat) has been invisibly sprayed with boar's pheromone, will be sought out by women in preference to all other vacant seats. Such are the mysteries of sexual attraction. The word is made from the Greek *pherein*, to convey + the *-mone* element of hormone, here explained as meaning 'to set up an urge'. So perhaps there is something to be said after all for the incorrect spelling 'feramone', if one relates it to the Latin *ferox*, meaning wild, savage, untameable + the Greek *-mone* for 'a wild urge'.

-PHILIA The 'love' suffix, from Greek *philos*, dear to, to love, to have an affinity with or, in the case of **H(A)EMOPHILIA**, a tendency towards. Homophilia is the opposite of **HOMOPHOBIA**, i.e. a fanciful description of the inclinations of homosexuals; the nonce-word **P(A)EDOPHILIA** feeds the pretence that pederasty and child-molesting are really manifestations of a love for children; **GERONTOPHILIA** means a love for old persons – and necrophilia is the final straw: see **NECRO-**.

PHIMOSIS Narrowness or contraction of the orifice of the **PREPUCE** of the **PENIS** so that it (the prepuce) cannot be retracted or the penis come forward; or paraphimosis when it is retracted over the glans with difficulty and gets stuck there. *Phimos* is the Greek word for a muzzle, a device which when put on a dog allows it to bark but not bite.

PHLEBOTOMY From the Greek *phleps* (see below) +*temnein*, to cut. The classical name for blood-letting. Nursing-staff who take blood-samples from patients are now called Phlebotomists. See also under **CUPPING** and **LEECH**.

PHLEPS Greek for vein, Latin *vena*. Hence numerous formations, e.g. phlebotomy, phlebography, etc. – and phlebitis, which sounds uncomfortably close to the English jocular 'flea-bitis'.

PHLOG- The fever or inflammation prefix, from Greek *phlox*, a flame (which is also the Greek name for a wallflower, because of its flame-coloured aspect, though modern phlox come in several colours); *phlogistos*, inflammable; *phlogopos*, fiery-looking.

PHLYCTEN Another name for a kind of **PINK EYE**, or conjunctivitis, from Greek *phlyctaina*, a blister, an inflammatory swelling.

PHOBOS Greek for fear, producing an almost endless list of phobias. But homophobia, as commonly used, i.e. 'a fear of or aversion to homosexuals' should not be admitted to this list as it is a nonsense formation: for an explanation look among the various **HOM-** prefixes.

PHOCOMELIA From Greek *phoke*, a seal, + *melos*, a limb (see also **AMELIA**): a condition in which one or both of the hands or feet, or all four limbs, or rudimentary semblances of them, are attached to the trunk like flippers without the existence of upper arms or legs. This is now widely associated with numerous tragic cases that followed the Thalidomide disaster but it was, of course known previously (the *Oxford English Dictionary* says it was first described in 1892). The term is only one of many examples of the crass thoughtlessness that lies behind many medical namings – or, more likely, indicates doctors' certainty that the patient does not understand what they are talking about. They would hardly say, 'Well, Mrs Jones, that's a right little seal you've given birth to...'

PHONE Greek for the voice (the final *e* is sounded).

PHOT(O)- From the Greek *phos*, *phot(o)-*, light. Photophobia, a fear of light (i.e. because it is painful to a sick person's eyes). See **PRK**.

PHRAGMA One of the **ARCHITECTURAL TERMS**: the Greek for a wall, partition, hence the diaphragm. See **DIA-**, and **PHRENIC**, below.

PHRASIS Another Greek word for speech, as in tachyphrasia, fast talking (as tachycardia is a fast heartbeat). See illustration on page 121, and also **-PHASIS**, above.

-PHRENIA The madness suffix, from the Greek word for the mind (see below), hence schizophrenia and other disturbances. It also produced the (non-clinical) words frenetic and frenzy, originally written phrenetic and phrenzy.

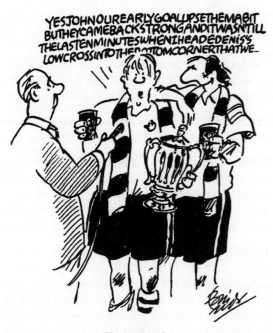

YESJOHNOUREARLYGOALUPSETHEMABIT
BUTHEYCAMEBACKSTRONGANDITWASN'TILL
THELASTENMINUTESWHENHEADEDENIS'S
LOWCROSSINTOTHEBOTTOMCORNERTHATWE...

Tachyphrasia

PHRENIC Of the diaphragm – and of the mind, thanks to a classical confusion.

PHRENOLOGY From Greek *phren*, mind + the *-ology* suffix denoting knowledge, which suggests that it should be the study, or science, of the mind. But the word was annexed by a pair of early 19th-century **CHARLATANS**, Gall and Spurzheim, who believed that the 'bumps' on one's head offered reliable information about the development of the human personality, of talents and mental faculties. When Ambrose Bierce started to write his *Devil's Dictionary* in the late 1870s phrenology was all the rage, and he defined it as 'The science of picking the pocket through the scalp'.

PHTHISIS The old-fashioned name for what is fortunately now an almost old-fashioned disease, i.e. pulmonary tuberculosis, also known as **TB**, the wasting-sickness or consumption, adjective *phthisic*. The Greek *phthisis* meant the waning of the moon, hence *phthinein*, to waste away, for which the Latin word **TABES** is also sometimes used. It has been familiar in English (imported not from Greek but the Greek-based French word *phthysique*) since the early 1300s, when it was written 'tyzyk'. The pronunciation 'tizzick' (also sometimes 'p'tizzik') remained current until the disease was almost conquered by **ANTIBIOTICS** during the middle of the 20th century (though with rapid population increase

and movement, especially in and from Third World countries, alarming outbreaks have been observed all over the world). In popular parlance the affliction was usually called 'the consumption', often preceded by 'galloping' because of the dramatic weight loss of the wasting-away process. Corpulence (see **BULIMIA**) was until the early 20th century considered to be a safeguard against it – that is, people supposed that being fat was to be healthy – and those who could afford it (and had the right metabolism) ate themselves to death – see under **BANTING**.

PHULAXIS/PHYLAXIS Greek for guard, hence prophylaxis, protection-in-advance.

PHYSICALLY CHALLENGED The euphemistic **PC** term for 'disabled', itself a euphemism for the now proscribed **CRIPPLED**.

PHYSIO Short for Physiotherapist' – see below.

PHYSIO- From the Greek *phusis*, nature, a much-used prefix, e.g. for

PHYSIOTHERAPY Literally, healing by natural means or, as the *Oxford English Dictionary* says, 'the treatment of disease, injury or deformity by physical methods, such as massage, exercise and the application of heat, light, fresh air and other external influences'.

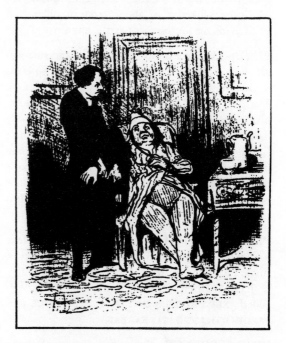

"Oh Doctor! I do believe I have the Consumption!"
Lithograph by Honoré Daumier

PICA Latin, via Greek, for a magpie ('a miscellaneous feeder', as ornithologists describe its eating-habits). In medicine pica is a perverted craving for non-nutritious or even harmful substances unfit for food, e.g. chalk, paper, coal, etc., symptomatic of certain diseases and often noted in pregnancy. When these substances include hair they may result in a **TRICHOBEZOAR**. See **BULIMIA** and cross-references for other eating disorders.

PID Abbreviation for Pelvic Inflammatory Disease, and formerly a euphemism for **GONORRH(O)EA**, a now rare cause of **PID**. Also Prolapsed Intervertebral Disc.

PIGEON CHEST Forward protrusion of the chestbone: the allusion is obvious and the condition harmless. See also **MENU CONDITIONS**.

PIGEON TOES More scientifically called **METATARSUS VARUS**, a congenital deformity of the foot in which the forepart rotates inward. I have seen many pigeons walking but fail to see the likeness.

PIGGYBACK PORT A coupling for the **IV** system to allow the addition of a supplementary solution to enter the system.

PILES The ancient English for **H(A)EMORRHOIDS** though both words coexisted from earliest times. A medical manuscript of about 1400–50 offers '...a good medicine for the pylys and ... emerawdys'.

PIL(O)- The hair prefix. In classical Latin *pilus* was 'the hair of the body', including pubic hair; whereas the hair on the head was *capillus* (see Adams, *The Latin Sexual Vocabulary*, Duckworth, 1982). Its removal is depilation – a slave employed to remove unwanted body hair was called an *alipile*; and French soldiers who, like British guardsmen, used to wear bearskin hats, are nicknamed 'the hairy ones', or *poilus*. In pre-pneumatic days hair was used for stuffing balls (see **BOL**) and thus produced a Latin name for the game of football: 'It is calde in latyn *pila pedalis*, a fotebal' (1486).

PILONIDAL SINUS An infected 'nest' of hair found on the bodies of the hirsute, or perhaps a single ingrowing (instead of 'outgrowing') hair, e.g. in the **NATAL** cleft of the sedentary, when it has been called **JEEP-DRIVER'S BOTTOM**. See **NIDUS** and **PSEUDOFOLLICULITIS BARBAE**.

PINGUESCENCE Fatness, obesity, or the process of becoming or growing fat. From Latin *pinguis*, fat – hence surely (though surprisingly even the *Oxford English Dictionary* fails to point this out) the corpulent, waddling penguin (the older and German spelling is *Pinguin*). See **LIP(O)-**; also **CELLULITE, OBESITY, PUPPY FAT** and **PYKNIC**. Also **BANTING**, if you would like to do something about your weight.

PINK EYE Conjunctivitis, for which see under **CONIUGARE**. Also **PHLYCTEN**.

PINNA (Plural *pinnae*) The external, protruding part of the ear or ears. It is the Latin word for a wing or feather (also pens, the ancient word for wings, as well as the pen, made from a wing-feather or quill – not to mention *penne*, one of the Italian pasta shapes).

PINNECTOMY From the Latin ear element (above) and the Greek **TOM-** denoting a cut: an operation which has figured in history. Poor, mad Vincent Van Gogh, on being taunted by a girl, gave himself a do-it-yourself pinnectomy in 1888: he severed one of his ears and sent it to her in the post. He was found lying on his blood-soaked bed, in a high fever, and was taken to a lunatic asylum, though some details of the story seem to be in dispute. An English severed ear provided the excuse for a small

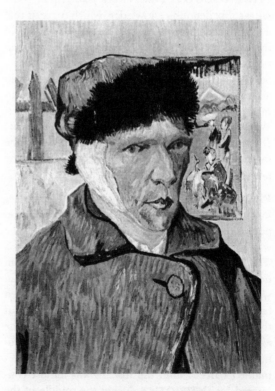

Vincent van Gogh, Self-Portrait with Bandaged Ear

colonising war between England and Spain. In 1731 Robert Jenkins, an English sailor, started a bar-room brawl with a Spanish customs officer in Havana and suffered a bad cut to an ear, which a local surgeon amputated. Jenkins kept the ear in his locker and took it home to England, where a Member of Parliament waved the object (doubtless looking by now more like a sun-dried tomato) in the House of Commons and demanded revenge for the alleged mistreatment of British smugglers and pirates (and see **SHROUD-WAVING**, also much in evidence in the British parliament). The Admiralty sent a force of six ships, under the command of Admiral Vernon, to the Caribbean islands, some of which he captured for Britain. See also **OT(O)-**.

PISIFORM Pea-shaped, from the Latin *pisum*, a pea. The word solved for me the mystery of the popular Austrian rice-and-pea dish *Risibisi*, whose origin cookery dictionaries always give as 'unknown' (*b* and *p* often sound alike in Austrian pronunciation). See also **PYRIFORM**.

PISS PROPHET Old English nickname for a doctor, especially one who set great store by the inspection of a patient's urine, and presumably one who kept a **CHAMBER-POT PRACTICE**. See also **STERCORARIAN**.

PITUITA Latin for slime, mucus or phlegm, related to Greek *ptuo* – hence the pituitary gland. This is so like the labial/lingual noise one makes when spitting (the initial *p* of *ptuo* was sounded) that one may assume it to be onomatopoeic: the Germans, incidentally, say *pfui!* when expressing disgust (sounding the *p* but giving Americans their 'phooey!'). Explosive-sounding *p*-words seem often to indicate things disgusting, just as *sp*-words tend to indicate wetness, see under **SPERMA**.

PLACEBO Latin for 'I shall please' (or 'I shall be pleasant') which some doctors probably murmur through clenched teeth when yet another patient asks them for 'a bottle of something'. In former times they might have given him or her a **TINCTURE** of (possibly coloured) water – either because the patient was not suffering from any (identifiable) disease of the **GOK** kind, or perhaps because the doctor did not know what to prescribe. Either way the patient probably felt better (an often-observed 'placebo effect'). My sensible old doctor used regularly to dispense placebos in the form of apples, which he kept in his desk and would give to patients who needlessly asked for medication ('An apple a day...'). The use of the placebo has been widened to include clinical trials or experiments in which certain patients are given real drugs while others take a placebo, or dummy, and they do not know which they are taking. This is a Blind Test; and when the doctor himself does not know which was which, it is a Double Blind Test. The origin of Placebo lies in the church, for it is short for *Placebo Domino in regionem vivorum*, i.e. part of the Vespers in the Office for the Dead in the Roman rites. In older and less scientific times doctors were expected to test medicines on themselves, though few did. In Wadd's *Nugae Chirugicae* (1824) he tells of Anthony Stork MD. 'Few medical people have acted so fairly by their patients as Dr Stork; who, before he advocated the use of the meadow-saffron, tried it upon himself in a crude state, until he was brought to the door of death. [He also] undertook some experiments on diet and prosecuted them with such imprudent zeal that they proved fatal to him, in his 29th year'. See also **PAREGORIC** and **PSYCHOSOMATIC**.

PLACENTA From *placenta*, the ordinary Latin name (adapted from Greek) for an ordinary, edible cake – hence the name for the afterbirth of mammals (which many female animals do indeed dispose of by eating it). In German, that often so prosaically literal language, the placenta is *Mutterkuchen* – 'mother's cake' (which one might almost expect to be followed by a recipe – 'just like mother used to make'): for an association with a sausage see **ALLANTOIS**. The normal way of stressing the word is on the middle syllable, placénta – so the medical student who stressed it on the first and thought it was 'a nursery' (i.e. 'play centre') was wrong on both counts. See also **AMNION** and **HYSTERECTOMY**.

PLAGIARISM *Plagiarius* in Latin is an abductor, a kidnapper (now probably also a hijacker), from which is derived the word for stealing someone else's work. Athough not strictly a medical term I include it in this book, whose contents I have of necessity compiled by plundering the wisdom of dictionaries, encyclopaedias and other reference-books (see *Bibliography*). But Dr Stephen Lock, for many years Editor of the *British Medical Journal*, says that plagiarism has reached epidemic proportions, largely because of the huge volume of often unchecked 'papers' being published.

PLAGUE From the Latin *plaga* (itself adapted from Greek *plege*), a blow or stroke (also figuratively, of fate), an affliction or scourge: see also **-PLEGIA**, below. See also **BUBONIC**. See also **PEST**.

PLANTA Latin for the sole of the foot: see under **BABINSKI**. The plantaris muscle at the back of the leg is that which flexes the foot and leg, and was put to some interesting uses by Roman soldiers: see **CONDOM**.

PLASMA From Greek *plassein*, to mould, shape. Hence the numerous *-plasia* words and those (see below) ending in *-plasty*. Also of course the **PLASTER**: the moulding substance as well as the stick-on dressing; also how the proprietary modelling substance Plasticene got its name. Blood plasma, a fluid in which blood cells are suspended, came to be named via a slightly different route, because of the plasma cell discovered towards the end of the 19th century.

PLASTER From Greek *emplassein*, to plaster on, Latin *plastrum*: originally an external curative dressing used for **TOPICAL** application in the form of a salve, paste or other medicament (which explains why the same word had for centuries been used also for builder's plaster). The older form 'plaister', which was used in the 18th century in Dr Johnson's writings, is perpetuated in the pronunciation still sometimes heard in Northern England and Scotland. What is now generally known as a plaster – a self-adhesive wound-dressing – has a connection with a different Johnson family. In 1876 Robert Wood Johnson heard an address by Sir James **LISTER** describing Lister's individually-wrapped sterile dressings. In the following year, with his brothers James Wood Johnson and Edward Mead Johnson, he took over part of a wallpaper factory in New Brunswick, NJ and with 14 employees started manufacturing self-adhesive pharmaceutical plasters with an india-rubber base – thus founding the firm Johnson and Johnson. The Johnson brothers had in fact been experimenting with a rubber-based adhesive plaster since 1874, before being reinspired by Lister.

-PLASTY The plastic-surgery suffix, e.g. mammaplasty, which combines Latin for the breast with the man-made substances known as plastics: Greek *plassein*, to mould, or form. Mastoplasty would have been all-Greek. The English word 'plastic' was itself named with due regard to Greek (the fount of so many beautiful words in modern languages).

PLEDGET The word is of uncertain origin but a pledget is a small plug or compress, or a flattened piece of lint (perhaps steeped in some medicament) for applying over a wound, a kind of widget, which is an undefinable word of uncertain origin for a gadget, which is an undefinable word for a small contrivance...

-PLEGIA *Plege* is Greek for a blow or stroke (both in the 'sword' and 'fate' sense). Hence the plague, as well as all the *-plegia* suffixes denoting paralysis, with which we are 'struck down'. See also **LEPSIS**, which attacks us, **ANGINA**, which strangles us, **VIRUS** which poisons our bodies, and the **SYNCOPE**, which may cut us off altogether. For a blow of the 'windy' kind see **VENTUS**.

PLETHORA Greek for a fullness.

PLEUR- The rib prefix, for which the Greek is *pleura*, hence pleurisy, etc.

PLOMBOSCILLOSIS Code description of the 'illness' of one pretending to be sick, invented by GPs (perhaps those who worked in the armed forces) and facetiously and artificially constructed from Latin *oscillare*, to swing, and *plombus*, lead. (For non-English readers it should be explained that 'swinging the lead' is an old military and nautical expression for the art of malingering and evading duty). See also **DAY TRIPPERS**, **MALINGERERS** and **MÜNCHHAUSEN**, as well as **SUPRATENTORIUM** and other diseases spread by the medico-legal industry, such

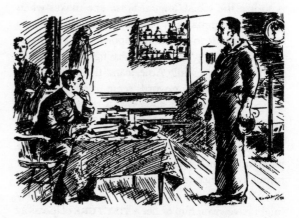

IN THE SICK BAY

Fleet Surgeon. "THERE DOESN'T SEEM MUCH WRONG WITH YOU, MY MAN. WHAT'S THE MATTER!"
A.B. "WELL. SIR, IT'S LIKE THIS, SIR. I EATS WELL, AN' I DRINKS WELL, AN' I SLEEPS WELL; BUT WHEN I SEES A JOB OF WORK – THERE, I'M ALL OF A TREMBLE!"

Punch, July 16, 1898

as **RSI**. Insurance companies have become wise to the ease with which successful claims can be made and have started a counter-industry: they employ under-cover camera crews to make videos of 'sufferers' who miraculously recover as soon as they have banked the cheque. And look for Abram-men under **BEDLAM**.

PLUMBERS Facetious (self-)description of those working in urinary **SPECIALTIES**.

PMT Premenstrual Tension (also PMS for Premenstrual Stress/Syndrome) from Latin *prae*, before + *menstrualis*, monthly + *tendere*, to stretch. It may manifest itself in nervous tension, irritability, (o)edema, headache, dysphoria, lack of co-ordination and concentration, irritability, loss of libido, excess of libido, frigidity, household breakages, road accidents, divorce, suicide and even murder. It was first named by Dr Robert Frank in 1931 but reached epidemic proportions – especially among the middle-classes – only from the 1970s/80s onwards, when women's magazines and pages in newspapers devoted to women began to give much space to it. They (as well as their menfolk) were doubtless always aware of it, but unable to articulate their difficulties or give a name to them, especially as the symptoms disappeared with the onset of the **MENSES**. Female ministers-of-state, high-ranking business executives, airline captains, surgeons, operational soldiers, etc., may also suffer from PMT but they never complain about it (at any rate publicly); and among African tribes it is said to be practically unknown. See also **MITTELSCHMERZ**.

-PNEUM- Word element denoting breath. The Greek *pneumon* means a lung; hence pneumonia, etc. dyspnea, difficulty in breathing, and other formations. The Latin equivalent is **PULMO, PULMINIS**.

PNEUMATURIA Literally, 'air-in-the-water', i.e. the presence of bubbles in the urine. It would be unwise to invoke a comparison with the *méthode champenoise* because any use of the word 'champagne' usually brings immediate sanctions from the French champagne growers, who have pursued successful lawsuits against even 'Champagne Hair Shampoo' and a non-alcoholic drink which was called – briefly – 'Elderflower Champagne'.

POCKETBOOK BIOPSY A doctor's discreet enquiries about a patient's financial status and ability to pay for the treatment he may be about to give him, or – perish the thought – withhold, if this preliminary examination were to be negative. As the actor Walter Matthau said after suffering a **CORONARY**: 'My doctor gave me six months to live but when I couldn't pay the bill, he gave me six months more'. The word

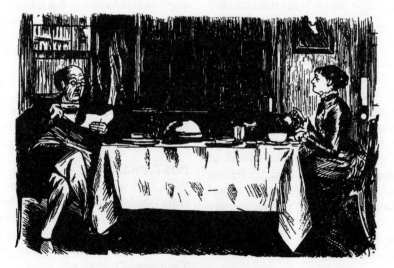

MEDICAL REMUNERATION.
Doctor. "Um! Most insolent!" *(To his Wife.)* "Listen to this,
my Dear." *(Reads Letter aloud.)* "'Sir, - I enclose a P.O. Order for Thirteen Shillings and Sixpence,
hoping it will do you as little Good as your two very small Bottles of "Physic" did me.'"

Punch, October 19, 1878

'pocketbook' reveals it to be an American coinage: the British equivalent would be Wallet Biopsy, which is not, as yet, common (or at any rate little talked about). See also **BIO-**. But, conversely, see **KERBSIDE CONSULTATION**.

POD- See **PED-**.

PODIATRIST The now usually preferred, and certainly more accurate, alternative word for what used to be called a **CHIROPODIST**. From the foot prefix, see **PED-/POD-** above, combined with part of **IATRO-**, a physician, in other words, someone who treats sick feet.

POETS' (DAY) Acronymic code for a shorter-than-usual round of hospital or surgery duties on a Friday, i.e. Piss Off Early, Tomorrow's Saturday, when doctors hope to have some free time.

POLIO(MYELITIS) Popularly and inaccurately called infantile paralysis – one of the great scourges of mankind until Sabin and Salk introduced their immunising vaccines: Sabin's taken orally and Salk's injected. From *polios*, grey (below) + *myelos*, marrow.

POLIOS Greek for the colour grey.

POLIOSIS Premature greying of the hair.

POLLEX Originally the Latin for both the thumb and the big toe but now used for the thumb only: 'of the thumb', *pollicis*. The big toe is the **HALLUX**. See also **DIGITUS**.

POLY- Greek-derived prefix denoting numbers: from several to many (and often to excess); or much, as in polydipsia, the urge to drink a lot, e.g. water in diabetes mellitus; and polyphagia, gluttonous over-eating. In some countries, medical group-practices with several doctors, or specialists in several fields, are called (as they have been in Germany and Austria for a century) polyclinics, after the model of polytechnics. Polyclinics could also be clinics serving 'the whole town'. Polyandry, incidentally, means having more than one husband, polygyny, more than one wife – and polygamy more than one marriage partner of either sex (the word 'marriage' being taken in a looser sense, as is the custom now).

POLYP Abbreviated form of *polypus*, a usually benign growth, often in the nose. The Greek word *polupos*, many-footed, originally denoted a cuttlefish, octopus, or other being whose eight or ten legs grew straight from its head.

POP Abbreviation of Plaster of Paris.

POPLITEAL, POPLITIC From Latin *poples*, ham (the kind that is inedible except to a cannibal), i.e. pertaining to the portion of the leg behind the knee. That part of the pig, the thigh, does indeed produce the finest roast ham.

PORTA Latin for a gate or door, producing various terms denoting an entrance of the body, or something situated at one. See also other architectural terms, from the **CLAUSTRUM** to the **FOCUS** and **FORNIX**, etc.

PORT-WINE STAIN See **N(A)EVUS FLAMMEUS**.

POSOLOGIST One who decides the quantity and dose of a drug, from Greek *posos*, how much + the all-purpose *-logy* or knowledge suffix, in other words a pharmacist. The *Oxford English Dictionary* dates its last recorded appearance in print 1876. Presumably it fell into disuse because a relationship might have been suspected with **CHARLATANS**, **QUACKS** or other poseurs.

POST- The 'after' prefix.

POSTCIBARIAN After eating, from Latin *cibaria*, things to eat. Numerous other *post* formations are self-explanatory.

POST COITUM OMNE ANIMAL TRISTE A much quoted Latin tag, but quoted from whom and where? Ovid? '*Post orgasmum...*' would be better, and the sadness probably afflicts the male animal more than the female, at least until he recovers his strength.

POST-NATAL As in *post-natal* depression, etc. A careless use of a common term. What is usually meant is *post-partum* – after parturition, or birth. Everything that happens to us after we are born is post-natal – and at the same time *pre-mortem*.

POST-PRANDIAL The same as postcibarian above, but specifically after dinner, although the Latin *prandium* means a late breakfast or early lunch (a 'brunch' before its time). Hence the old English word 'prandicle' (L. *prandiculum*) for a small, light meal taken at any time of the day – a snack or 'Continental' breakfast?

POST-TRAUMATIC STRESS DISORDER/ SYNDROME Better, surely, Post-Trauma Stress Syndrome as it is not the stress that is traumatic (for another such misnaming see **AIDS**). Gibson and

Potparic in their *Dictionary of Medical and Surgical Syndromes* (Parthenon Publishing) describe this recently discovered condition as '...a response to a life-threatening or very dangerous situation, such as a battle, a large disaster, or a physical or sexual assault...' etc. but it is also informally described as the Something Nasty in the Woodshed Syndrome. Sceptics take the view that (like **RSI**) PTSD may be an infection spread by trades-union representatives and compensation lawyers – in other words, a product of the litigation industry and **AMBULANCE-CHASERS**. This opinion is shared by retired ambulance-drivers, firemen, rescue workers, police and others whose work necessitates their exposure to dangerous missions, gruesome sights and generally unpleasant assignments such as the recovery of the injured and dead persons' remains. In truth, all who enter those dedicated professions know what to expect. After the football disaster at Hillsborough, Sheffield, in 1985, at which 95 people died, a television viewer – who had no friends or relatives at the scene – sued the TV companies for damages because, he said, he suffered long-term distress after seeing the tragedy unfold on the screen. He was evidently too stupid to turn off the television, and deservedly lost his case. In the two world wars of the 20th century (especially that of 1914–18) people suffered from shell shock, but PTSD was unknown; or else called **LMF** – Lack of Moral Fibre. See also **GULF SYNDROME** and **STRESS**.

POSTUM See **INSTANT POSTUM**.

POTATO TUMOUR See under **CAROS/CARUS**.

(THE) POX An early wilful plural of 'pock' (*cf* sox for 'socks') which gradually became the standard form. At first it indicated *any* disease resulting in pocks, or eruptive pustules on the skin, but later came to be used specifically and solely for syphilis, or 'the great pox', to distinguish it from the smallpox, the chicken pox, cowpox and other kinds. The syphilitic pox is not to be confused with **(THE) CLAP**, which is **GONORRH(O)EA**. Both clap and pox have been given French associations ('the French Pox' and the 'French Evil') because nations tend to blame foreigners for their ills, e.g. **INFLUENZA**, which was initially described in Italy and therefore claimed to have been 'caused' by Italians; more recently, Asian Flu to the Chinese and other oriental people (though some influenza strains are genuinely **ADVENTITIOUS**). **PRUNELLA** began as the

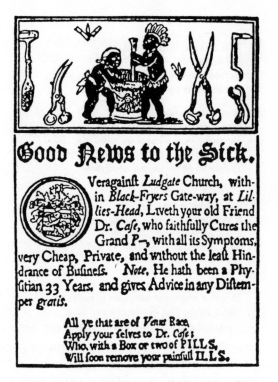

Visiting-card of a 17th/18th-century London Pox Doctor

'Hungarian Camp Fever', and **BUGGERY** was claimed to be the favourite pastime of Bulgarians. Because of the explosive noise of 'pox' the word has always been good for exclamations and oaths, e.g. 'A pox on you!'.

POX DOCTOR Informal – and ancient – name for a venereologist. In Liverpool slang any elegantly dressed man may be described as 'Got up like a pox-doctor's clerk'.

PR Non-medically, 'public relations', but in clinical terminology the abbreviation of *per rectum*, e.g. for the administration of a pessary (for which see under **PESSOS**) or when performing a rectal examination. As the wise teacher–physician says to his students, 'If you don't put your finger in it you'll put your foot in it'.

PR(A)E The 'before' prefix.

PRAECOX Latin for earliness, prematurity, ripeness before time, etc. Hence *ejaculatio praecox* (literally 'throwing out before time') for a premature male **ORGASM**. The poet John Dryden (1631–1700) offered an effected remedy for this distressing condition:

Whilst Alexis lay prest
In her arms he loved best,
With his hands round her neck,
And his head on her breast,
He found the fierce pleasure too hasty to stay,
And his soul in a tempest just flying away.

When Celia saw this,
With a sigh and a kiss
She cried, 'Oh, my Dear, I am robbed of my Bliss!
'Tis unkind to your love, and unfaithfully done
To leave me behind you and die all alone'.

The youth, though in haste
And breathing his last,
In pity died slowly, while she died more fast;
Till at length she cried, 'Now, my dear; now let us go;
Now die, my Alexis, and I will die too!'

Thus entranced they did lie,
Till Alexis did try
To recover more breath, that again he might die:
Then often they died, but the more they did so,
The nymph died more quick, and the shepherd more slow.

Curiously enough the name of the delicious apricot (in the past variously written abrecox, abrecock, apricock, etc.) is also derived from *praecox*, because of its 'early ripening'. See also **APRICOT SICKNESS**.

PRAYER'S KNEE Akin to **HOUSEMAID'S KNEE** but suffered by priests, monks and nuns. Praying muslims wisely pray little but often, thus lessening the risk of damage. Heaven knows what happens to the knees of those Mexican pilgrims who shuffle to their shrines for miles on unprotected knees.

PREPUCE Also written praepuce: the foreskin, on both the penis and the clitoris. From Latine *pr(a)e* before + a word which, regrettably, seems to be related to *putidus*, rotten, stinking, putrid (see **SMEGMA**): no wonder that about one-sixth of the world's population cuts it off in the **CIRCUMCISION** of boys – usually for religious reasons, although the original purpose was one of hygiene. See also **INFIBULATION** and **PHIMOSIS**.

PRESBYS Greek for an old man, creating words with the prefixes *presby-* or *presbyo-*, hence presbyopia, the eyesight of the old, usually inclining to long-sightedness, and presbyotic, dull of hearing in consequence of old age. The Presbyterian church is governed by elders.

PRESÉNT In ordinary usage this is a transitive verb, in that someone presents something or some-body to someone else. Medical people, however, like to use the word (usually followed by 'with') intransitively, in the sense of a patient's 'presenting', i.e. being present in a surgery and telling his or her medical adviser of the complaint or condition from which he or she believes to be suffering. This is a comparatively recent usage, a new-fangled and to some objectionable noun-into-verb formation introduced into British English during the 1960s from the United States. While it rolls easily off medical tongues, patients still prefer to speak their simple, ordinary – and no less precise – language: 'I went to the doctor with ...' Perhaps such trade-talk is intended to allow the practitioners to remain aloof from their customers. For another of the many noun-into-verb formations see under **ORGASM**.

PRIAPUS The Greek and Roman god of procreation, vineyards and gardens, where his statue was often placed to encourage plant-growth and fertility. It was represented by either a man with a huge, erect penis or just the penis on its own. In medicine, priapism means persistent and prolonged male erection, caused either by sexual excitement or, more often, a condition of the urinary or nervous sytem.

PRIMARY HEALTH CARE The provision of early diagnosis, advice, usually in general practice and by team-work, helped perhaps by the publication of leaflets and advertisements outlining a desirable lifestyle which may reduce the call on secondary health care. 'Don't smoke, Don't drink, Don't eat too much – and Take Plenty of Exercise and Fresh Air' are the most important elements in such advice. The Anglo-Irish satirist Jonathan Swift (1667–1745) wrote, in *Dialogue 2, Polite Conversations*: 'The best doctors in the world are Doctor Diet, Doctor Quiet, and Doctor Merryman', and he was paraphrasing a similar utterance made earlier by Dr William Bullein in his *Government of Health* (1558). John Dryden revealed that he knew about the quest for a **MACROBIOTIC** kind of regimen.

Better to hunt in fields for health unbought
Than fee the doctor for a nauseous draught,
The wise for cure on exercise depend;
God never made his work for man to mend.

PRIMUM NON NOCERE An ancient medical precept meaning 'First, do no damage'. From Latin *nocere*, to hurt. See **NOXA**.

PRK Photorefractive keratectomy, an operation performed with an **EXCIMER** laser on the cornea to correct deficiencies in the eyesight. See **KERAT(O)-**.

PRN Pharmacists' abbreviation for Latin *pro re nata*, 'when required' (not, as the finals examination candidate claimed, *'per rectum nocte'*).

PROBATUM (EST) Latin for 'it has been proved' – meaning tested and approved – formerly often added to prescriptions as an indication of their alleged efficacy. Hence a probatum, a well-tried, possibly **PATENT**, medicine. The saying 'The exception that proves the rule' (as well as the allegation that the proof of the pudding is in the eating) means 'proved' in this sense, i.e. the exception which *tests* the rule.

PROCEDURE Usually short for 'surgical procedure', meaning an operation, a meant-to-impress term imported from America and now often copied in Britain.

PROCTOS The Greek word for the Latin *anus* or *rectum*. When combined with some of the standard medico-verbal building-blocks, endings like -algia, -cele, -ectomy, -itis, -scopy, etc. (all of which please see) different conditions in that part of the body can be described. But whatever students at the older British universities may say, those stout disciplinarians the *proctors* are unrelated to proctos: their name is derived from a contraction of the Latin *procurator*; but in the days when Greek and Latin were still standard items on the educational menu medical students bearing the family name Proctor must have had a hard time of it.

PRODROMAL Relating to the period of time preceding a clinical event, e.g. the incubation between onset of the first symptoms of an infectious disease and the development of rash or fever, etc. From the Greek *pro* + *dromos*, running or travelling forward. See also **DROMOMANIA**.

'PROFESSIONAL' DISEASES/SYNDROMES See under **BREWER'S DROOP**, **DERBYSHIRE DROOP**, **CELLIST'S NIPPLE**, **DRUMMER'S THUMB**, **COFFEE–WASHER'S LUNG**, **FARMER'S LUNG**, **FLAUTIST'S CHIN**, **FIDDLER'S NECK**, **GAMEKEEPER'S THUMB**, **HANGMAN'S FRACTURE**, **HOUSEMAID'S KNEE**, etc. Also **RSI**, **PLOMBOSCILLOSIS** and other suspected 'lead-swinging' conditions.

PROGNOSIS Literally, 'knowing in advance': the likely outcome of a disease assessed by the condition

of the person as well as observations of the course it took in similar situations. A handbook published in 1655, *Institutiones Chirurgicae*, suggests that 'To know if a man shall live or dye, Take the Sickmans water and let a woman drop in her milk, and if it mingle with the water he shall dye, and if it swim above the water he shall live'. In 1994 a computer program was announced which claimed to do the same thing. See **GNOSIS**.

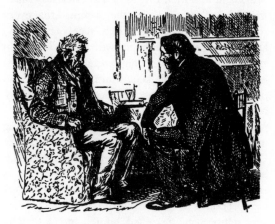

A SINE QUA NON
Patient. "DO YOU MEAN TO SAY MY COMPLAINT IS A *DANGEROUS ONE*?"
Doctor. "A *VERY* DANGEROUS ONE, MY DEAR FRIEND. STILL, PEOPLE *HAVE* BEEN KNOWN TO RECOVER FROM IT; SO YOU MUST NOT GIVE UP ALL HOPE. BUT RECOLLECT *ONE* THING: YOUR *ONLY* CHANCE IS TO KEEP IN A *CHEERFUL FRAME OF MIND*, AND AVOID ANYTHING LIKE *DEPRESSION OF SPIRITS!*"

Punch, October 4, 1879

PROLAPSE See under **LAPSUS**.

PROLES Latin for offspring (pronounced 'proelez', not rhyming with 'holes' as in George Orwell's *Nineteen Eighty Four*) from which comes the word proliferate as well as proletarians (see below). According to Servius Tullius, a *proletarius* was 'a citizen of the lowest class who served the state not with his property, for he had none, but only with his children (proles), to be turned into soldiers' (later called 'cannon-fodder'); to which end the Roman state fed, housed and clothed him. Now that the state-supported underclasses are proliferating as they have not done since the fall of the Roman Empire, the word may yet come into its own again, in the sense outlined below.

PROLETARIANS Every **GP** with a city practice has his share of them. Otiose in the true meaning of the word (Latin *otiosus*, at leisure, unemployed) most proletarians are caught in a poverty trap and rely on the **WELFARE STATE** for subsistence. Their unfortunate situation (which they blame on **THE SYSTEM**, often with justification) makes them more prone to illness than those who lead fulfilled lives. They are a far cry from the working-man idealised by Karl Marx and Friedrich Engels in *The Communist Manifesto*. Like all early socialists they assumed that every worker would be a thoroughly nice person who knew his place and was happy with his lot. He would extend his education at night-school after a day's manual work (which kept Marx and Engels and others of *their* class in their privileged positions) and, having improved himself, would rule the world – presumably in his spare time and while continuing to toil in the mills and factories: *somebody* had to. Unfortunately it was a romantic fantasy dreamed up by a couple of middle-class political theorists, as even the most unreconstructed Marxist now accepts. Today's proles are, like their Roman precursors, self-perpetuating – fed, housed and clothed by the state; uneducated (apart from what knowledge they absorb from almost continuous television-watching) and easily manipulated by commerce, their interests and pursuits almost exclusively orificial: sex, drugs, food, drink and tobacco, much of it consumed irresponsibly, with the risk of excess-related sickness and a significantly lower life-expectancy than the middle-classes. Mind-numbingly loud music (see **TINNITUS**) addles their ears (its beat recalling the drums that kept Roman legions in step) and they reproduce their kind – mostly out of wedlock – at such a rate that they will soon be the democratic majority. A Dictatorship of the Proletariat indeed, but not what Marx and Engels had in mind. At the other end of the Roman social scale were the *patricii*, or patricians, the noble families, who were themselves divided into the *patricii majorum* and *minorum gentium*, who formed the upper and ruling classes. It was they who brought doctors to Rome from Greece and Egypt.

PRONATION Assumption of a prone position, i.e. face-downwards. The opposite is **SUPINATION** – but 'prone' and 'supine' are often confused. 'I fell prone on my back, doctor' is a confusing statement. The difference may be memorised by recalling that when lying supine on the spine one can see the sky.

PROPHYLACTIC A substance or action taken to prevent, or as a precaution against, disease. In pre-1980s American usage both prophylactic and preventive were euphemisms for a **CONDOM** – not unreasonably: see below.

PROPHYLAXIS Preventive treatment: literally, 'advance protection', from Latin *pro-* + Greek *phulaxis*, guard, see **PHYLAXIS**. But see also **(GA)LACT-**.

PROSTATE From Latin for 'one who stands before'. The general public and many journalists insist that this is a misspelling of 'prostrate' – a mistake doctors and health workers should not take lying down.

PROSTHESIS Greek for 'addition or attachment to...' but also, in practical terms, a replacement, now generally an artificial limb or other part of the body, fitted to correct a deficiency. The true meaning comes from *pros*, next to + *thesis*, a placing or setting, i.e. an addition. It would therefore be more appropriate for a *third* leg, not a replacement. Prosthetics is now often coupled with **ORTHOTICS**, and universities offer combined degree courses in these two subjects to train health technicians. British sailors speak of a 'jury-mast' or 'jury-rig', a prosthetic emergency mast or rig lashed to one that is damaged: 'jury' is here short for 'injury'.

PROTEIN From Greek *proteios*, first rank.

PROTO Latin prefix denoting something that is first in time, original; earlier, and therefore perhaps primitive.

PROXIMAL From Latin proximus, for next, next to, close to or intimate. See also **DISTAL**.

PRUNE BELLY SYNDROME In this, also known as the Eagle Barrett Syndrome, the lax skin of the belly looks like that of a prune – see Gibson and Potparic's *Dictionary of Medical and Surgical Syndromes* and the illustration on page 131. See also **MENU CONDITIONS**.

PRUNELLA Another pretty name for a girl (see **AMELIA, CANDIDA**, etc.), which actually means a 'little plum (tree)' as well as an infectious disease that causes sore throats and turns the tongue brown – a corruption of the Latin word *brunella*. From the 16th century the condition was known also as Hungarian Camp Fever, until infectious diseases began to be more scientifically classified in the 19th century. A

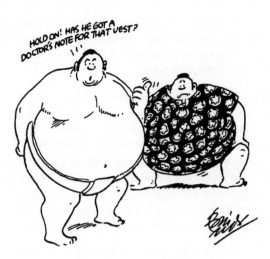

HOLD ON! HAS HE GOT A DOCTOR'S NOTE FOR THAT VEST?

Prune Belly Syndrome

form of **QUINSY**, perhaps. If girls are named Anastasia, why not also Quinsy, Aphasia, Amnesia – and the perhaps smothered-at-birth Euthanasia?

PRURITUS From Latin *prurire*, to itch, usually on the surface of the skin; hence also prurience: the latter originally a polite name only for a physical itch but later also a liking for impure or lascivious thoughts of sex, or curiosity about it. See also **PSORA** and **PUPPY PRURIENCY** below.

PSEUDO- The prefix of falseness or of a superficial resemblance which is not a real one, from Greek *pseudos*, a falsehood. Thus *pseudoleukemia*, apparent *leukemia*; and *pseudocyesis*, a phantom pregnancy. As the limerick has it:

> *A worried young girl from New York*
> *Was expecting a call from the stork.*
> *By the mercy of Jesus*
> *It was pseudocyesis*
> *So now she is back at her work.*
> [Dr Erich Geiringer]

FLATULENCE, perhaps?

PSEUDOFOLLICULITIS BARBAE One of the disadvantages a man may suffer for having a nice curly beard. According to Dr Thomas Stuttaford of *The Times* hairs may grow back into the skin before they have left the follicle, and grow beneath the surface, where they instigate a foreign-body inflammatory action. It is, he says, particularly common in naturally curly-haired Black races, making the beard

appear to grow in small clumps. See also **PILONIDAL SINUS**.

PSITTACOSIS From Latin *psittacus*, a parrot. A disease from which this bird suffers and which it can pass on to humans – who become, literally, sick as a parrot. See also **BIRD-FANCIER'S LUNG** and other recreational or occupational complaints, as listed under **BREWER'S DROOP**; also **HANGMAN'S FRACTURE** and **HATTER'S SHAKES**.

PSORA Greek noun, adopted into Latin, meaning an itch, hence psoriasis. Latin noun **PRURITUS**, verb **PRURIRE**, above. Where there is an itch there is sure to be a scratch – for which see **SCABERE**.

PSYCHO- The 'mind' prefix, from the Greek *psyche*, breath, life or soul. It appears in numerous words, including illnesses described as **PSYCHOSOMATIC** – see below.

PSYCHOLOGICAL PROFILING A chance for psychologists to turn an honest penny by making deductions or drawing conclusions – or simply speculating – about criminals, prospective employees, or others of whom insufficient is known. If this is done in a suitably convincing manner, police and employers will provide a ready market.

PSYCHOSOMATIC A word used to describe physical disorders thought to be caused or aggravated by mental or emotional factors. See also **SOMA**, Greek for the body.

PSYCHROLUSIA You are unlikely nowadays to hear this word in your doctor's office or GP's consulting-room but it was formerly a recommended treatment for strengthening the body: cold bathing, from Greek *psychro-*, cold + *louein*, to wash or bathe (*cf* Latin *ablutio*, a washing-off). One who is given to taking cold baths is a psychrolute or psychrolutist. Victorian England had a *Society of Psychrolutes* who hoped to remain healthy (or, more likely, to keep impure thoughts at bay) by 'bathing out of doors between November and March'. Exposure between April and October was presumably not uncomfortable enough. See also **THALASSOTHERAPY**.

PTARMIC A substance that induces sneezing. Not much prescribed today, and more often dispensed by snuff-merchants than chemist–druggists.

PTOMA Greek for a dead body – one of the 'fallen' – see **PTOSIS**, below. Hence *ptomaine*, a word formerly much used by the general public (before such infections were properly understood) for the 'poison' in food which had 'gone bad' (the culprit often being shellfish). 'Ptomaine poisoning' was once almost synonymous with food-poisoning. See also **NECRO**.

PTOSIS A drooping eyelid – the Greek for a fall, so literally a 'fallen' eyelid (see **BREWER'S DROOP** for a different kind of downfall). From *ptosis* comes also the symptom, literally a 'falling-together' of circumstances. The German for a case (e.g. of sickness) is indeed *Fall*.

PTS See **POST-TRAUMATIC STRESS DISORDER/ SYNDROME**.

PU Passing Urine. See also **OB**.

PUBES/PUBIC The first meaning of the Latin *pubes* was 'signs of adulthood', i.e. the signs of *hair* that covers the *mons veneris* or *mons pubis*, 'the pubic mount', and not the place the hair grows on, though it later widened its meaning to include the groin and 'private' parts generally. The Greek word for the pubic region is *episeion*. Hence **EPISIOTOMY**.

PUBLISH OR PERISH Given in *Mosby's Pocket Dictionary* as 'a practice followed in many academic institutions in which a contract for employment is renewed at the same or higher rank only if a candidate has demonstrated scholarship and professional status by having had work published in a book or in a reputable professional journal'. Some of my friends whose duties include the reading and checking of academic papers report that by sheer bulk the practice has reached Sorcerer's Apprentice proportions.

PUBOCOCCYGEUS EXERCISES A kind of beneficial aerobic exercise that a woman can perform without loud music which might disturb the neighbours, or dressing up in a leotard (which might amuse them). It is, as *Mosby's Pocket Dictionary* puts it, 'A regimen of isometric exercises in which a woman executes a series of voluntary contractions of the muscles of her pelvic diaphragm and perineum in an effort to increase the contractility of her vaginal introitus or to improve her retention of urine. The exercises' (whose benefits need hardly be rehearsed here), 'involve the muscular squeezing action ordinarily required to stop the urinary stream while voiding; and that action is performed in an inten-sive, repetitive, and systematic way throughout each day'. And all the while, bystanders, fellow-passengers – even your dinner-guests – are none the wiser. See **COCCYX/COKKYX**.

PUDENDA From Latin *pudentia*, shame, *pudere*, to make or be ashamed, hence this word for the genitals (see **GEN-**) or sexual organs – almost literally 'the bits-to-be-ashamed-of'. A poem privately circulated during the 1930s and 40s was attributed to the English writer, humorist and Member of Parliament, Sir Alan Herbert, and indeed it follows his favourite metre and rhyme-scheme. Although he never acknowledged its authorship, neither did he deny it.

> *The portions of a woman that appeal to man's depravity*
> *Are constructed with considerable care;*
> *And what first appears to be just a simple little cavity*
> *Is in fact a most elaborate affair.*
>
> *Physicians of distinction have examined these phenomena*
> *In numerous experimental dames;*
> *They have tabulated carefully the feminine abdomina*
> *And given them some fascinating names.*
>
> *There's the vulva, the vagina and the jolly perineum,*
> *And the hymen, in the case of many brides,*
> *Lots of different little things that you would like if*
>   *you could see 'em:*
> *The clitoris and other things besides.*
>
> *So isn't it a pity, when we common people chatter*
> *Of these mysteries to which I have referred,*
> *That we use for such a delicate and complicated matter*
> *Such a very short and ordinary word.*

Herbert forgot the simple and euphonious English word **FANNY** (which is included under its own heading because of the honourable nursing associations it carries), although in American usage this means the buttocks, or **GLUT(A)EUS** maximus.

PUER Latin for a boy, often widened to mean a child of either sex (the specific word for a girl is *puella*). Puerperium is the period immediately following the birth of a child, adjective puerperal – and puerile, the word for anything childish and, by association, trivial. See also **P(A)ED-** and **PROLES**.

PUGE/PYGE Greek for the buttocks – see the Latin equivalent, **NATES**; also **GLUT(A)EUS** and **CALLIPYGIAN**.

PULMO Latin for the lung. The Greek is **PLEUMON** or **PNEUMON** – hence pneumatics.

PULSUS ALTERNANS A pulse with an alternate strong and weak beat. Mr Michael Reilly recalls a Professorial Teaching-round at St. Mary's Hospital, Paddington, London. 'The Consultant in charge stopped at the bedside of a patient with such a condition. "What do you feel, boy"?, he asked a student; who replied, "Pulsus interruptus, sir". The Great Man did not hesitate: "Are you sure that you do not mean coitus alternans?", he said'.

PUNCH-DRUNKENNESS A person is said to be suffering from this when stupefied from severe and frequent blows to the head, which bring about reduced muscular co-ordination, hesitant speech and slowness of thought. The term refers to the punches exchanged in boxing, the only sport (sport?) in which the avowed intention of the participants is to knock each other unconscious. The Punch-Drunk Syndrome will be found in *A Dictionary of Medical and Surgical Syndromes* by Drs Gibson and Potparic (Parthenon Publishing). Punch-drunkenness is not related to drunkenness induced by alcoholic punch, a beverage whose name was brought to England from the West Indies in the 17th century. Some of the symptoms may, however, be similar. But then, 'hesitant speech and slowness of thought' have been observed also among proponents of the Noble (noble?) Art of Boxing who have never entered a boxing-ring.

PUO Pyrexia of Undetermined/Unknown Origin.

PUPIL The name of the circular, central part of the iris of the eye comes from the Latin *pupilla*, a little girl. The ancient poets used to speak of 'babies in their eyes', meaning the small image one sees, of oneself, reflected when gazing into another person's eyes – whether romantically or otherwise. Galen called the pupil of the eye *glene*, Greek for a mirror. See also **BELLADONNA**.

PUPPY FAT Excessive fat or plumpness in children and adolescents which usually disappears in time. On the other hand, **OBESITY** may continue into adulthood.

PUPPY PRURIENCY Nickname for signs of early sexual curiosity in children, sometimes manifesting itself (especially in single-sex schools) in behaviour that might be interpreted as homosexual. Unfortunately some prurient puppies do grow up into gay dogs (or, since we must not be sexist, into bitches). See **PRURITUS**.

PURSY/PURSINESS Old word for breathlessness, short-windedness, and asthma, from French *pousser*, 'to breathe with labour or difficulty'. It has fallen into disuse but is still sometimes heard when heavily breathing horses are described. It was also a word for fatness and corpulency: Shakespeare's *Hamlet* (1602) 'In the fatnesse of these pursie times, Vertue it selfe, of Vice must pardon begge, and an *Oxford English Dictionary* quotation from an author of 1654: 'Our short legges and pursie hearts cannot hold out here...' Also: 'An elderly fat gentleman, pursy, scant of breath...', in *History of Frederick the Great* by Thomas Carlyle (1795–1881). Thus are prettily evocative old words forgotten. For more about **CORPULENCE** see under **BANTING** and **PINGUESCENCE**.

PUS, PURIS Latin for the viscous, purulent matter emanating from a sore or wound, called suppuration. The Greek word for *pus* is **PYON**, hence empyema, etc.

PUSTULA Latin for a blister or other eruption on the skin.

PVS Persistent Vegetative State. Popular journalism equates this – often wrongly – with 'brain-death'.

PYKNIC Greek for thick, shrunken, close-packed (remember the picnic or packed lunch). A pyknic type of human frame is one of stocky, **PINGUESCENT** physique, rounded body and head, thick-set trunk and a tendency to be fat. The picnic (or picnic lunch) was first mentioned in foreign countries (Germany, Sweden and France) from the early middle of the 18th century, but did not become known as a typically English institution until about 1800. The *Oxford English Dictionary* appears not to have noticed any connection between *pyknic* and the picnic: food that is packed, eaten – and probably also fattening... just as it has drawn no parallels between pinguescence and the penguin. See also **BANTING, BULIMIA, CELLULITE, OBESITY, OREXIS**.

PYON See under **PUS**.

PYR- The heat or burning prefix, hence:–

PYREXIA Fever, from Greek *pyretikos*, fire, therefore antipyretics, drugs which subdue fever. See also **CAUSIS**. Not to be confused with:–

PYRIFORM From *pirum*, Latin for pear: Latin *pirus*, a pear-tree, so it should really be piriform, but the misspelling with a *y* arose in medieval Latin, risking confusion with fire. Pyriform breasts are pearshaped, not fiery. But better pyriform than **PISI-FORM** ones.

PYROMANIA Not so much a mania as a **LAGNIA** – a morbid desire to set things – sometimes even people – on fire, to gain some kind of sexual satisfaction. Sometimes the pyromaniacs' activities contain an element of the **MÜNCHHAUSEN SYNDROME-BY-PROXY**: being first on the scene of the fire they have started, they report it and like to watch the emergency services arrive and put it out. Pyromaniacs make good fire-fighters, as they are dedicated to and interested in their work (and when there is a fire-raiser at large, the police tend to make their first discreet enquiries in the fire service). But is this not part of the psychology of job-choice? Child-abusers are often found among those working with children; designers of women's shoes appear to be haters of the female foot; those who shape the seats for railway-carriages seem to hate the human neck; men who design the clothes to be worn by women are seldom lovers of them; and some journalists, to judge from their prose, have a deep-seated hatred for the English language. Even W.E. Gladstone (1808–98), the apparently saintly British Prime Minister, derived vicarious pleasure from his nightly street-walks among London prostitutes, though his avowed aim was their reform and redemption. But, as you will see under **HIPPOLAGNIA**, there is no accounting for the ways people get their kicks. And has there ever been a pyromaniac who is also a slave to **UROLAGNIA**?

Qq

QUACK An ignorant pretender to medical or surgical skill and hence a general and derisive term of abuse for a doctor, short for 'quacksalver'. The *Oxford English Dictionary* suggests that such a mock-doctor might have cried up, or quacked, his salves (but does not find a possible parallel with mercury, or quicksilver, a substance often used for quack 'cures'). A quack is the same as a charlatan, but whereas the quack has retained his strictly medical connotations, charlatans can be pretenders to any kind of skill or knowledge, scientific and technical. Quacks were first mentioned in early 16th-century literature and soon became stock characters in plays and operas. Operatic doctors, too, are legion, and are usually figures of fun. See **MEDICASTER, MESMERISM** and **STERCORARIAN**.

QUAD Medics' abbreviation for a quadraplegic. See **-PLEGIA**.

QUARANTINE Originally a legal term dating from feudal times which meant a period of 40 days when a widow had the right to remain in her deceased husband's house (see also **DOWAGER'S HUMP** for another manifestation of English widowhood). Then the word was applied to ships carrying sailors suffering from contagious or infectious diseases for up to 40 days (Samuel Pepys, Secretary of the English Navy, mentions ships' quarantine in his *Diary* in 1663) and later to persons themselves.

QUININE From the Spanish *quina*, itself from *quichua kina*, the bark of the Peruvian Quichua or Cinchona tree (also called Jesuit's Bark) which yields this white, bitter crystalline alkaloid used in preparations against **MALARIA**. Sir Kenelm Digby, in his Letters (1656) reported, 'I haue made knowne ... in these partes, a barke of a tree that infallibly cureth all intermittent feauours. It cometh from Peru, and is the barke of a tree called by the Spaniardes Kinkina'. It is also an important ingredient in the **TONIC** water that accompanies gin and other alcoholic drinks.

QUINSY Like **PRUNELLA**, quinsy is a pretty name for an ugly condition, viz. a peritonsillar abcess, or throat infection. The origin of quinsy is, however, more sinister: from Greek *cuon, cunos*, a dog + *anchein*, to throttle: like a dog straining at one of those constricting chain-leashes which tighten round its throat. For a different form of 'strangling' see **ANGINA**.

QS Pharmacists' abbreviation for Latin *quantum sufficiat*, sufficient quantity.

Q-SIGN The mouth with the tongue hanging out: see **O-SIGN**.

R*r*

R Short for 'Roentgen', when used as a measurement of radiation.

R Physicians' and pharmacists' abbreviation of 'take' or 'to be taken'.

RABELAIS François (c. 1494–1553). Doctor and writer: he entered a Franciscan order at Fontenay-la-Compte in 1520 but was drummed out for his addiction to the Greek language, became a Benedictine instead and, helped by his knowledge of Greek, studied medicine so successfully that he eventually left the religious life. Rabelais was in his time celebrated first and foremost as a physician, practising and teaching medicine at Lyons and in Rome. He published *Pantagruel* in 1532 and *Gargantua* comparatively late in life – between 1534 and 1552 – proving to be the first of numerous doctor–authors to have a Rabelaisian sense of humour. We also owe to him the word 'gargantuan'. His name is mentioned also under **CLITORIS**.

RABIES The Latin word for rage or madness, *rabere*, to rage. The Greek **RHEXIS/RHAGIA** denotes a raging, bursting or bursting-out.

RADI(O-) *Radius* is one of those multi-purpose Latin words that have left their mark (or rather their root – see **RADIX**, below) on and in many terms. It can mean a spoke, ray, beam or even staff or rod. Hence the radius of a circle (i.e. a line, or in a wheel a spoke) drawn from the centre to the circumference, radio transmission, *radiotherapy, –graphy, –logy*, etc, some of which suffixes will be found under their own headings.

RADIOGRAPHER/RADIOLOGIST The first is a person, e.g. **NURSE**, qualified to operate radiographic equipment; the second a medically qualified practitioner of the diagnostic use of **X-RAYS**: see the **-GRAPH(O)/(IA)** and **-(O)LOGY** suffixes. Both are skilled in their particular field, but if you must confuse the two it is better to address a radiographer as a radiologist than the other way round.

RADIUS Latin for a staff or stake, a measuring-rod or spoke, a ray: one of the bones of the forearm.

RADIX Latin for a root, hence words like radical. The Greek word is *rhiza*, prefix *rhizo-*.

RALE From French *râle*, rattle (*râle mourant*, death rattle). A perceived chest noise, which may be sibilant or sonorous. See also **FREMITUS**.

RANULA A large mucocele on the floor of the mouth, from Latin *rana*, a frog. Literally, a little frog. This kind of frog is clearly better in the mouth than the throat.

RECTUM From the Latin rectus, straight, i.e. the final, straight bit of the bowels. See also **ANUS** and **PROCT-**.

RECUPERATE Had this dictionary been compiled a century ago, this word might have been included as an unwelcome Americanism requiring an explanation. A 19th-century complaint about it will be found under **CONVALESCE(NT)**.

REDCURRANT JELLY STOOLS The same as **CRANBERRY JELLY STOOLS** – a certain bowel condition involving the presence of blood in the **FAECES**. See **MENU CONDITIONS**.

REEKER Doctors' slang (especially in the casualty ward) for a patient with a strong body-odour.

REGIMEN Latin for guidance or direction, from *regere*, to rule. Now a rather old-fashioned word, it meant the regulation of such matters as have an influence on the preservation or restoration of health; a particular course of diet, exercise, a **MACROBIOTIC** mode of living, prescribed or adopted to this end: all mostly ignored by those meant to benefit from it. The English satirical magazine *Punch* in 1883 printed a poem entitled '*That Dreadful Doctor!*':

> *He warns us in eating, he warns us in drinking,*
> *He warns us in reading and writing and thinking;*
> *He warns us in football, footrace, eight-oar 'stroking';*
> *He warns us in dancing and cigarette-smoking;*
> *He warns us in taking champagne, and canoeing;*
> *He warns us in wearing red socks and shampooing;*
> *He warns us – of drains – in our snug country quarters;*
> *He warns us – of fever – in mineral waters.*
> *He warns us in - everything mortals may mention.*
> *But – what gives rise*
> *To but little surprise –*
> *Nobody pays him the slightest attention!*

The first real health warning about smoking did not appear until 1945, when in an address at Duke University (which had been endowed with a fortune derived from tobacco sales), the New Orleans surgeon

Alton Ochsner reported 'a distinct parallelism between the incidence of cancer of the lung and the sale of cigarettes. The increase is due to the increased incidence of smoking and ... smoking is a factor because of the chronic irritation it produces'.

RELEASE INTO THE COMMUNITY A British government programme implemented (often with tragic results) by the **GREY SUITS** of the **NHS** in the 1990s, under which **LUNATICS** were turned out on the streets because it was cheaper than caring for them in hospitals. See also **CARE IN THE COMMUNITY, COMMUNITY** and **HOSPITAL NAMES** – and especially Abram-men under **BEDLAM**.

REMEDY/CURE Two words with different meanings, a distinction which advertisers during the 19th century were able to ignore, offering infallible **PANACEAS** for incurable conditions.

REMISSION A decrease (often temporary) in the severity of an illness or the pain it brings. From Latin remittere, to send back. See also **EMESIS**.

RENES Latin for the kidneys, hence renal matters and **ADRENALIN**. The Greek is *nephros*.

REP Pharmacists' abbreviation for Latin *repetatur*, 'let it be repeated'.

REP Abbreviation for a Medical Representative, employed by pharmaceutical companies.

REP AMBO Pharmacists' abbreviation of 'Let both be repeated'.

REP BAITERS Family physicians (British **GPs**) who enjoy being rude to medical representatives.

REPETITIVE STRAIN INJURY/SYNDROME A condition supposedly caused by repetitive work activity. It appears seldom, if ever, to be caused by repetitive leisure activities, and some authorities maintain that it is one of the conditions created by the medico-legal compensation industry (see also **AMBULANCE-CHASERS**). An editorial in the *British Medical Journal* in 1992 described it as 'An infectious disorder of recent recognition acquired in the workplace and usually transmitted via a union representative'. So far no claim for **RSI** has been made by any side-drum player in a symphony orchestra who when playing Ravel's Bolero is required to repeat the same rhythmic figure for 340 bars non-stop with absolute concentration and iron rigidity of posture (apart from his hands and wrists); but the day cannot be too distant, especially as an existing, recognised condition, **DRUMMER'S THUMB**, awaits their attention. See also **LIBIDO** (loss of), **POST-TRAUMATIC STRESS DISORDER, DAY TRIPPERS, WHIPLASH** and cross-references.

REP OMNIA 'Let everything be repeated'.

RESECTION Literally, 'cutting again' but, in practice, usually cutting and rejoining, e.g. a piece of gut.

RESIDENT The American and Australian equivalent of the British **HOUSE OFFICER**.

RESIDENT HOUSE OFFICER As above, but in the USA.

RESURRECTIONIST A passionate believer in the Resurrection of Christ; also a racehorse which has recovered the early form it lost for a prolonged spell; and in addition, since about 1776, an exhumer and stealer of corpses which were later (or perhaps better, sooner) sold to anatomists for dissection and research. The Resurrection Men found that they had to strip the corpses naked, as disturbing a grave and taking its occupant was in English law merely a misdemeanour, whereas taking its clothes as well would have constituted theft and therefore a felony. The most notorious British Resurrectionists were Burke and Hare, a partnership consisting of William Burke, an Irish navvy (in 19th-century Britain a kind of guest-worker) and his Scottish accomplice, William Hare, with the connivance of the Edinburgh surgeon Robert Knox. Mr Knox, asking no questions and therefore being told no lies, made good use of the cadavers in his anatomy practice. Burke and Hare eventually created so great a demand that they would not only exhume existing corpses but create new ones: having, with the help of their wives (Mrs Burke and Mrs Hare), lured their victims to their deaths. They were caught and successfully prosecuted after Hare turned King's Evidence (that is, became an informer by plea-bargaining). This saved his neck, but Burke was hanged in 1829. It led to the Anatomy Act of 1832, after which the supply of **CADAVERS** was regulated.

RETINA The name for this part of the eye is probably derived from Latin *rete*, a net. See also **CATARACT**, for a 'grating'.

RETRO Latin for behind, backward, reversed, or back into the past.

RF The standard abbreviation for rheumatic fever.

R(H)ACHIS Greek for the spine (Latin **SPINA**), hence rachitis, which would usually mean inflammation of (or at any rate 'a condition of') the spine, but was used as early as 1650 for what in English-speaking countries is popularly called rickets. There is also the colloquial word 'ricking', meaning to sprain or twist, e.g. 'I've ricked my neck' – originally written 'wricking': compare 'wrenching' and numerous other *wr-* words denoting movement and often violent or wrecking action; just as *sp-* words usually indicate some kind of wetness.

RHAGIA A raging, bursting or bursting-out, e.g. of an illness or, in bleeding, a **H(A)EMORRHAGE**.

RHAPHE Greek for a seam, hence the *-rrhaphy* suffix – e.g. **PERINEORRAPHY**. The Latin equivalents come from *suo*, I sew, *sutura*, a sewing-together, c.f. **SUTURE**. See also **-PEXY** – for making do and mending.

RHEIN/RHEUMA/RH(O)EA Greek for flow, flowing, hence rheumatism, diarrh(o)ea, h(a)emorrhoids, etc. See also **GONORRH(O)EA** and **(THE) CLAP**.

RHEXIS Greek for a bursting or breaking out. Also applicable to -rhagia words: e.g. menorrhagia, an excessive flow of blood during the menses.

RHINOPHYMA A permanent and often progressive enlargement and reddening of the nose, or **ROSACEA**, also (often unfairly) called **GROG BLOSSOM**. See **RHIS/RHINOS**, below.

RHIS, RHINOS Not for nothing is the rhinoceros so called, for rhin(o)- is the nose prefix – and the -ceros syllable refers to *ceras*, or horniness (please don't misunderstand but turn to **KERATIN**). Rhinoplasty (see **PLASTY**) is plastic surgery on that organ; rhinoscopy looking down (or up) it; the rhino **VIRUS** causes rhinitis, which is an uncommon name for the common cold; and rhinology in general is that branch of medicine which deals with nasal disorders and conditions. There are also many naso- words, from *nasus*, the Latin word for the nose. See also **OLERE**.

RHIZO- From the Greek *rhiza*, a root, e.g. in rhizotomy. See also the Latin equivalent, **RADIX,** giving us 'radical'.

RHONCHUS A beautifully echoically descriptive word for snoring, from Greek via Latin. Was there ever a better one to describe the clearing of **MUCUS**? **BORBORYGM(US)** and **ERUCTATION** are two other echoic words that describe their particular activities by the sound they make.

RHT See **HRT**.

RHUBARB This plant of the genus *Rheum* no longer figures in medical books but was extensively used for various medicinal purposes from earliest times: it 'drawys the fleume from the mouth of the stomake' (c.1400). Being both purgative and astringent ('The phisicions with a lyttell Rubarb purge many humours of the body' (c. 1533) it can still play a valiant role in **PERISTALTIC PERSUASION**. Because of this it was for centuries one of the stock joke-sources about the medical profession. See also **HOMEOPATHY**.

RICE WATER STOOLS Description of the evacuations of cholera patients, and one of the unappetising **MENU CONDITIONS**.

RICKETS See **R(H)ACHIS**.

RICTUS Latin for the expanse or gape of the mouth. See also **O-SIGN** and **Q-SIGN**.

RIGHTS WORKERS Employees of the **NHS** whose task is to acquaint members of the public of their rights – as claimants, patients, and potential litigants, etc. Significantly there are no 'Duties Workers'. See also under **EQUALITY OFFICERS, GREY SUITS, COUNSELLING, WELFARE STATE**, etc.

RIGOR Latin for stiffness – any kind, not only *mortis*.

RIMA Latin for a fissure or cleft, usually short for *rima glottidis*, the passage in the glottis between the vocal cords and the arytenoid cartilages. But it is also part of the Latin sexual vocabulary – in classical literature the exterior aspect of the female **PUDENDA**.

RINGWORM See under **TINEA** and **DHOBI ITCH**.

ROCET Contrived acronyms are now inescapable, especially among pressure-groups. This one, (pronounced 'rocket') stands for Reproductive Organs Conservation Trust, which co-ordinates legal action on behalf of women who claim to have had hysterectomies, or ovaries removed without their consent. Where the 'conservation' comes in is anyone's guess.

ROSACEA A form of reddening of the skin: see also **RHINOPHYMA**.

ROSE COTTAGE Coded hospital euphemism for the mortuary. A doctor enquiring about the whereabouts of a patient may be told 'He's in Rose Cottage'. Compare this with the fictitious code-names used by stores to summon their detectives and security-men over the public-address system; and by certain English theatres and concert-halls to let staff know of an outbreak of fire without causing panic among the audience.

ROUNDHEADS AND CAVALIERS Nicknames, probably invented in British public-schools, for the circumcised and uncircumcised penis, respectively.

-RRHAPHY The sewing suffix.

-(R)RH(OE)A Combined with other words, both Greek and Latin, denotes an excess of, or too great a, flow – of whatever is prefixed.

RSI See **REPETITIVE STRAIN INJURY**. Then pull the other one – it's got bells on.

Ss

SACRUM Latin for a sacred or holy thing: in anatomy, one of the pelvic bones – which, in some ancient civilisations, was used for sacred, ritual purposes, though if used for drinking, the wine – or blood – would have leaked out through the *foramina* – see under **FORAMEN**. As it is the last bone to decay after death it was believed that when the last trumpet (see **BUCCINATOR**) sounds and we are resurrected, the new body would form round it.

SAD Seasonally Affective Disorder (sometimes called 'Winter Depression') – one of the newer **SYNDROMES** from which many people now claim to suffer and many more think they suffer after having read about it in the newspapers and women's magazines. I suspect that the disorder (if disorder it is) was named to fit its appropriate acronym, which helps to make people naturally given to sadness the more certain that they have it; unlike **TATT**, which sounds less glamorous. Perhaps the winter sunshine holiday trade is behind it all. Not to be confused with **CHRISTMAS DISEASE**. See also **NEURASTHENIA**.

ST. VITUS'S DANCE Properly known as **CHORE(I)A**, this term for involuntary, rapid and

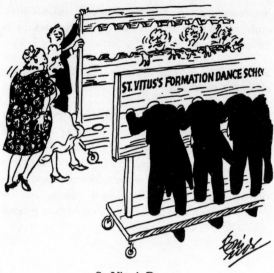

St. Vitus's Dance

purposeless movements is derived from what was in the Middle Ages thought to be a religious dancing-mania, also called St. Guy's or St. John's Dance.

SALIVA The Latin word for spittle. Salivarius means slimy. But see **SPUTUM**, below, which is worse.

SALMONELLA A rod-shaped bacterium whose connection with salmon, smoked or fresh, is entirely

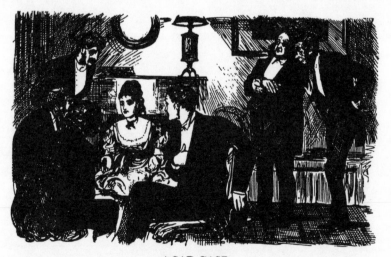

A SAD CASE

Mr. Killjoy. "I'm so glad you've come, Dr. Bland! I want to consult you about my poor wife." *Dr. Bland.* "What's the matter with her?"
Mr. Killjoy. "Such fearful depression of spirits!"
Dr. Bland. "Depression of spirits! Why, she's the life of the party!"
Mr. Killjoy. "Ah, she always bears up in company, poor thing! But you should see her when we are together alone!"

Punch, November 30, 1872

fortuitous: it was so named in 1900 after its discoverer, the American pathologist Daniel Elmer Salmon. In spite of its plural sound *salmonella* is the singular form: the plural is *salmonellae*. Unlike **CANDIDA**, **PRUNELLA** and **AMELIA**, salmonella has never been used as a name for a girl; but there is a reported sighting in the South of England of an Italian restaurant bearing the pseudo-Italian and rather unfortunate name 'Valmonella'.

SALTUS EMPIRICUS An important element in research – see **EMPIRICUS**, and under **IMMUNISATION**.

SALVARSAN Also called Compound No. 606, a drug patented in 1910 and based on a previous discovery by Paul Ehrlich (1854–1915) in his search for a cure for syphilis. The name is constructed from the Latin *salvare*, to save + Greek *arsenik*. Ehrlich, who is also mentioned under **MAGIC BULLETS**, was a German Jew considered by many to have been the father of haematology, immunology, chemotherapy and pharmacology. Within five years his drug, arsphenamine, reduced the incidence of syphilis in England and France by 50%, but was attacked on the grounds that it 'encouraged sin'. After 1933 his memory was reviled by the Nazis, who persecuted his widow and confiscated her property, though they nevertheless continued to reap the benefit of this and Ehrlich's other discoveries when they caught the **POX** or **DIPHTHERIA** and other illnesses. Frau Ehrlich was saved through the joint efforts of Ehrlich's English pupil and disciple Sir Almroth Wright (for more about him see under **ALLERGY**) and funds provided for her by the pharmaceutical industry.

SANGUIS Latin for blood – competing with the Greek **HAIMA**.

SANGUISUGA Also **HIRUDO**, the generic names of the blood-sucking **LEECH**, which please see.

SANITARY/SANATORY The two words are often confused. Sanitary comes from Latin *sanitas*, health, and is applied to matters pertaining to good health and **HYGIENE**, from rules for safe, antiseptic procedures and healthy practices like meticulous hand-washing, neat, glazed sanitary fitments and efficient sewage-disposal (for which see **CLOACA** and **CLOACINA**). Sanatory, from *sanare*, to heal, refers only to the healing process.

SANITARY In addition to the true meanings, above, the word has also become a euphemistic word denoting anything to do with **MENSTRUATION**, i.e. sanitary towel, sanitary tampon, etc. See also **TAMPAX**.

SANITARY INSPECTOR Until the late middle of the 20th century this was a low-ranking but formidable figure in British local government whose duties included the inspection of facilities outlined in the previous entry, including restaurant and food-shop hygiene. His office is now endowed with grander titles which vary from one borough to another and are bureaucratically subdivided into different categories and disciplines.

SARC(O)- The flesh prefix, from the Greek word *sarx*, flesh, hence sarcoma, a fleshy growth. The Greek word for a coffin, *sarcophagus*, came from the belief that stone 'ate' flesh: *see* **-PHAG(E)-**. The Greek flesh word also gave us sarcasm – a 'cutting' or 'biting' remark. See also **EXCORIATE**.

SARTORIUS The muscle used in crossing the legs – the longest muscle in the body, crossing the thigh obliquely in front and extending from the pelvis to the calf of the leg; and acting to flex the thigh and rotate it laterally, and to flex the leg and rotate it medially. The name comes from the Latin *sartor*, a tailor, because members of that craft traditionally sat – and in England many still sit – cross-legged, and *on* a table, not by it (and are prone to **TAILOR'S ANKLE**). See also **BUCCINATOR**.

SATURDAY NIGHT PALSY Temporary paralysis caused by drunkenness, as when someone in a drink-induced stupor falls asleep in a chair with one or both of his arms hanging over the side. He may wake next morning with one or both 'paralysed'. Unfortunately it does not happen only on Saturday nights. See also **ARSD** and **HOLIDAY HEART SYNDROME**.

SAWBONES This old nickname for a surgeon has a ring of Shakespeare about it but was in fact first noticed in Charles Dickens's *Pickwick Papers* (1837): 'What, don't you know what a sawbones is, Sir,' enquired Mr Weller; 'I thought everybody know'd as a Sawbones was a Surgeon'.

SCABERE Latin, to scratch, hence *scabies*, etc. For the itching that usually precedes it, see **PRURITUS** and **PSORA**.

SCALPERE Latin, to cut or carve. *Sculptor*, a stone-cutter or carver, who would use a *scalprum*, and the Roman surgeon a *scalpellum* – hence the modern scalpel – and sculptor.

SCAPEGOATING A favourite word among British trades union leaders, who use it as an inelegant variation of 'victimisation'. But it was clinically defined as long ago as 1943 in *The Journal of Abnormal and Social Psychology* to mean the action of shifting blame onto someone else so as to avoid self-confrontation, and is therefore a recognised term in that branch of healing.

SCAPHOCEPHALIC Having a long, narrow head, from Greek *scaphe* a boat (hence the skiff) + *kephale*, head. As opposed to **DOLICHOCEPHALIC**.

SCAPULA Latin *scapula*, the shoulder, plural *scapulae*, the shoulder-blades.

SCARF SKIN Old English word for the **EPIDERMIS**.

SCARIFICATIO Late Latin for 'a scratching', scarification, used in some methods of vaccination.

SCHIZO- Prefix derived from the Greek *schizein*, to split (*cf* schism) and therefore also:–

SCHIZOPHRENIA Literally, split mind: the above prefix with the suffix derived from *phren*, mind. See also the madness suffix, **-PHRENIA**.

SCIATICA A medieval corruption of *ischiacus*, which is Latin for 'one who has gout in the hip'. Shakespeare must have been familiar with it, for in *Troilus and Cressida* he calls it the 'incurable bone-ache' and in *Measure for Measure* asks, 'Which of your hips has the most profound sciatica?'; and goes so far, in *Timon of Athen*, as to wish it on the senators (see under **CRIPPLE**). See also **LUMBAGO**.

SCLER(O)- Prefix denoting hardening or thickening, e.g. in *sclerosis*, from Greek *skleros*, hard. See the **BASIN** mnemonic.

SCOLIOSIS From Greek *skolios*, crooked, bent. Lateral curvature of the spine. Distinguished from **KYPHOSIS** and **LORDOSIS**. And see **DOWAGER'S HUMP**.

-SCOPE, -SCOPY The 'looking, seeing or visually examining' suffix, from Greek *skopeein* to view, look, look at. Hence the numerous – and self-explanatory – words with -scopy endings: arthroscopy, cystoscopy, laparoscopy, laryngoscopy, proctoscopy, etc., each combined with the appropriate prefix (all of which please see). The -scopy ending denotes the procedure and -scope the instrument used for it. But the suffix is also used in the context of more general examination, e.g. stethoscope (Greek *stethos*, the chest).

SCREEN Noun and verb. Until recently the only screen a physician would have in his room would be made of wood, metal or fabric, and enable the patient to undress and dress without being seen doing so (a convention of etiquette, as the doctor might have to see him naked anyway). Today a doctor's screen is more likely to be one displaying computer data or a patient's notes. Patients, too, may be screened. The verb is comparatively recent (first noted in the USA in 1943) and means to examine a person (especially one of a large group) for disease or defects, or to assess his suitability for possible treatment or other benefits.

SCROGGS In English hospitals, occupational therapists' slang for patients, either elderly or inept, who are unable to attempt the tasks set for them as part of their therapy.

SCROTUM Medical Latin for the bag containing the **TESTES**. Some linguistic authorities say it is a corruption of *scortum*, a skin or hide or a bag; and, as these were often made from a leathern substance, perhaps a kind of 'wrinkled old retainer'? In classical Latin *scortum* was also used figuratively for a harlot or a strumpet ('old bag'?) and *scortator* for a whoremonger or fornicator.

SCRUBBING UP In medical – usually surgical – use, the action of antiseptic washing, dressing in sterile gowns, etc., and generally attaining as germ-free an environment as possible.

SEBUM (SEVUM) Latin for grease, tallow. Hence for the *sebaceous* secretion which lubricates the hair or skin through the openings that contain the hair follicles. See also **ADEPS** for the softer kind of adipose fat.

SECRETION See **-CRET-**.

SECTION The verb to section means to cut through something, usually a specimen of tissue so as to present part of it, i.e. a section, for examination or analysis; also visual cross-sections obtained from a living person by a **CAT** scan. More recently it has become possible in Britain to 'section' people in an abstract manner, as in 'he was sectioned by a psychiatrist', which means the person in question was compulsorily detained under the provision of the relevant section of the Mental Health Act of 1983. Previously a person would have been 'certified insane', but that is now considered unacceptable (and rightly so) for reasons of accuracy, compassion and **PC**. See also under **RELEASE INTO THE COMMUNITY** and **HOSPITAL NAMES**.

SELLA Latin for a seat, or saddle; and for a saddle-shaped bone.

SELLA TURCICA A shallow depression in the body of the sphenoid bone that encloses the pituitary gland. The Turkish allusion is not clear, but might be explained after further research. Maybe the Turks, who invaded much of Europe during the 17th and 18th centuries, used shallower saddles?

SEMEN The Latin word for seed, of any kind, human, animal and botanical, and the sperm of the male, from Latin *serere*, to sow. See also **SPERMA**.

SEMINAR A German word, first used in German universities, where it still means a select group of advanced students associated for special study and original research under the guidance of a professor or teacher. Now often used to mean a conference or **SYMPOSIUM** of specialists in a particular field or discipline; also a course of instruction for managers or **GREY SUITS**. The word comes from the Latin *seminarium*, a nursery, seed-nursery, seed-plot or seminary for the young (see **SEMEN**, above).

SEPSIS Greek for putrefaction, hence antiseptics, septic(a)emia, etc. Classical writers described a venomous serpent called *seps*, whose bite or sting made the wound 'go bad', so they called this a 'septic' effect. Other Greek poison-words are *pharmakon* (see **PHARMACY**) and **TOXICOS**, the latter meaning specifically poisoning resulting from an arrow-wound.

SEPTUM A partition, hedge or fence: ancient Roman neighbours would discuss the latest news over their dividing *septum*. *Septum nasi* (also *imbrex narium*) is the partition between the nostrils. *Imbrex* was a rain-tile or gutter such as used on a roof; a

possible allusion therefore to a dripping or 'running' nose. The septum lucidum or pellucidum is a thin double layer of tissue forming a partition between two parts of the brain. See also **VOMER**.

SERUM Latin for whey, or any watery animal fluid, especially that exuded from clotting blood.

SHARPS As in 'Discarded Sharps': a warning of the presence of needles, scalpels and other dangerous hospital or laboratory equipment – an abbreviation which might cause momentary confusion to some of the many doctors who are also practising musicians.

SHINGLES From Latin *cingulum*, belt or girdle – *zoster* in Greek, or *herpes zoster*. The Germans, who usually try to transliterate Latin terms into vernacular constructions, call this complaint *Gürtelrose*, literally, 'belt-pinkness'. See also **HERPES**.

SHROUD-WAVING The citing of tragic cases said to have been brought about by cuts in funding or shortage of money.

SIAMESE TWINS The popular name for conjoined twins, after two natives of Siam, Chang and Eng (1811–74) who were united by a tubular band in the region of the waist. They were first described (in *The Times* of 25 November 1829) as 'the Siamese United Twins'. On the following day the same paper reported a two-headed birth from Sardinia, so if this event had preceded the birth of Chang and Eng, we might now be speaking of 'Sardinian Twins'.

SIBILUS A hissing noise in the ears, perceived internally, by the sufferer only, not by bystanders. It comes from the Latin *sibilare*, to whistle or hiss. An English handbook of surgery of c. 1400 quoted in the *Oxford English Dictionary* described 'Greet sownynge [sounding] in the eeris & sibillus & defaute of heeringe & deefnes'. For other noises see under **SUSURRUS**.

SICK BUILDING SYNDROME Like other carelessly named syndromes, this invites the question of how a building could fall sick. Perhaps a good architect should be called in. In truth, some modern buildings do pose health-hazards, either by the ventilation-system or because they were built on an unhealthy site.

SICKLE-CELL AN(A)EMIA Named after the characteristic crescent-shaped red cells found in the blood of affected people – mostly African or Afro-Caribbean. For other selectively-racist diseases see **FAVISM, KURU, TAY-SACHS DISEASE** and **THALASS(ANA)EMIA.**

SICU Surgical Intensive Care Unit.

SIDS Sudden Infant Death Syndrome (also known in Britain as Cot Death) – acronymic abbreviation which shares with **AIDS** a confusion arising from the modern, almost endemic, resistance to putting hyphens where they ought to go. A Death Syndrome affecting Sudden Infants? No; to make it clear it should be Sudden Infant-Death Syndrome.

SILICON/SILICONE *Silex* means flint, hence also other 'stony' substances, e.g. sand, which produced the word silicon. Silicone is, among other things, a material used for certain body implants or **PROSTHESES.** For a more considered explanation see a real textbook.

SILVER HOUR See **GOLDEN HOUR.**

SINISTER Relating to the left side of the body and left-handedness (see also **LAEVUS** and **MANCINISM**). According to some ancient and primitive superstitions, left-handed people were supposed not only to lack **DEXTER**ity but also to be more disposed towards evil and corruption – in other words to possess more *sinister* attributes than right-handers. This bias is enshrined in European culture, e.g. in music, which always favours the right hand, and which in turn influenced the design of instruments (right-hand = tune, left-hand = accompaniment). Some cultures still reserve the left hand for 'sanitary' bodily purposes, regard a left-handed handshake as an insult and view left handers with suspicion.

SINUS As every mathematics student known, this is Latin for a curve; also for a bend, or a bay closed at one end; therefore for any natural hole or cavity in the substance of a bone or other tissue. The layman thinks of the sinuses solely as something in the nose that gets blocked.

SITZBATH From the German *Sitz*, a seat; *sitzen*, to sit. A 19th-century English euphemism for a hip-bath, or, more specifically, one to wash the lower parts of the body or **PUDENDA.** This kind of bath was used by over-delicate English people in the middle of the 19th century (probably by those who had had experience of German spas) and reflects an age when bathrooms were rare, when bathing was considered a danger to health and as little as possible of the body was actually immersed: a **BIDET** would do the trick today. It has been said that an English lady travelling abroad could keep herself fragrant with a single saucerful of water a day (which is perhaps the reason why no English gentlemen sips his tea from a saucer. The German word *Sitz* seems to appeal to the English. Among operatic artists a *Sitzprobe* (literally translated, a seated rehearsal) is a sing-through without costumes or actions; and among ski-ers (anglicised) a *sitzmark*, the impression made in the snow by the bottom of a skier unable to stop in any other way than by sitting down. The first few months of the Second World War, a period of relative inactivity when Hitler's threatened lightning-war, the Blitzkrieg, failed to materialise, were nick-named *Sitzkrieg*. This is an example of a German wartime joke.

SKELETON From Greek *skeletos*, dried up – dry as a bone, indeed. See also **ETIOLATED.**

SKILL Mnemonic for the excretory organs: Skin, Kidneys, Intestines, Liver, Lungs.

SKIN FLICKS Slides used by dermatologists to demonstrate various skin conditions (in English slang a skin flick is a film prominently featuring nudity).

SKIN GAME Junior doctors' nickname for dermatology – hence also **SKIN FLICKS**

SLIDER A form of **FLATULENCE.**

SLIMMING See **BANTING.**

SMBD(D) **GPs'** abbreviation for a patient's plea that 'Something Must Be Done (Doctor)'. See also **GRANNY-DUMPING.**

SMEGMA Although the chemical compound we know as soap, with its abundant cleansing lather, was unknown to the ancients, *smegma* is the Greek word for a soap-like unguent. The Romans used the same word for a cream 'for making the hands smooth'. In medicine, however, it means the secretion which accumulates under an unwashed prepuce and around the analogous place in the female. This (the *Concise Oxford Medical Dictionary* says) 'becomes readily infested by a harmless bacterium that resembles the tubercle bacillus'. Recent research has, however, shown that it may be carcinogenic and therefore

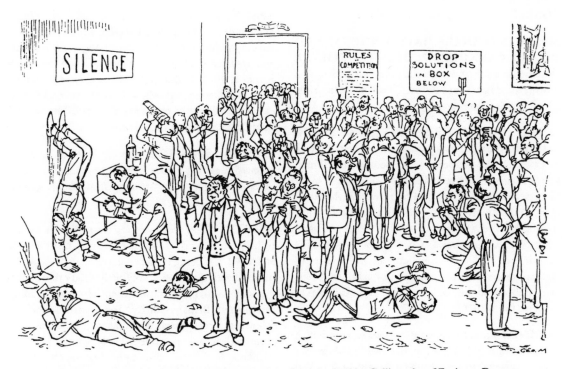

Competition Night at the Pharmaceutical Society. Deciphering the Calligraphy of Eminent Doctors

harmful not only to uncircumcised men but also, more significantly, to their female sexual partners. In the First World War the substance was also used as an ingredient for a simulated **BLIGHTY**. The doctors' informal name for it is Foreskin Cheese – better omitted from my list of **MENU CONDITIONS**.

SMOKER'S FACE Described a *British Medical Journal* article in 1985 by Dr Douglas Model, who found that the faces of those who smoked developed more and heavier wrinkles (as well as a 'pigmented grey appearance of the skin with skin wasting [and/ or] a flushed orange, purple and red complexion...') than those of non-smokers; and that they developed them earlier in life. It was also discovered that fear of wrinkles caused more female smokers to abandon the habit than fear of cancer and other killer-diseases caused by it. A lined but characterful face that was always held up as a warning was that of the 40–60-a-day poet W.H. Auden, whose complexion would probably have been even worse had he had more **TESTOSTERONE** in his make-up.

SNEERING MUSCLE See under **LEVATOR**.

SNELLEN CHART The eye-test chart consisting of type-letters of different sizes arranged in unfamil-

iar, i.e. gibberish, combinations so that they cannot be memorised – except by the **OPTOMETRIST**, who soon knows them by heart. Its inventor, the ophthalmologist Hermann Snellen (1834–1908) probably not only knew them by heart but could make sense of them, as he was Dutch. His test is not to be confused with the **BLIND TEST** or **DOUBLE-BLIND TEST**.

'SOCIAL' DISEASES Delicate euphemism for any one of the **VENEREAL** diseases (except **AIDS**), a term devised by social workers and the 'caring' welfare state in the belief that unpleasant conditions are somehow alleviated when given a more acceptable name. However, the euphemisers are, for once, nearer the mark than they suspected. 'Social' comes from the Latin *socius*, sharing, companionship, being together (hence society, socialism, etc). For more about VD see under **POX** and its cross-references.

SODA An archaic medical term for a headache. It is an Arabic word meaning 'splitting' – hence a splitting headache. See also **MIGRAINE**.

SODOMY See **BUGGERY**.

SOMA Greek for the body, Latin *corpus, corporis*. A psychosomatic illness is therefore a contradiction in terms, unless explained as a 'mind–body' illness.

SOMAT- The 'body' prefix, see above.

SOME CRIMINALS HAVE UNDERMINED ROYAL CANADIAN MOUNTED POLICE Mnemonic for the bones of the upper limb: Scapula, Clavicle, Humerus, Ulna, Radius, Carpals, Metacarpals, Phalanges.

'SOME FOLKS ARE WISE AND SOME OTHERWISE' This epigram on patients (as well as doctors) was penned by the Scottish physician, ship's surgeon and later full-time novelist, Tobias George Smollett (1721–71), in his novel *The Adventures of Roderick Random* (1748). (He also seems to have pioneered the alliterative title: *Roderick Random; Peregrine Pickle; Ferdinand, Count Fathom*, etc.). Like Arthur Conan Doyle, Smollett put his powers of clinical observation to good use in his books: 'Facts are stubborn things', he wrote. See also his observations on the **BIDET**.

SOMNUS Latin for sleep; also *somnium*, a dream. A somnambulist (+ Latin *ambulare*, to walk) is therefore a sleepwalker (but see also **NOCTAMBULIST**). And see below.

SOPOR Latin: a deep sleep – deeper than **SOMNUS** but less deep than a **COMA**. See also **HYPNOS** – and **CAROS**.

SOS Nothing to do with the international distress signal but the pharmacists' abbreviation for Latin *si opus sit*, 'if necessary'.

SOUP See under **BROTH**.

SPAMMIE The reddish-pink **STIGMA** left on, usually, the neck (of teenagers, normally) after over-enthusiastic kissing/sucking by a partner. It is often used as a showing-off signal to school-mates and others of a peer-group that the wearer is sexually active. The slang name comes from Spam, the trade-name (acronym of '*sp*iced *ham*') of a popular and long-established brand of canned pork product of a reddish-pink colour, which when sent to Britain from the USA in large quantities between 1939 and 1945 helped to win the Second World War. The British are faithful to their friends and Spam is still available to this day, made in Liverpool under licence to Geo. A. Hormel & Co, Austin, Minnesota, USA. *See other* **MENU CONDITIONS** and **PORT-WINE STAIN**.

SPANISH FLY See **CANTHARIDES**.

SPANSULE On 14th March, 1884 Sir Henry Wellcome patented the **TABLOID**, which please see. Seventy years later, on 2nd March, 1954, the Spansule was registered in the US Patent Office by Smith Kline & French Laboratories – a capsule which when swallowed releases a drug for several hours, either steadily or at prearranged times. The word is made from [time]-span + [cap-]sule.

SPASMA, SPASMOS Greek (leading to Latin *spasmus*) meaning to draw or tug, hence also for an involuntary, jerky or twitching movement, spasms or convulsions.

SPASTIC The word comes from the Greek for tightly stretched. Like the words **LEPER** and **MONGOL** it is being replaced in popular parlance by more specific descriptions of the disability that causes a particular kind of disablement. In 1994 a long-established British charity, the Spastics Society, following a recognised trend (as well as a liking for meaningless, snappy, one-syllable words) changed its name to 'Scope', thus annexing an established word and giving it a spurious meaning. Now its officials have to say, 'Scope formerly the Spastics Society', so they are no better off.

SPECIAL CLINIC Common euphemism for an out-patients' department specialising in venereal diseases – or 'social' diseases – another euphemism. See also under **HOSPITAL NAMES**.

SPECIALTY/SPECIALISM A special line of (medical or other) work. English doctors used to say 'speciality' but the American 'specialty' has now almost replaced the British form (though 'specialty' was an English word before America was even discovered). Today the American spelling is accepted: the former Editor of the *British Medical Journal* Dr Stephen Lock, has written that 'specialty' is for medicine, 'speciality' for chefs.

SPECULUM Originally meant a looking-glass in Latin (which in Roman times was not really a mirror in the modern sense, but a piece of polished metal). The 'looking' element was borrowed by medics, so that they now understand by a speculum a metal instrument for looking into a cavity, e.g. the rectum, vagina, etc. by inserting it in such a way as to keep the walls apart. One of these instruments is called a 'duck bill', because of the way its two halves open like the beak of a bird.

SPERMA Greek for seed, related to the Latin *spargere*, to sprinkle, or to scatter it, whether in a garden, field or ditch – see **FOSSA**. For some unexplained reason many words denoting wetness: splashing, spitting, sprinkling, spewing (and indeed 'spunk', the vulgar word for semen) begin with *sp-*. See also **SPUTUM** and **SPOROS**.

SPHINCTER From Greek *sphingein*, to bind tight, to strangle – hence the closable, contractile, ring-like muscle by which an orifice in the body is kept normally closed (and not only the one everybody knows). Remember the mythological strangler the Sphinx, that tight-lipped, enigmatic monster with the head of a woman, the body of a lion and the wings of a bird, who set difficult riddles to passers-by and strangled those who failed to solve them. Only Oedipus got the answer right and escaped, but he later experienced other troubles, as Sigmund Freud never tired of telling us.

SP(H)ONDULOS/(-DYLOS) The Greek for a **VERTEBRA**. Could this be the origin of the American slang word for money, spondulicks – as vertebrae were used by some primitives in place of coins?

SPHYGMOS/SPHUGMOS Greek for the pulse, hence the sphygmomanometer, which measures blood (i.e. pulse) pressure. It should be noted that Greek *manos*, meaning thin or rare, refers to pressure, and is not to be confused with *manus*, the hand.

SPIN DOCTOR Not a medical doctor but a hired expert who teaches politicians to 'doctor' the facts and spin yarns to the electorate. More information under **DOCTOR**.

SPIR- Prefix or word-element which can indicate either a spiral form or respiration.

SPINA The Latin word for a thorn, hence also for the backbone or spine, which – with a little imagination applied – resembles a long thorn. The Greek is **RHACHIS**.

SPLEN Greek for the spleen, which is **LIEN** in Latin.

SPOONERISM The accidental transposition of the initial sounds, or letters, of two or more words, e.g. 'well-boiled icicles' for well-oiled bicycles; or 'the meeting will be hauled in the hell below', etc.

It is named after the Reverend Dr W. A. Spooner (1844–1930) but was surely not 'invented' by him. The *Oxford English Dictionary* says the word 'spoonerism' was in colloquial use from about 1885 in Oxford, where Spooner was a teacher; and after he became known for such transpositions they were soon turned into a game by his students. This helped to keep the Spoonerism (and Dr Spooner's name) alive. It has been suggested that his linguistic lapses were due to a form of **DYSPRAXIA** or **DYSARTHRIA**, especially as he also suffered from **DYSGRAPHIA** (*see What was the matter with Dr Spooner?* by J.M. Potter, in *Errors in Linguistic Performance*, ed. Fromkin, San Francisco, Academic Press, 1980). In addition, Spooner was an **ALBINO**; and his verbal confusions are thought to have been related to one or all of his conditions (see another article entitled *What was the matter with Dr Spooner?* by Barrie Jay, Professor of Clinical Ophthalmology, Moorfields Eye Hospital, London, *British Medical Journal*, 17 October 1987). Perhaps the true answer is that he was afflicted by a wicked sense of humour, or worse, the traditional professorial absent-mindedness: after the First World War he met one of his former students on the street and, peering intently at his face, enquired, 'Let me see. Was it you or your brother who was killed in the war?' The spoonerism has never been unique to Oxford and is a great deal older than Dr Spooner. Metaphrasis, as it might be called (reviving an existing old word), also works well in German, where it is called *Schüttelreim* ('jumbled-up rhyme') and often presents possibilities of multiple, yet meaningful, transposition; and in France, too, the *contrepèterie* is alive and well. A famous example is attributed to General Charles de Gaulle who, in a speech in which he meant to speak of *'la population du Cape'* he said instead, *'la copulation du Pape'*.

SPORADIC From Greek *sporaden* (see also below) meaning scattered. Of an illness, one which occurs at scattered, intermittent and apparently random intervals. See also **ENDEMIC** and **EPIDEMIC**.

SPOROS Another Greek word for seed, giving us spores – and 'scattered', **SPORADIC** illnesses described above.

SPUTUM The Latin word for **SALIVA** or, more usually, for matter brought out from the lower air passages or the lungs. *Spuo*, to vomit (*cf* English 'spew').

Spitting was one of many insanitary habits the ancients indulged in, and they even had a Latin word for a habitual spitter, *sputator*. See also **SPERMA**, above.

SQUAMA Latin for scale, at first applied to those of fish as well as to the articulated metal leaves of body-armour. In medicine squamation refers to scaly skin and, in anatomy, to a thin, scaly portion of bone.

$\overline{\text{SS}}$ Pharmacist's abbreviation for *semis*, half.

STACCATO or DRUM BEAT A form of **FLATU-LENCE**, which please see.

STAPES Latin for stirrups, hence the name of the small, stirrup-shaped, innermost of the three *ossicles* (see **OS**) of the ear. The *Oxford English Dictionary* suggests that it is a medieval Latin word as the ancients did not use stirrups when riding horses and therefore had no word for them.

STAPHYLO- From the Greek *staphyle*, a bunch of grapes, hence staphylococci, i.e. **COCCI** arranged as if in bunches. See also **STREPT(O)-**.

STD Sexually Transmitted Diseases; also, for some years, when a new technology was introduced into telephone systems, Subscriber Trunk Dialling. The two could not have existed side-by-side, but when telephone STD became the normal method of making calls and operator-connected ones all but obsolete, the field was left to the Sexually Transmitted Diseases. A change may, however, be imminent, as STD Clinics relied on the public's ignorance of what the initials stood for. Now that public awareness has increased a new euphemism will probably be called for, e.g., the already existing Special Clinics. See **HOSPITALS**.

STEAT(O)- The fat prefix – see below; also **ADIP(O)-** and **LIP(O)-**.

STEATOPYGIA The Greek *steat-*, *stear-*, *steato-* prefixes always denote fat or fatty tissue, from the Greek *stear* meaning tallow. Steatopygia means an accumulation of unusual amounts of fat in the buttocks, a normal condition in women of some black races, whose natural steatopygiousness is considered both **CALLIPYGIAN** and a useful method of fat-storage that does not impede heat-loss from the rest of the body.

STEATORRH(O)EA The prefix above, with the

-ORRHEA 'flowing-out' suffix denotes too much fat – in this usage fat flowing out – in the stools, which then show a resistance to being flushed away and are popularly called 'floaters'. See **RHEXIS** and **-RHEIN**.

STENOSIS An abnormal narrowing, e.g. of a blood vessel, or opening. Think of stenography – the now rather old-fashioned word for shorthand writing, i.e. the contraction of words.

STERCORARIAN A doctor of the old-fashioned school who is too lazy, or refuses, to keep abreast of advances in the practice of medicine – from **STERCUS**, below: perhaps one who maintains a **CHAMBER-POT PRACTICE**. The *Oxford English Dictionary* is very clear in its definition of the word: 'A derisive appellation for a physician following obsolete methods of practice'. The Greek for dung is **COPROS** (leading to copro- formations); and more waste matter will be found under **FAEX, FAECIS**.

STERCUS The Latin word for excrement and much used in old English (adjective: stercorous). 'Oh, stercus!' might be worth reviving, and would make a change from the more vulgar cry now so widely heard (and incidentally, my antipodean medical friends inform me that in Australia and New Zealand the word shit has been rehabilitated into their standard English usage and can be uttered anywhere, in the politest company and even – or perhaps especially – in their parliaments). Stercus also occurs in combination: e.g. stercolith, a stone formed of dried, compressed faeces, (which is also known as a faecolith). The Stercoranists were a Christian religious sect whose members believed that the consecrated elements in the Eucharist remained sacred even after digestion and evacuation: surely a perfectly logical view, since the Scriptures make no assertion to the contrary. See also under **BORBORYGM(US)**.

STERNUM Latin for the breast-bone, from Greek *sternon*, the chest.

STEROID One of a large group of naturally-occurring or synthetic organic compounds – many of which have important pharmacological uses. From the Greek *stereos*, solid. (See under the headings **ANA-** and **BOL** for anabolic steroids).

STERTOR A kind of heavy, noisy breathing, especially in very sick patients; but also plain snoring in the healthy. From Latin *stertere*, to snore.

STETHOS Greek for the chest, Latin *pectus, pectoris*, making chest-related words containing the steth(o)- or pect- syllables.

STETHOSCOPE From Greek *stethos*, the chest + *skopein*, to view. It originally meant looking at, not listening to, the chest. **AUSCULTATION** was always intended, so it is difficult to imagine what its inventor, a Dr Laennec, would have seen though it in about 1819. No wonder that by 1858 a Dr S. S. Alison tried to put things right: 'An instrument which I have invented ... and which, as it is specially adapted for the auscultation of differences of sounds of different parts of the chest, I have named the Differential Stethoscope, or Stethophone'. (*Proceedings of the Royal Society* of that year, IX). But stethoscope it remained, absurd as the name is. Observant hypochondriacs may have noticed that junior doctors have for some time treated this indispensable diagnostic instrument as a fashion-accessory. In former days it was worn in a, so-to-speak, Y-shaped configuration, i.e. with the ear-pieces resting on either side of the wearer's neck. Today the U-shaped look is preferred, the whole stethoscope being folded in half and draped round the neck like a victor's wreath. As medical soap operas proliferate on TV, and younger doctors become more senior, the fashion has spread to all strata of the profession. See also **AEGOPHONY, GREY SUITS, VOCAL RESONANCE** and **WHISPERING PECTRILOQUY**.

STIFF NECK This genuine, old-fashioned complaint, also called 'a crick in the neck' and often attributed to 'a draught', and which can have many causes, is now often attributed to **WHIPLASH** and frequently features in insurance claims and other forms of **PLOMBOSCILLOSIS**.

STIGMA A mark or marks, such as certain spots on the skin, which to a doctor characterise a certain disease. In Greek the word means a mark made with a pointed instrument, e.g. Christ's stigmata (the plural) on hands and feet; also a branding-mark or spot, perhaps where rays converge through a lens. Astigmatism in the eye is imperfect focusing. A **SPAMMIE** is also a kind of stigma, though one that is gladly borne.

STOMA Greek for the mouth, hence an opening or hole – producing the -stomy suffix. From stoma came also the English word stomach – via Greek *stomachos*. The Latin for a mouth is *os, oris* (not to be confused with *os, ossis*, a bone) hence orifice, etc.

STRABISMUS Greek *strabismos*, twisted, later adapted into Latin, *strabo*, I squint, I look askew. Many English readers of a certain generation will be familiar with 'Dr Strabismus of Utrecht, whom God preserve', a character made famous by the writings of the satirist 'Beachcomber'. See also **NUSTAGMUS**.

STRAWBERRIES This fruit figures, metaphorically, in the names of several conditions because of an alleged likeness in some of its aspects, e.g. Strawberry Gallbladder, Strawberry Nevus, Strawberry Nose, etc. For other unappetising namings see **MENU CONDITIONS**.

STREAM TEAM The urology department.

STREP(TO)- From Greek *streptos*, twisted (i.e. like a chain). See also **COCCUS**, making streptococci, bacteria in which the cocci are arranged in chains. See also **STAPHYLO-**.

STRESS A good old English word for what is now a fashionable illness of epidemic proportions. Almost as soon as a **SYNDROME**, real or imaginary, has been given a name, newspapers and magazines devote articles to it, to its causes and symptoms, and more and more people begin to suffer from it. This in turn inspires the creation of alleged cures and remedies, from vitamins to **ELIXIRS** and even prerecorded, soothing audio-tapes. To the diagnostician certain symptoms masquerading as stress may,

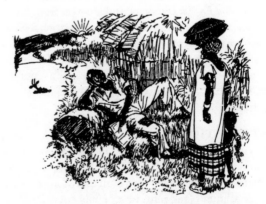

"I AIN'T GONNA WORK - I'M ILL. DE ADVERTISEMENTS IN DIS PAPER SAY DAT I AM SUFFERIN' FROM NOORUSTEENIA CAUSED BY DE RUSH AN' STRESS OF MODERN LIFE."

Punch, June 21, 1933

however, provide pointers to an identifiable or curable condition. Dr Rob Briner, Lecturer in Occupational Psychology at the University of London, in a lecture reported in the press in the spring of 1994, described stress as a 'national obsession' and 'modern myth', pointing out that specific mood descriptions, e.g. tension, anxiety, frustration and anger, were more helpful. The stress on a modern, Western man and his wife is hardly comparable with that experienced by their Victorian forebears, subject to TB, 'blood-poisoning' and perinatal death, and whose infants died like flies; or (as the distinguished British cardiologist Professor Sir Melville Arnott remarked), the stress suffered 'by a tribesman in Equatorial Africa, tortured by the taboo and sanction of primitive belief' (quoted in The *Medical Risks of Life*, by Stephen Lock and Tony Smith, Penguin Books); or indeed by a family under siege in some strife-stricken, war-torn city. Of the many forms of stress which are said to be the result of eating-disorders, only one is observed among African tribesmen – hunger. There was neither **OBESITY** nor **ANOREXIA** in German wartime concentration-camps. See also **ANGST, RSI, SAD, PTS, WHIPLASH**, etc.

STRIATION From Latin *stria*, a furrow (plural *striae*): a streak, line or linear scar on the skin, e.g. a **CLEAVAGE LINE**; or what are popularly known as 'stretch marks' seen on the abdomen after pregnancy or dramatic weight-loss.

STUPOR 'A disorder characterised by great diminution or entire suspension of sensibility', says the *Oxford English Dictionary*, and it comes from Latin *stupere*, to be stunned. People who are in such a state, perhaps after an injury, appear to have their faculties dulled or deadened and may be taken for being 'stupid' – a word which has the same origin – but see **PUNCH-DRUNK**. Also **COMA, TORPOR** and cross-references.

STUPRATION The old medical word for rape, forcible deflowering, violation or defiling, from the Latin *stuprare*, to violate. Constupration, with the intensifying prefix *con-*, is an even more forceful kind of ravishment (and must be carefully enunciated, to avoid confusion with its near-soundalike constipation). 'The good gostlie father that constuprated ii hundred nonnes in his tyme!', wrote an incredulous author in 1550; and in Burton's *Anatomy of Melancholy*

in 1621: 'Their wives and loveliest daughters constuprated by every base cullion...'). Masturbation is a corrupted form of *mastrupation*, from the Latin *manu stuprare*, to defile with the hand, i.e. 'hand-rape'.

STYPTIC A kind of **PLEDGET** to control bleeding, or a substance used as an astringent, from Greek *styptikos*, a contracting or pulling-together.

SUCCUBUS The difference between this and an **INCUBUS** has more to do with Freudian analysis than medicine, but is dicussed under **INCUBATION**. See also **DECUBITUS**.

SUCCUSSION The action of shaking; the condition of being shaken up; a splashing noise heard when a patient has a large quantity of fluid in his body, e.g. the pleural cavity (see **PLEUR-**). From Latin *succus*, juice or gravy – hence 'succulent'.

SUDOR Latin for sweat. Hence also **EXUDE**, from *ex-sudare*, literally to sweat it out. The Greek is *hydros*. I have seen a women's dress-shop in an English county town whose proprietresses, named Susan X. and Dorothy Y., acronymically called it and their products 'Sudor'.

SUITS Short for **GREY SUITS**.

SUPER/SUPRA- The Latin equivalents of **HYPER**.

SUPINATION To turn someone on his or her – or oneself on one's – back, the opposite of **PRONATION**.

SUPPOSITORY A medicated plug for administration by insertion, usually into the rectum but also other possible canals. From Latin *sub + ponere*, to put below. This also, by a circuitous route, gave us the word 'supposition' , which in turn may throw light on the prescribing-practices of a 'Dr' Mohammed Sayeed, an unqualified impostor who for 30 years until the early 1990s instructed his patients 'to swallow two suppositories before meals'. As a patient said, 'For all the good they did me, doctor, I might as well have ....' But everyone knows this folk-joke.

SUPPURATION See **PUS**.

SUPRATENTORIUM Doctors' code-word for 'this patient is imagining things', a reference to the upper part, the **TENTORIUM** (*supra*, above) of the brain, where thought-processes are formed. See also **PLOMBOSCILLOSIS, MÜNCHHAUSEN** and **RE-PETITIVE STRAIN INJURY**.

SURGEON The word has nothing to do with 'cutting' but means, literally, one who practises the healing arts by *manual* operation – originally chirurgeon: for the 'hand' connection see under **CHEIR**. It is the fashion for modern dendrologists who cut down trees – however skilfully or painlessly – to describe themselves as 'tree surgeons' (though so far there is no Royal College of Tree Surgeons). This fad goes back at least as far as Shakespeare, who, in *Julius Caesar* (i, l, 27), makes a cobbler say 'I am, indeed, sir, a surgeon to old shoes'.

SURGEON FISH A brightly coloured tropical marine fish 'having one or more sharp, erectile spines' – and many a junior **HOUSE OFFICER** has encountered one. The name is derived from the fact that the spines may be lancet-like.

SUSURRUS The Latin – echoic – word for buzzing, humming, muttering or whispering – in medical parlance a low-pitched humming in the ears. For other kinds of in-the-ear noises see **BOMBUS, BRUIT, SIBILUS** and **TINNITUS**. Further terms which echo the actions they denote will be found under **BORBORYGM(US), ERUCTATION, MUCUS, RHONCHUS, SIBILUS, TINNITUS**.

SUTURE From the Latin word *suo*, I sew, *sutura*, a sewing-together, or seam. Most of the Latin references apply the word to cobblers or tailors – none to doctors or surgeons: as Pliny said, '*Sutor, ne supra crepidam (judicaret)*', Let the cobbler stick to his last. The Greek counterpart is *rraphe*, which also produced many medical terms, e.g. **PERINEORRAPHY**.

SWAB From the Swedish *svabb*, a mop – also *svabba*, a dirty person.

'SWALLOWING THE TONGUE' A mishap apparently requiring urgent first aid but seems to be unknown outside sports (especially soccer) fields and newspaper offices. The question must be asked, how can one swallow it while it is attached to the mouth? And what happens to it when it reaches the stomach? The tongue can, however, obstruct the **TRACHEA** or windpipe without being swallowed.

SYMPOSIUM A grand old name for a conference, usually one convened for the dissemination

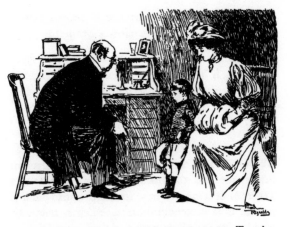

Doctor. "NOW, MY BOY, SHOW ME YOUR TONGUE. THAT'S NOT ENOUGH. PUT IT RIGHT OUT."
Small Boy. "I CAN'T -'COS IT'S FASTENED AT THE BACK!"

Punch, November 20, 1907

and exchange of specialist knowledge. The original purpose of such symposia was, however, the consumption of alcoholic drink, and such conversation as it might incidentally have generated. The word is Latinised from the Greek, *symposion*, from *syn*, together + *posis*, drinking. Roman *symposia* provided not only drink (water and wine mixed) but also musical entertainments. Today's conferences, meetings or symposia often combine both activities – and more often than not take place in pleasant localities or countries that have a good climate and other attractions to offer. But they usually lack the musical entertainments (see, however, the compiler's Medical Muse mentioned in the introduction). See also **DROMOMANIA** and **SEMINAR**.

SYMPTOM Greek for, literally, a conflation or 'falling-together' of circumstances. Several symptoms can make a **SYNDROME**. See also **PTOSIS**.

SYN- (also **SYM-**) Prefix from Greek meaning togetherness, union, similarity, likeness, simultaneity; hence the syndrome, now so popular with journalists and other laymen, synalgia, a sympathetic ('referred') pain in one part of the body caused by an injury to, or condition in, another; synesthesia, a sensation induced in one part of the body when a stimulus is applied to another; or synethnic, belonging to the same race. And numerous other combinations.

SYNCOPE Failure of the heart's action, resulting in unconsciousness and sometimes death. From the Greek for a cutting-off, a striking. See also **-PLEGIA**.

SYNDROME A concurrence of several **SYMP-TOMS**, or a set of such concurring symptoms.

SYNOVIA A word which, says the *Oxford English Dictionary*, is 'probably an invention of Paracelsus (d. 1541), applied by him to the nutritive fluid peculiar to the several parts of the body, and also to the **GOUT**, but limited by later physicians to the fluid of the joints'.

SYNOVITIS The inflammation of a synovial membrane (see also **GAMEKEEPER'S** or **DRUMMER'S THUMB**). It is important to spell this word with a y, not an *i*, as is sometimes seen, when it might be taken to mean 'inflammation of the Chinese'.

SYPHILIS It is no coincidence that this disease, which for centuries caused such ravages, which changed the course of music, art, science, politics and history, but which is now under control, thanks to **ANTIBIOTICS**, sounds like the name of a classical character. Its name comes from that of Syphilus, a fictional shepherd, supposedly the first sufferer and chief character in an extended poem by Girolamo Fracastoro of Verona (1483–1553), *Syphilis, sive Morbus Gallicus* ('Syphilis, or the French Disease'). The poem was published in 1530 and probably marks the earliest recorded instance of blame for venereal diseases being put on the French – see **(THE) (FRENCH) POX** and **(THE) CLAP**. (But under **MENSES** will be found a different examples of international abuse).

SYR. Pharmacists' abbreviation for Latin *syrupus*, syrup.

SYRINGE Related to the Greek *syrinx*, a nymph whom the god Pan turned into a pipe and played upon. A syrinx is often also the name of the pipe itself, or a bundle of reeds of graduated size bound together like **FASCES**, blown at the top and also known as pan-pipes.

(THE) SYSTEM This, according to many **WELFARE STATE** claimants, carries the blame for most of our troubles. The Third World, curiously enough, has many more troubles but no System to blame them on.

SYSTEMIC In medicines, a substance which affects the body system in general, usually introduced into the blood-stream, not one given in a specific place, which is a **TOPICAL** administration.

SYSTOLE The contraction of the heart walls and arteries, from Greek *sustellein*, to contract. See also **DIASTOLE**.

T*t*

TAB INOCULATION See under **IMMUNIZATION**.

TABES Latin for a wasting-away. See also **PHTHISIS** and **TB**.

TABLOID A word invented by the 19th-century chemist and seller of patent medicines Sir Henry Solomon Wellcome (1853–1936). The word was registered by him as his intellectual property (i.e. declared copyright) on 14 March 1884 and is technically still owned by his company, though the company does not pursue its rights (unlike the **CHAMPAGNE** industry, which wages a relentless and undignified campaign against anyone who sells bubbles and hints at the name of the drink). 'Tabloid' is a combination of the first syllable of 'tablet' and the Greek suffix -**OID**, 'in the shape of'. Wellcome's invention related to a process of compressing medicinal tablets (previously often in the form of a **BOLUS** – that is, large and unpalatable) into a small and compact form that could easily be taken by mouth. Not only was the Wellcome Tabloid an instant commercial success but it became a general vogue-word which was applied to other things small and compact, much in the way 'mini' has been used more recently. Thus when Sir Thomas Sopwith built a small and agile fighter-plane at the beginning of the First World War he named it the 'Sopwith Tabloid'. Then, in 1925, the newspaper-owner Lord Northcliffe announced that he was introducing a compact, small-format newspaper about half the size of normal-size papers (now called 'broadsheets', though this 18th-century word had a different meaning). In the course of a speech informally announcing these plans to his employees and colleagues, Northcliffe described it as a 'tabloid' paper – much as today he might have said a 'mini' newspaper. And so the newspapers that bring you the most sensational revelations, punning headlines, crashing clichés, misprints and half-naked women – not to mention ideas compressed into bite-sized, easily swallowed, jerky sentences – owe their name to a patent-medicine with a Latin–Greek trade-mark. Sir Henry's patent Tabloid also laid the foundation of a huge and successful pharmaceutical drugs and research industry as well as a charitable trust and research foundation. A later patented formation is the **SPANSULE**.

TACHY- The prefix denoting speed, or quickness, from the Greek *tachys*, quick, fast, *tachos*, quickness, speed: tachycardia, an abnormally fast heartbeat, tachypnoeia, rapid breathing, tachyphrasia, rapid and voluble speech, etc. See also the opposite, **BRADY-**. The tachometer, familiar to every motorist, is therefore really a *speed*ometer and measures miles-travelled only because someone discovered that it was convenient to combine the two functions on one instrument. The proper word for the distance-measuring instrument in a car, etc., is odometer, from Greek *odos*, way + the 'measuring' suffix, but is now seldom seen.

TACTUS Latin for touch, from *tangere*, to touch.

TAILOR'S ANKLE An occupational disease (for others see **BREWER'S DROOP** and cross-references) suffered by tailors from sitting cross-legged. See also **SARTORIUS**.

TAMPAX The proprietary name registered by the New York firm which invented it in 1936 of a sanitary tampon for use by menstruating women. The name is now, however, loosely applied to any variety of tampon. It probably comes from the first syllable of tampon + Latin *pax*, peace, i.e. peace of mind.

TARSUS/TARSALS Greek *tarsos*, the sole of the foot.

TASE *Aide-mémoire* meaning Told About Side Effects. Like **UAG** it may be produced in court if the advice was ignored and the patient suffers harm.

TATSP GPs' code abbreviation: 'Thick As Two Short Planks', that is, stupid.

TAT Abbreviation of tetanus antitoxin.

TATT In GPs' notes means 'Tired All The Time'. The patient himself (more often herself) will probably claim to be suffering from **SAD**, especially after having read about it somewhere. See also **NEURASTHENIA**.

-TAX- The prefix/suffix for order, orderly arrangement, function, etc., so that **ATAXIA** denotes a lack of it. Greek *tassein* has also given us such words as tactics, taxonomy and syntax (the arranging-together of words), taxidermy (arranging skins when stuffing animals). But taxes or taxi-cabs, both related to tax-gathering, which comes from a Latin word.

TAXIS The returning to their normal position of displaced bones by manipulation. See above.

TAY–SACHS DISEASE For a comprehensive book of **SYNDROMES** see the works by Firkin and Whitworth and Gibson and Potparic listed in the Bibliography at the front of this book. Tay–Sachs is included here because it helps to define the difference between 'racism' and 'racialism', a distinction blurred by popular usage. In the strict dictionary sense, *racialism* is 'a belief in the superiority of a particular race leading to prejudice and antagonism...' – which every decent person condemns – whereas *racism* merely means that different races have different human characteristics and may be visited by different illnesses. Tay–Sachs (Amaurotic Familial Idiocy) afflicts 100 times more Jews than any other ethnic group, whereas **SICKLE-CELL ANAEMIA** affects mostly Africans and Afro-Caribbeans, and **THALASS(ANA)EMIA** and **FAVISM** Mediterranean peoples. Twice as many American Black males develop prostate cancer as do white Americans. On the other hand, cystic fibrosis is rarely seen in West Indians. Dr Stuart Marshall-Clarke says 'the Epstein–Barr virus is the causative agent of glandular fever in Caucasian people but appears to cause the much more serious Burkitt's Lymphoma and nasopharyngeal carcinoma in people of African and Oriental origin'. See also **KURU**, the 'Trembling Disease', which is even more narrowly selective, affecting only members of the Fore tribe in New Guinea; and Polynesians are thought to have a genetic predisposition to **OBESITY**: their monarchs (remember the giant Queen Salote of Tonga?) breaking all 'heaviest monarchs' records.

TB Short for tuberculosis, 'the consumption' or **PHTHISIS**.

TBF Hospital abbreviation for Total Body Failure, e.g. in the very old or calamitously sick; (and facetiously, when used of a colleague, 'Total Brain Failure').

TDS Pharmacists' abbreviation for Latin *ter in die*, three times a day.

TECTUM The Latin word for roof, and hence the roof of the mid-brain: another **ARCHITECTURAL TERM** put to medical use by the Romans (the very word 'architecture' means 'arched roof').

TEN-/TON- The tension, stretching or straining elements. from Greek *teino*, I stretch, Latin *tonus*, *tendere*. Hence tensor, extensor, tendon, hypertonic, hypotonic, peritoneum (literally 'stretched around') etc. See more about it under **TONIC**, and below.

TENDO ACHILLIS Or Achilles' Tendon: the tendon by which the muscles of the calf are attached to the heel. From the mythological story of the infant Achilles being held by the heel and dipped in the River Styx by his mother Thetis, to render him invulnerable; but part undipped proved his undoing. Had Thetis used a bit of string and dipped the whole child she might have preserved many footballers from their most common injury. In its medical application it is a modern term which, according to the *Oxford English Dictionary*, first appeared in 1900 in *Dorland's Medical Dictionary*. For an often mythical footballing complaint see **THIGH STRAIN**.

TENESMUS Straining in def(a)ecation, or the sensation preceding it; or a sense of incomplete evacuation possibly caused by a rectal tumour. One of numerous words derived from Greek *teino*, I stretch. See also under **TONIC**, below, and the entries above.

TENNIS ELBOW Just as housemaid's knee does not necessarily affect only floor-scrubbing housemaids so can tennis elbow strike even those who have never wielded a racket. It is tendonitis (sometimes erroneously tendinitis), a painful inflammation of the tendon at the outer border of the elbow.

TENO-/TENDO- The tendon prefix. Tenosynovitis may manifest itself as **DRUMMER'S, TRIGGER** or **GAMEKEEPER'S THUMB**.

TENTORIUM Latin for a tent, hence the name for the membranous partition between the cerebrum and the cerebellum. See also the doctors' code-word **SUPRATENTORIUM**.

TERATO- The Greek 'monster' prefix, usually indicating some kind of deformity: e.g. teratogenesis, giving birth to a misshapen offspring; teratogen, an element or factor thought to cause deformities in the embryo; teratoma, a tumour – though the likeness of the two words is coincidental. Also, non-medically, teratologist, one who tells tales of marvels or monsters; teratology, a discourse or treatise on such; and teratoscopy, which is the observation (not medical!) of, or augury from, the aspect of monsters. But when the Thalidomide disaster was first described, teratology was once more pressed into medical service in the study of that deformity-producing drug.

TESTIS A testicle, but as these usually come in pairs, the plural, *testes*, is more common. In Latin *testis* also means a witness, one who attests, either in speech or writing. Under Roman law no man was permitted to testify in a dispute unless in possession of a pair of descended testicles (a qualification later applied also to those wishing to be ordained priests in the Church of Rome – see **CASTRATION**). The Greek equivalent is *orchis*: both forms are used in a number of medical terms. And for good measure, here is some useless information: the name of that delicious fruit the avocado is derived from the Aztec *ahuacatl*, meaning testicle, because of its shape. See also **GONADS** and cross-references.

TESTOSTERONE A steroid hormone that stimulates the development of male secondary sexual characteristics and is produced in the testes (and also, to a much lesser extent, in the ovaries). The word was first formed in German as *Testosteron* in 1935, from **TESTIS** (above) + the -sterone suffix, and later anglicised.

(THE) TEST-TUBE OBSERVATION TEST A favourite, old and well-known trick played by professors and lecturers on students to test their powers of observation (see both **EMPIRICUS** and **SALTUS EMPIRICUS**) goes something like this:

> *Professor*: 'Today, ladies and gentlemen, I should like to talk to you about the importance of developing your powers of observation. Let us conduct a little experiment. I have here four test-tubes, each containing human urine. The first, produced by a six-week-old infant, fed solely on milk, tastes bland, almost neutral. (*Dips finger in test-tube, tastes, and passes the phial down the rows of students. Students taste, nod sagely*). And here we have the urine of a 14-year-old girl. Puberty has set in, and there is a distinctly stronger taste. (Dips in finger, tastes, and passes phial to students). Next, that of a 29-year-old woman, twenty-four weeks pregnant... (*Dips finger, licks it, describes the taste and passes test-tube along. Students do likewise*). Finally, the urine of a man aged

78, a chronic alcoholic – need I say more? (*Phial passed down, each student tastes and some show signs of queasiness*). And that ends our little experiment.'

Student (raising hand diffidently): 'Er – Sir. You said that the experiment, interesting as it was, would help us develop our powers of observation'.

Professor: 'Oh yes. I was coming to that. The more *observant* among you will have noticed that I dipped *this* finger into the first test-tube, and licked this one'.

TETANUS From Greek *tetanos*, a muscular spasm which, in its extreme and often calamitous form, is *lock-jaw*. See **TONIC**.

TETTER An Old English general term for any kind of skin eruption, from **ECZEMA** to **IMPETIGO** and **LUPUS**. It seems that the word fell into disuse in the 19th century, when more precise descriptions came into being. The latest (CD-ROM, 1993) edition of the *Oxford English Dictionary* still defines vitiligo as 'tetter', without further explanation. Tetters, it explains under its heading, came in various forms, crusted, pustular, humid, running, honeycomb... and 'eating' – see **NECROTISING FASCIITIS**. In Shakespeare's *Hamlet* the Ghost reports (Act I Scene 5) that when Hamlet's uncle dropped the poison into his father's ear, the result was immediate: '...a most instant tetter bark'd about, Most lazar-like, with vile and loathsome crust, All my smooth body'. See also under **LAZAR**.

THALAMOS/THALAMUS In a Greek house the *thalamos* was an inner chamber, usually the bedroom. Hence the *epithalamion/epithalamium*, a bridal poem, hymn, song or other composition, performed outside or by (see **EPI-**) the bedroom. It was the celebrated physician Galen who, in the 2nd century AD, applied the word to an inner part of the brain. The brain, too, has an epithalamus. For other architectural origins see also **ATRIUM, FORNIX, VESTIBULUM, CLAUSTRUM, FASTIGIUM, FAUCES, FOCUS, FORNIX, PHRAGMA, PALATUM, PORTA, TECTUM, TENTORIUM, TRABECULUM, VESTIBULUM**, etc. Even **FORENSIC MEDICINE** owes something to buildings.

THALASS(ANA)EMIA A form of hereditary anaemia found among Mediterranean, African or South East Asian people (or their descendants) who 'live by the shore'; *thalassa* is the Greek word for the sea. The abbreviation to *thalass(a)emia* is American and, like many simplified spellings, makes the word slightly less self-explanatory: the difference, indeed, between **(A)EMIA** (generally concerned with blood) and **AN(A)EMIA,** lack of it.

THALASSOTHERAPY A fancy word for 'bathing in seawater'. From the early 19th century this was thought to be beneficial to health and usually done under medical supervision. The therapy was conducted from a 'bathing machine' – which was a horse-drawn, covered wagon or cabin on wheels, towed to a shallow part on the shore until partly-submerged. With its door facing decently out to sea, the subject, naked and attended by a bathing-woman, would carefully submerge all but his head. Even today some cruise-lines crow about their 'Thalassotherapeutic Baths', forgetting to mention that *all* liners fill their swimming-pools from the limitless water-supply that surrounds them: 'therapeutic' only by default, provided they are not filled while the ship is in harbour or near a leaking oil-tanker. Thalassotherapy makes a change from **BALNEOTHERAPY** and **PSYCHROLUSIA**.

THANATOS The Greek word for death, and a Freudian term for the death instinct. Euthanasia (see **EU-**) means a good death; thanatophobia (see **-PHOBIA**), a fear of death, thanatopsy is (with **NECROPSY**), a better word for an **AUTOPSY**, and a thanatophoric dwarf is an infant with severe **MICROMELIA**. During the Second World War the Germans developed their own form of thanatology, the art of murdering the greatest number of people as cheaply and economically as possible. See also **NECRO-**.

THEATRE The surgeons' operating-theatre was at first intended for public dissection, that is, for teaching students anatomy on dead bodies only: 'I was much pleased with a sight of their Anatomy schole, theater and repository adjoyning...' wrote John Evelyn in his *Diary* in 1642. The term 'operating-theatre' (note the hyphen) for a room specially set aside for surgery on living persons seems to have been coined not earlier than the middle of the 19th century – an apt term, as most operations were performed before a class of students.

THERAPY From the Greek *therapeuein*, to heal, to cherish or cosset.

THERME Greek for heat, a word which gave us among other things the thermometer. See also its Latin equivalent, **CALOR**.

'THEY SHOULD DO SOMETHING' A demand frequently heard from **NHS** claimants who blame the **SYSTEM**.

THIGH STRAIN A usually imaginary complaint invented by football managers as an excuse for not fielding one of their players – either for reasons of tact (when it can mean anything from a disciplinary offence to a **SOCIAL DISEASE**) or as a tactical ploy. Backache is a condition often feigned by **MALINGERERS**: 'Me back's gone'.

THIXOPHOBIC A person who cannot bear to be touched, from *thix-*, the Greek 'touching' prefix. Apparently this does not include the ticklish, though it should do. There is more about the mysteries of tickling under **CLITORIS**.

THORAX The Greek word for chest, though the ancients often used the word as much for the emotions as for anatomy, and sometimes as an alternative to **ABDOMEN**.

THROMBOS(IS) Greek for a plug, an obstruction, hence thrombosis. Latin and Greek words also gave us **INFARCT(ION)**, **CORONARY** and **EMBOLISM**.

THRUSH A songbird of the *turdus* group, and also the informal medical term for candidiasis, usually of the mouth, which might make singing painful. Probably from the Old English *thrusc*, and Danish *trøske*, rotten or decayed wood. The *OED* also points to the Norwegian dialect word *trausk*, for a frog, and the fact that in cattle a disease of the mouth is called 'frog', and hoarseness 'a frog in the throat'.

THYMUS Latinised, from Greek *thymos/thumos*, a warty excrescence, hence the thymus gland, thought to resemble a bunch of thyme.

TIBIA Latin for the shin-bone, and a pipe or a flute – but which came first, the anatomical or musical term? Certainly many ancient flutes were made from this bone, which is of convenient length, though it would need a giant to produce a 'baroque' concert flute in D (my own tibiae look as if they might make a pair of piccolos in E flat). For another flute-derived term see **SYRINGE**; also **FIBULA**.

TIC A spasmodic, involuntary twitching of certain

muscles, often called a 'nervous' tic. See **GILLES DE LA TOURETTE**. Compare **NICTARE**, to wink, though the connection may be fortuitous.

TIGHT PANTS SYNDROME Described in the *Journal of the American Medical Association* in 1994, by Dr Octavio Bessa, from Stamford, Connecticut, who said he saw about ten male patients a year who presented with symptoms such as abdominal pain and bloating. After putting them through various tests he discovered that they had one thing in common: they all wore trousers which were at least three inches smaller than their waistline. The cure: bigger trousers held up by braces. Sir John Christie, the English landowner and founder of Glyndebourne Festival Opera, achieved a long and healthy life – perhaps because he insisted on having his trousers made to a generous chest (not waist) measurement. He suspended them with braces (suspenders) from a point just below his nipples, and the garments had to be of such generous width that he could step into them in the morning without unfastening and refastening any buttons.

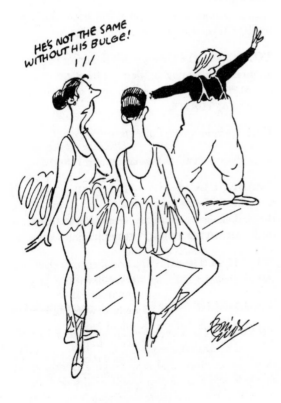

Tight Pants Syndrome

TIMOTHY DOTH VEX ALL VERY NERVOUS HOUSEMAIDS Mnemonic for the order of tendons, vessels and nerves in a part of the ankle.

TINCT. Pharmacists' abbreviation for Latin *tinctura*, a tincture, a solution in alcohol. See also **TR**.

TINCTURE A medicinal substance dissolved in a liquid, from Latin *tinctus*, a dye. It was thus originally a coloured ('tinted') solution or mixture, the dye being harmless and functionless – apart from making the patient believe a coloured mixture to be more effective than one looking like plain water.

TINEA Latin for a bookworm, a gnawing worm or larva of the clothes-moth. Also the medical name for **ATHLETE'S FOOT**, i.e. *tinea pedis*, or ringworm of the foot, a condition by no means confined to athletes. Nor to the foot. Other forms include *tinea corporis*, of the body, and *tinea cruris*, of the crotch – for which see **DHOBI ITCH**. Textbooks reveal that the 'ringworm' is not in fact a worm.

TINNITUS From the Latin word for bells: a ringing in the ears. Also used to describe a hissing sound (i.e. without a musical note being perceived) although this should strictly be called **SIBILUS** – from the Latin word for hissing. See also **BOMBUS, GARGARISMA, GARGLE, SUSURRUS** and **BRUIT**. The loud pop music to which many young people and immature adults are addicted (see under **PROLETARIANS**) has caused a great increase in tinnitus and early deafness.

TMA GPs' notes code for Too Much Alcohol. With an increased litigiousness on the part of patients many doctors find it advisable to disguise adverse comments, so that TMA might be replaced by 'Might be worth checking LFT'. According to the American physician Alvan L. Bachrach (1895–1977) 'An alcoholic has been lightly defined as a man who drinks more than his own doctor'.

TODDY Also a Hot Toddy. One of the most pleasant medicines to have come out of Scotland. ℞: A large glass, half-filled with whisky and topped up with hot water, to which is added sugar or honey. It is the only reasonably effective remedy so far discovered for the **COMMON COLD**, under which heading you will learn how it should be administered.

TOE-TAGGED Hospital slang for a patient ready for burial.

TOKEN Something serving as evidence, or a proof or fact, hence used for a spot or macule on the body indicating disease, especially the **PLAGUE**.

-TOM- Greek prefix/suffix for cutting: from *-tomia*, cutting. Hence **ANA**tomy, cutting-up, **-OSTOMY** for cutting a hole, **-OTOMY** for simple cutting (i.e. into), and **-ECTOMY** for cutting out (i.e. removing), and their numerous familiar formations in combination with other Greek, Latin and English words.

TONIC Those who ask their doctor to give them 'a tonic' may be surprised to hear that in its proper meaning the word does not imply a relaxing substance, e.g. drink or medicine, but something that stretches and tenses the muscles. The original ancient tonics seem to have been a kind of balm or rub, used in the way oil is applied to leather to give it stretch. 'Tonica, those things which being externally applied to, and rubb'd into the Limbs, strengthen the Nerves and Tendons', says a medical dictionary of 1693. The word is derived from Greek *tonikos*, of and for stretching – and *tonos* (Latin *tonus, tendere*). In tonic contraction the stretching of the muscles is sustained, whereas its opposite, *clonic*, denotes alternate contraction and relaxation. Numerous derived words include tensor and extensor, atonia, hyper- and hypotonic and tetanus, or lock-jaw. **ISOTONIC** is a bogus word much bandied about by the soft-drinks industry; perhaps reminiscent of the carbonated, non-alcoholic water which, since the 1920s, taken with ice and a slice of lemon and accompanying a generous quantity of gin, has helped the British (especially colonials) to relax in hot climates. Tonic water used to contain appreciable quantities of quinine (it still includes some, but augmented and probably swamped by unspecified 'flavourings') which since the 17th century has helped to alleviate **MALARIA** in certain parts of the world – properties which were in fact discovered many centuries ago by the ancient people of Peru. For pink gin (formerly a drink favoured particularly by naval officers) see under **AMBULANCE**. The British also drink much 'Tonic Wine' – which the *Oxford English Dictionary* defines as 'weak, flavoured wine sold as a medicinal tonic'.

TOPICAL In general, everyday use, topicality means up to date, up to the minute. But in medicine it refers not to the time but the locality, from Greek *topos*, place. It means a remedy externally applied, specifically to a certain place, e.g. adhesive tape or ointment. The opposite is **SYSTEMIC**. See also **ECTOPIC**, for something that is out of place.

TORPOR Latin for numb, numbness, but the word is now so loosely and often facetiously used by the population at large that it is of little medical use – like **STUPOR**.

TOURETTE See **GILLES DE LA TOURETTE**.

TOURNIQUET From French *tourner*, to turn. A bandage or other device for stopping or checking the flow of blood through an artery by compression. It may also be tightened by the insertion and twisting of a rod or bar in the bandage – when strictly it ceases to be French and becomes a 'Spanish windlass', though this is more a nautical than medical term.

TOXI-/TOXO- The poison prefix.

TOXIC SHOCK SYNDROME A severe infection caused by a strain of *Staphylococcus aureus* which has affected people of both sexes and all ages but came into prominence after it was associated in particular with tampons used by menstruating women. This dealt a powerful blow for old-fashioned protection and against tampons, whose sales fell dramatically as a result of adverse exposure in the media.

TOXICOS The Greek word meaning poisonous, originally arrow-poison, derived from *toxon*, a bow. See **SEPSIS**, which was originally a serpent-poison. See also **ANTIDOTE**.

TPR Temperature, Pulse, Respiration.

TR. Pharmacists' abbreviation: see **TINCT**.

TRABECULUM Latin for a little beam, the diminutive of *trabs*, which is a full-sized one. Hence the trabecula in anatomy. See also **FAUCES** and under **ARCHITECTURAL TERMS**.

TRACHEA The windpipe, so called after the Greek *trachus, trachea*, rough: for the windpipe is ridged.

TRACHELOS Greek for the neck. See also **CERVIX**.

TRAUMA The Greek word for a wound, but now misused by almost everybody, especially journalists, to mean an emotional hurt ranging from a severe shock to slight disappointment or discomfort, e.g. 'After the trauma of three League defeats in a row...' It should, however, be said that the word was officially adopted (and subsequently mishandled) by psychiatrists themselves long before newspapermen got their hands on it. The anglicised plural is 'traumas', the Greek *traumata*. See also **INJURIES/WOUNDS**.

TREMBLING DISEASE See **KURU**.

TREPAN From the Greek *trupanon*, via Latin *trepanum* a drill-bit, or hole-borer. Trepanning is the boring of a hole, usually in the skull, and was supposed to allow evil spirits to escape from the brain. People usually needed such an operation like they needed a hole in the head. The trepan also had an early military application, as an instrument for drilling holes in fortifications: compare with the *petard*, for blowing holes in defences, which you will find under **FLATULENCE**.

TRIAGE From the French *trier*, to pick, sort or choose, used in English (often in the anglicised pronunciation 'try-age') since the 18th century: the action of assigning relative degrees of urgency to the treatment of wounds or injuries (originally on the battlefield). The term is now increasingly heard or seen in hospital casualty departments, where there may even be a door grandly labelled 'Triage Nurse'. She assesses the relative needs of those waiting to be treated.

TRIBADE Latin *tribare*, to rub, from Greek *tribas*. Hence a tribade, a homosexual, Lesbian or **'GAY'** woman, and tribadism (both coined by the French in the 16th century, taken into English usage and still pronounced in the French manner), meaning female homosexuality or sexual activity between women, since it was supposed that rubbing each other was about all they could do (but see **DILDO**). *Chambers's Twentieth-Century Dictionary* still quaintly defines a tribade as 'a woman homosexualist'. (See also **CLITORIS** for the tickling connection.)

TRICHOBEZOAR A hairball, a coalesced mass of hair in the stomach, perhaps present as a result of **PICA**. See **BEZOAR** and various eating-disorders cross-referenced under **BULIMIA**.

TRICHOS Greek word for hair. See also the Latin **PILUS**, also **CRINATE** – and **ALOPECIA** for baldness or manginess.

TRIGGER THUMB The trigger of a gun is usually pulled with the first finger (some may remember the Duke of Edinburgh's diplomatic illness described as 'a whitlow on his trigger finger') so why trigger thumb? The name is derived from the distinctive click heard and felt after initial resistance when the thumb is bent or straightened, just like the action of a trigger. The condition in question is a form of teno**SYNOVITIS**.

TRIPPER see **DAY TRIPPER**.

TROCAR A sharp, pointed rod that fits inside a **CANNULA** or tube and is used for the aspiration of fluids or instillation of medication. From French *troquart*, *trois-quarts* – or *trois*, three + *carres*, sides. The spellings have varied down the centuries: 'Trochar, a Cane, or Pipe made of silver, or Steel, with a sharp-pointed end, us'd in tapping those that are troubled with the Dropsy' (1706).

TROCH. Pharmacists' abbreviation for Latin, from Greek, *trochiscus*, a lozenge.

TROCHLEA Latin *trochlia* via Greek, a pulley – which is precisely the function of that anatomical part.

TROPHE Greek for growth (originally nourishment, which results in growth), hence hypertrophy, excessive growth; dystrophy, bad growth; atrophy, no growth – or shrinkage.

(THE) TROTS Popular name for **DIARRH(O)E(I)A** (also short for a communist faction called Trotskyists who are now almost extinct): see under **(THE) TURKEY TROTS** below as well as various cross-references. The equally popular 'Doctor I've got the runs' would be doubly descriptive: of the constant need of 'running' (i.e. 'trotting') to a place where the sufferer can empty his bowels as well as to their looseness.

TSS Abbreviation of **TOXIC SHOCK SYNDROME**.

TTFO GPs' code in patient's notes, recording the refusal of treatment or prescription asked for by a **MALINGERER**. The abbreviation stands for 'Told (him/her) To F... Off'.

TUBERCULOSIS Or **TB**: the consumption or **PHTHISIS**, from Latin *tuber*, a swelling + Greek *osis*, a condition.

TUMESCENCE Chiefly applied to sexual excitement, from Latin *tumescere*, to swell, and (see also the **-ESCENT** suffix). *Tum-* is the prefix of enlargement – whether benign, malignant, beneficial or pleasurable, and has also produced the tumulus, or burial-mound, i.e. the ground 'enlarged' by a heap of soil. See also **ONCOLOGY** and below.

TUMO(U)R Latin *tumor*, a swollen state or swelling.

TUNNEL VISION Loss of peripheral vision, for the causes of which see a medical or ophthalmological dictionary. In non-medical usage the term has become a favourite but meaningless **KNEEJERK** press and headline cliché (see also **PAVLOV'S DOG**) relentlessly flogged in Britain ever since the Channel Tunnel was begun and showed little sign of abating even after it was opened in 1994.

TURISTA South American Spanish-speakers' name for the stomach/bowel upset traditionally suffered by tourists, caused by the travellers' lack of tolerance to mildly contaminated drinking-water and the generally poor personal hygiene of many local inhabitants. See also **DELHI BELLY, BOMBAY CRUD, GIPPY**

TUMMY, MONTEZUMA'S REVENGE and the **TURKEY TROTS**.

(THE) TURKEY TROTS Travellers' **DIARRH-(O)E(I)A** – when contracted in Turkey – and a reference to a dance-step, the Turkey Trot. See above.

TUSSIS Latin for a cough. *Tussiculis* is a small cough, the merest 'ahem'. See also **OAC**.

TYMPANUM The Latin word for a drum, as played in bands and orchestras; also the name of the ear-drum in the middle-ear: too much noise from the first kind tends to damage the structure of the second, especially in people who listen to too much rock music.

TYPHLITIS Also perityphlitis. See under **CAECUM**.

TYPHOID/TYPHUS Fevers resulting from an infection of the digestive system: both come from the Greek *tuphos*, smoke, vapour.

U*u*

UAG Usual Advice Given: *aide-mémoire* in doctors' notes which, like **TASE**, may be crucial in case of subsequent court proceedings.

ULNA The large bone on the little-finger side of the fore-arm. The word is Latin for the elbow and also gave us the ell as a measurement. See also **FUNNYBONE**.

UMBILICUS Latin for the navel, from *umbo*, the round, central boss of a shield. For more interesting information on the subject please turn to the related Greek word for the navel, **OMPHALOS**.

UNG. Pharmacists' and dermatologists' abbreviation for unguentum, an ointment, from Latin *unguere*, to anoint – hence also the oily, greasy quality of unctuousness attributed to a person.

URETHRA From Greek *ourethra*, Latin *urethra*, but used in English as early as the 16th century as ureter, which some may consider a simpler and more sympathetic word. See also **MEATUS** and some of the 'wetness' words beginning with *sp-*.

-URIA The often uneasy urine-denoting suffix, e.g. **NOCTURIA**, whose 'real' meaning should really be 'night urine' but which is applied to a frequent passing of it during the night. Formations like **H(A)EMATURIA** and **PNEUMATURIA** are, however, linguistically sound and self-explanatory.

URINE From Greek *ouron*, Latin *urina*. We all know what it is, but the *Oxford English Dictionary* has given us a neat definition: 'The excrementitious fluid secreted from the blood by the kidneys in man and the higher animals, stored in the bladder, and voided at intervals through the urethra'. The Greek and Roman words were also used for plain water, making it perhaps an early euphemism, e.g. 'passing water'. Icelandic, too, has an apparently related word for water, *ur* – so the Urals may have more in common with urinals than schoolboy-jokers imagine. A diuretic is a substance that induces the passing of urine. Nocturia (a comparatively modern, manufactured word, invented to describe a condition) means the frequent need (usually by men) to pass urine during the night. For an interesting practical use which the Romans made of urine see **LOTIUM** and **LYE**.

UR(O)- Prefix denoting urinary matters, urine.

UROLAGNIA Sexual stimulation or lust (see **LAGNIA**) derived from urine or urination, often involving unusual acts and practices. Perhaps urolagnists (has a female one ever been reported?) might be encouraged to combine with those (also invariably men, it seems) who are driven by **PYROMANIA** – to their own and everyone else's advantage?

UTERUS The Latin word *uterus* denotes the womb but is related to *uter*, a bottle or container, which in ancient times would be made from leather or some other animal substance. In medieval English the uterus was called a **BIT**, the same word as was used for a butt, a leathern bottle or flask. See also **VAGINA**, originally a container, or sheath, e.g. for a sword.

UTRICULUS Latin for a small bag, from which is named the utricle, the larger of the two membranous pouches in the ear.

UVULA The diminutive of Latin *uva*, grape, or a bunch of grapes, hence the name of the small, soft extension which dangles down from the soft palate and is agitated when one gargles. As it is always damp it may be related to the other meaning of uva, which is moist or humid. More about this under **GARGLE**.

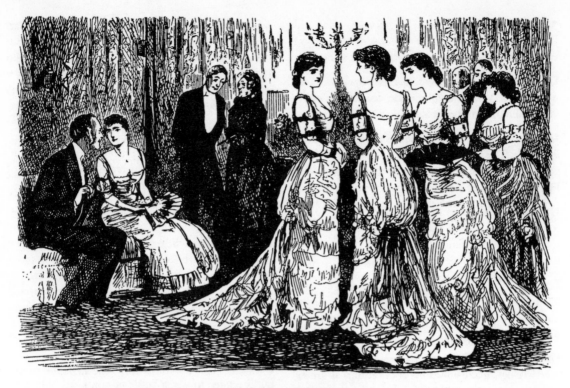

THE NEW SLEEVE

Granny (from the Country). "BUT WHY DO THEY ALL SHOW THE TOPS OF THEIR ARMS IN THAT RIDICULOUS MANNER?"
Facetious Youth. "THE FACT IS, GRANDMA, THEY'RE ALL GOING TO BE VACCINATED AFTER SUPPER!"

Punch, May 8, 1880

V*v*

VACCINATION The inoculation with the virus of the cowpox as protection against the smallpox, introduced at the end of the 18th century. *Vacca*, Latin for a cow.

VAGINA Latin for a sheath or scabbard, e.g. of a sword, and one of many originally suggestive Latin words for the female sexual organ, thought of as a container for the male (*cf* Henry Purcell's song, *Man is for the Woman made / As for the scabbard is the blade*). But females have no monopoly of the word: for example, vaginalitis is not a female complaint but the inflammation of the vaginal coat, or tunic, i.e. sheath, of the **TESTES**. See also **PENIS** and **VULVA**.

VAGITUS The (first) cry of an infant.

VAGUS Latin for wandering, straying or strolling about, with a pre-classical parallel Sanskrit word. Hence vagrants – who may be genuine sufferers from

DROMOMANIA. The vagus is one of a pair of cranial nerves which 'wander' all over the body, vagabond-like, impinging on many sensibilities and functions.

VALETUDINARIAN Old-fashioned name for a person who is – or thinks he is – always ailing, and who might be a pessimist, a **HYPOCHONDRIAC**, or a genuine sufferer from the **MÜNCHHAUSEN SYNDROME**. From Latin *valetudo*, state of health.

VARICELLA See **CHICKENPOX**, for which it is the Latin name, and the diminutive of **VARIOLA**.

VARIOCELE Dilated veins in the spermatic cord – see **VARIX**, below + the **-CELE** ending, which denotes a swelling.

VARIOLA Smallpox, the Latin word for a pustule or pock, from *varius*, spotty or speckled. Perhaps that is why it is called *chicken* pox – a speckled *hen*?

VARIX Latin for a distended or distorted vein, 'especially in the thighs', say the classical Roman authors, possibly relating it to *varicare*, to spread the legs apart – 'in an obscene fashion', says *Lewis and Short*.

VAS Latin for a vessel. The *vaso-* prefix, with angio-, phlebo-, arterio- and veno-, denotes blood-vessels. But the **VAS DEFERENS** transmits rather than contains.

VASCULUM A small vessel, diminutive of the above. To the Romans a *vascularius* was not a kind of vascular surgeon but a tinsmith, whitesmith or gold-smith, a man who made small metal containers.

VAS DEFERENS There is nothing 'deferential' about this vessel, which carries spermatozoa *down* from the **EPIDIDYMIS**: the operative word is Latin *deferre*, to carry down or away through the **URETHRA**, which the – surely better – spelling *vas deferrens* would make clearer.

VASELINE A proprietary name (now used generi-cally in some countries, although still a trade-mark in Britain) for an emollient substance, a kind of petro-leum jelly, introduced by the American chemist Robert A. Chesebrough in 1872. The name is derived either from the German *Wasser*, water and Greek *elaion*, oil or, according to another story, from the English vase + *elaion*, because Chesebrough was said to have borrowed some of his wife's flower vases for his experiments. Take your pick.

VEN(E), VEN(I) The prefix relating to veins, from Latin *vena*. Hence **INTRA**venal, etc. Not to be con-fused with the venereal prefixes relating to the God-dess of Love, below.

VENEREAL, VENERIS, VENUS Relating to sexual activity or **CARNAL** love, Venus (genitive *Veneris*, of Venus) being the Roman Goddess of Love – and venereal diseases, for which **MERCURY** was once an often unsatisfactory cure: as they used to say, 'Spend a night with Venus and months with Mercury'. She gave her blessing also to the prettily named **MONS VENERIS** or **PUBES**. See also **EROS, LIBIDO, CUPID-ITY** and **CONCUPISCENCE**, etc. Also under **APHRO-DISIAC** for the lady's Greek equivalent.

VENTR- The prefix denoting the belly or any other hollow, from Latin *venter, ventris*, belly. In the literal German language a ventriloquist is a *Bauchredner*, or belly-talker. (See also under **AEROPHAGY**.) The Romans had a good word for a glutton, *ventricola*, 'one who makes a god of his belly' *(Lewis and Short)* which would make a useful addition to the secret vocabulary of GPs' patient-notes. Not to be confused with matters of wind and breath:–

VENTUS Latin for a blow (in the sense of blowing like the wind). **HYPERVENTILATING** is a more im-pressive way of saying 'breathing hard', and is a recent favourite among English sportsmen. For a 'blow' in the sense of striking someone or something, see **-PLEGIA**.

VENUS At first she was merely the Roman goddess of vegetation but was identified from the 3rd century BC with the Greek Aphrodite, goddess of sexual love, female beauty and fertility. In imperial times she was also worshipped as Venus Genetrix, mother of Aeneas; also as Venus Felix, bringer of good fortune; Venus Victrix, bringer of victory; and Venus Verticordia, protector of feminine chastity. Her son **EROS** did even better as a sex-symbol.

VERMIFORM Long, thin, and more-or-less cylindrical: from Latin *vermis*, worm. Another *vermis* is the median lobe of the **CEREBELLUM**, a worm-like structure. See **APPENDIX** and under **CAECUM**.

VERMIFUGE A preparation or agent that causes the evacuation of worms from the intestine. From *vermis*, above, and *fugare*, to chase or flee.

VERRUCA The Latin name for an unsightly ex-crescence on precious stones, also for a wart on the body. Pliny used the word in both senses.

VERTEBRA Latin for a joint, in particular the joint of the spine, from *vertere*, to turn. The equivalent Greek is **SPHONDULOS**, which also has several de-rived formations, like spondylitis. Vertebra is singu-lar in spite of the *-a* ending, so that those who insist on 'vertebrum' are both pedantic and wrong. The plural is *vertebrae*.

VERTIGO Latin for 'a whirling round', from *vertere*, to turn. The standard pronunciation of the word used to be 'ver*teego*', which now sounds quaint but at least gave no rise to feeble puns.

VESICANT Latin *vesica*, a bladder, also a blister; hence vesication, blistering – formerly used as a cure for various conditions but which often killed the patient.

VESTIBULUM The ante-chamber of a Roman house which, like the inner chamber, the **ATRIUM**, was turned to medical use. For other **ARCHITEC-TURAL** terms see **CLAUSTRUM, FOCUS, FORNIX, PHRAGMA, PORTA, THALAMOS, TRABECULUM** and similar cross-references under **FAUCES**.

VESTIGIUM Latin for a footprint, mark or trace, hence the word for something surviving in a degenerate or **ATROPHIED** form. Also an investigation, which means 'tracking something down by the evidence left'.

VIMTO A strengthening carbonated fruit drink formulated by J. N. Nichols early in the 20th century – a beverage not unlike Lucozade (though the respective makers of the two products would probably disagree) and, like it, favoured by convalescents regaining their strength. It was originally called Vimtonic, from *vim*, accusative singular of the Latin *vis*, strength or energy, plus **TONIC**, but shortened by a syllable – perhaps somewhat unfortunately as it produces an **EMETIC** anagram.

VIOL-HIPPED A recognised, serious medical term describing a woman's figure, after the shape of the body of that instrument (which is different from that of the cello); and furthermore, the shape of the renaissance, not the baroque, viol is meant.

VIRILISM In a woman, the state of being (or process of becoming) masculine, with increased body-hair, a lowering in pitch of the voice, reduction in the size of breasts, growth of extra muscles, etc. – all of which describes a typical mannish woman-athlete surreptitiously pumped full of illicit **STEROIDS** in the name of 'sport'. But a male virilist is one who excessively cultivates masculine (or supposedly masculine) activities, like muscle-building, beer-swilling, wife-beating, etc. These and other words come from the Latin word *vir*, a man. Another Latin word, *vis*, *vires*, strength, doubtless also helped to shape the virile terminology.

VIRULENCE See below.

VIRUS Originally a Latin word for poison, or for slimy, nasty liquids or evil-smelling substances, now the name for a specific kind of disease-producing organism. Hence **VIRULENCE**, although this refers to extreme malignancy or violence of *any* kind, caused by any organism, not necessarily viral. Viruses have nothing to do with **VIRILISM** (above) nor with the other derivations from *vir-*, a man or male. And they differ from **BACTERIA**, being smaller (the smallest of **MICROBES**) and at present unaffected by **ANTIBIOTICS**.

VISIT/VISITATION The first generally implies the arrival of a relative, friend – or the doctor: the second suggests a higher being, but also the **PLAGUE**.

VITAMINS From Latin *vita*, life + the combining suffix *amin(e)*. Organic compounds needed in the diet for their biochemical role, a function best explained by specialised textbooks. But the following anonymous rhyme might help.

> *Vitamin A keeps the cold-germs away*
> *And tends to make pale people nervy.*
> *B's what you need when you're going to seed,*
> *And C is specific to scurvy.*
> *Vitamin D makes the bones in your knee*
> *Tough and hard for the Service on Sunday,*
> *While E makes hens scratch and increases the hatch,*
> *And brings in more profits on Monday.*
> *Vitamin F never bothers the chef, for this vitamin never existed;*
> *G puts some fight in the old appetite and you'll eat all the foods that are listed.*
> *So now when you dine, remember these lines,*
> *If long on this earth you will tarry:*
> *So try to be good and choose most of your food*
> *From the orchard, the garden and dairy.*

VITILIGO From Latin *vitium*, blemish. A skin pigmentation fault which appears in the form of irregular patches of various sizes totally lacking in pigment, and most often affecting exposed areas of the skin. A case has been recorded of a dark-skinned Indian actor whose face turned white with advancing years, thus diminishing his ability to play character roles. See also **ALBINO**.

VITRUM Latin for glass, related to *video*, *videre* to see – hence the idea of transparency, and by extension a test-tube. See **IN VITRO**. Also **HUALOS (HYALOS)**.

VITUS See **ST. VITUS'S DANCE**.

VIVISECTION Anyone who has read as far as this will not need to be told that the word comes from *vivus*, living + *sectio*, cutting, that is to say, the cutting up or dissecting of a living being. This is now understood to mean experiments on animals (with strict safeguards to regulate the practice), but ancient doctors were able to procure convicted criminals, taken from jails as 'volunteers' and systematically taken apart in the interest of medical research. The doctor who in about 270 BC found and named the **DUODENUM** (which see) discovered this and other organs by gruesome vivisection. According to a report in *The* (London) *Times* dated 11 February 1995, six veterans of the Japanese Medical Unit 731 confessed after 50 years that during the Second World War they had performed vivisection experiments on prisoners-of-war; and the world needs no reminding of the notorious pseudo-scientific vivisection conducted on concentration-camp inmates in the 1940s by the evil Dr Josef Mengele. See also under **DONOR**.

VOCAL RESONANCE The sounds the doctor hears through a stethoscope when a patient speaks, and which tell him something of his condition, e.g. **AEGOPHONY** or **WHISPERING PECTRILOQUY**.

VOMER Latin for a ploughshare – and yet another everyday object appropriated by the early doctors, this one to describe the partition between the nostrils. See also **SEPTUM**.

VOMIT From Latin *vomere*, related to Greek *emeo* (hence **EMETIC**). See also nausea and cross-references to **(THE) WOMBLES**, etc.

VORARE Latin, to devour. See also the Greek 'eating' pre/suffix **-PHAG(E)-**.

VULVA The Latin word for a wrapper or envelope, hence its use for the external organ of generation in the female, especially the opening or orifice of that organ. Clearly a male-invented term, for as with the word **VAGINA**, which is Latin for a sheath or scabbard, the implications are that its chief purpose is to receive the male organ. **VULVA** is also the acronymic name unwittingly chosen by the Vintners' and United Licenced Victuallers' Association. See also **FICA**.

VWF Vibration White Finger. Any practical householder who has wielded a hand-held power-tool knows that the continuous depression of a 'dead man's switch', combined with the continuous vibration of the implement, may produce numbness in the operative finger or thumb. The phenomenon (also called the Dead Hand Syndrome) may appear also when compensation is in the offing. Outbreaks of VWF among professional users of electrical equipment appear to be epidemic, whereas the home handyman may spend many happy hours with his power-tools without suffering any ill-effect. (A 'dead man's switch' is one which when released cuts off the current and stops the machinery – or a railway train). See also **TRIGGER FINGER/THUMB** and **DRUMMER'S THUMB**.

Ww

WALLET BIOPSY See **POCKETBOOK BIOPSY**.

WARD A hospital room or hall containing one or more beds. The word is derived from an old Teutonic one related to guarding, watching, observing or keeping safe. Hence also the prison warder.

WASSERMAN(N) TEST/REACTION A test for **SYPHILIS** devised in 1909 by August Paul Wassermann (which is how his name should be written, not 'Wasserman'). He lived from 1866 to 1925. See also **AMELIA** and **SALVARSAN**.

WATERBRASH A good English word meaning the sudden filling of the mouth with dilute saliva, often as an accompaniment to **DYSPEPSIA**.

WATERWORKS In British family physicians' slang this euphemism usually forms part of the question 'How are your waterworks?' – meaning the functioning or otherwise of the kidneys, bladder (prostate if male) and urethra.

WEB (IN THE EYE) The early English medical name, first recorded in 1387, for a **CATARACT** or other gradual impairment of vision. A writer of 1387 advises '...to voyde the webbes of thyne eyen, to make thee clerely to see the errours thou hast ben [sic] in'.

WEBER'S TEST A certain kind of test employing a musical tuning-fork. It is named after the 19th-century German physiologist and anatomist E. H. Weber (1795–1878) and not, as might have been apt, after his compatriot Carl Maria von Weber (1786–1826), the composer of the opera *Der Freischütz*, a story based on the use of **MAGIC BULLETS**.

WELFARE STATE Welfare is defined by the *Oxford English Dictionary* as 'The state or condition of doing or being well; good fortune, happiness or well-being (of a person, community, or thing); thriving or successful progress in life, prosperity' – that is to say, a *state* of being well, not a *State*, with its constitution and laws. When the term Welfare State (in the State sense) first came into use in the 1940s it had only a positive, beneficial meaning, as given above by the dictionary, a State which concerns itself with the wellbeing of all its citizens. Its coining has been ascribed to the historian and political scientist Sir Alfred Eckhard Zimmern (1879–1957), who is said to have been the first to use it in the 1930s; but the *Oxford English Dictionary* says that 'it has not been traced in his published writings'. Today it is often used opprobriously to describe a something-for-nothing society, both in the UK and America, with the suggestion that 'the state will provide for everyone's needs'. It has been said that the transformation of the UK into a Welfare State immediately after the Second World War, when the British were exhausted by five years of superhuman struggle for survival, helped to sap the nation's self-reliance and speeded her decline. The **NHS** forms the largest part of the Welfare State.

WEN A rare thing: a short, simple old English word a thousand years old, for a bump, or protuberance, or a certain kind of swelling or cyst under the skin.

(THE) WEREWOLF SYNDROME A popular name, favoured by sensationalist newspapers when a case occurs, for hypertrichosis or hirsutism, a condition in which the patient's body is covered entirely with a thick growth of hair.

WHILE I'M HERE, DOCTOR... Well-known opener from a patient, usually a **DOORHANDLE**, who has 'just remembered' another complaint he is suffering from, though it may well have been the reason for his appointment in the first place.

WHILE YOU'RE HERE, DOCTOR... When a physician is on a home-visit and has concluded his assignment a relative is likely to say, 'Oh, and while you're here, doctor, granny upstairs has got this awful boil...' See also **DOORHANDLES**.

WHIPLASH An injury often suffered by occupants of an insured motor vehicle which has come into contact, however slight, with another, especially one which has attracted the attentions of **AMBULANCE CHASERS**. It used to be called a stiff neck and, like **RSI**, is often exacerbated by the pleasing prospect of prolonged absence from work and financial compensation. The popularity of 'whiplash' injuries is self-evident on crowded city streets, where the informal statistician may observe numerous **CERVICAL** collars.

WHISPERING PECTRILOQUY See the prefixes **PECT-** and **VENTR-**, for chest and talking, respectively. When a patient with a pleural effusion whispers '99' it is the upper level of the effusion at which the sounds heard through the stethoscope adopt a 'thrill'. Hence the size of the effusion can be estimated. See also **AEGOPHONY**.

WHITLOW The homely English name, going back to about 1400, for **PARONYCHIA**. Spelling variations given in the *Oxford English Dictionary* include whitflow (supposedly the original, possibly derived from the Dutch), whitflaw, whyte flaw, white flow, whickflow, quickflaw, whitblowe, whytelowe, whitloe and even whitloaf. The most memorable whitlow was diplomatic, suffered by the Duke of Edinburgh when he was on a visit to an African country. Its President invited the Duke, who was then President of the World Wild-life Fund, to accompany the presidential party on a big-game hunt to shoot the very animals the Duke was protecting. He could hardly offend his host, but on his next appearance in public he had a heavily-bandaged forefinger. A bulletin was issued announcing 'His Royal Highness is suffering from a whitlow on his trigger-finger'. See also **DIGITUS** and **TRIGGER THUMB**.

WIDGET Any kind of multi-purpose or improvised gadget, which you will find mentioned under **PLEDGET**.

WOMBLES A useful old English word (also wambles), which the *Oxford English Dictionary* says is 'A rolling or uneasiness in the stomach; a feeling of nausea'. 'Our meat going down into the stomacke merrily, and with pleasure, dissolveth incontinently, all wambles...' wrote an author in 1603. Surely a much prettier (if echoically less descriptive) word than **BORBORYGM(US)**. Dr Andrew Boorde called them **GURGULACIONS**. In 1685 a London doctor in Maiden Lane advertised an alleged cure for 'the Wambling Trot, the Moon-fall and Hockogrockle'.

WOOS Abbreviation sometimes seen in patients' case-notes meaning 'Work Out Own Salvation'. Other GPs' abbreviations include **GOK, TATSP** and **TTFO**.

WOUNDS See **INJURIES**.

X

XANTHOS Greek for yellow, hence the *xanth-* prefix, as in xanthoma, xanthinuria, xanthopsia, etc. From the descriptions of some of these conditions it may be supposed that the ancient Greeks used the word for a darker yellow shade, tending towards orange (though they had no word for orange as they had yet to import this fruit from the Far East: see also **CIRRHOSIS**).

XENOGRAFT See under **HETERO-** and below.

XENOPHOBIA From the Greek *xenos*, foreign, + **PHOBIA**, fear: therefore literally 'fear of foreigners'. It often manifests itself in the way nations blame each other for the spread or origin of diseases: see under **BUGGERY, FRENCH POX, INFLUENZA, SPANISH FLU, SPANISH FLY, HUNGARIAN CAMP FEVER, MENSES, SYPHILIS**, etc. Not to be confused with certain apparently 'racist' diseases prevalent among ethnic groups, like **FAVISM, KURU, TAY–SACHS DISEASE** and **THALASS-(ANA)EMIA**, etc.

XENOS Greek for strange, foreign, hence xenograft (formerly **HETEROGRAFT**), a graft between different species (see also **ALLO-** and **AUT(O)-**), etc. See also under **ADVENTITIOUS** diseases.

XIPHOID Sword-shaped, e.g. the lower end of the **STERNUM**. From the Greek *xiphos*, a sword + *-OID*, in the shape of. See also the Latin **GLADIOLUS**.

Y*y*

YARD The cliché headline often seen in English newspapers, 'Man Held by Yard', refers to Scotland Yard, the London police department, but would have had a different meaning for Chaucer. For 'yard' is an ancient, facetiously or optimistically exaggerated, name for the **PENIS**. 'The urine passith out by the yerde', says a medical manuscript of 1379 quoted by the *Oxford English Dictionary;* and Wyclif's translation of *Genesis* xvii, 11 has: 'Ye shulen circumside [sic] the flehs [sic] of the ferthermore parti of youre yeerde' – apparently suggesting do-it-yourself surgery. See also under **CLITORIS**.

Zz

(TO) ZAP Medics' informal slang for the action of giving a patient **ECT** – Electro-Convulsive Therapy.

ZEUS The name of the supreme deity of the ancient Greeks, also called Jupiter and Jove. He was the God of Thunder, who hurled **FULMINANT** lightning strikes at mankind, yet those born under the planet named after him are supposed to be 'jovial' – and that word was coined by that jolly and learned physician **RABELAIS** in about 1550. See also under **HERMES** and **MERCURY**.

ZIMMER The proprietary trade-name for a patent walking-frame for the infirm or elderly which made the surname of its inventor and his firm, Zimmer Orthopaedic Ltd., London, into a household word (not to be confused with Sir Alfred Zimmern, who appears under **WELFARE STATE**). It is also facetiously used, in the same way as **GERIATRIC**, for anybody or anything elderly or obsolete, e.g. 'He belongs to the zimmer section of the firm'.

ZIT See **MACULA**.

ZOSTER Greek for a girdle. See under **HERPES** and **SHINGLES**.

ZYGOMA The bony arch on each side of the skull. It comes from the Greek word *zygon*, a yoke, because the arch is thought to look like one. Numerous 'look-alike' names and references will be found in the preceding pages.

ZYGOTE From Greek *zygotos*, yoked together. A body of living protoplasm, cell or cell-nucleus, formed by the fusion of two such bodies in reproduction. For the related words applied to like and unalike twins yoked together (sometimes yolked together – the soundalike is coincidental as the two words are etymologically quite unconnected) see **DZ** and **MZ**.